Sustainable Construction

Sandy Halliday

AMSTERDAM • BOSTON • HEIDELBERG • LONDON • NEW YORK • OXFORD
PARIS • SAN DIEGO • SAN FRANCISCO • SINGAPORE • SYDNEY • TOKYO

ELSEVIER

Butterworth-Heinemann is an imprint of Elsevier

Butterworth-Heinemann is an imprint of Elsevier
Linacre House, Jordan Hill, Oxford OX2 8DP, UK
30 Corporate Drive, Suite 400, Burlington, MA 01803, USA

First edition 2008

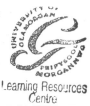

British Library Cataloguing-in-Publication Data
A catalogue record for this book is available from the British Library

Library of Congress Cataloging-in-Publication Data
A catalog record for this book is available from the Library of Congress

ISBN 978-0-7506-6394-6

For information on all Butterworth-Heinemann publications
visit our website at www.books.elsevier.com

Typeset by Charon Tec Ltd (A Macmillan Company), Chennai, India
www.charontec.com

Printed and bound in Slovenia

08 09 10 11   11 10 9 8 7 6 5 4 3 2 1

Contents

About the author

Sandy Halliday is Principal of Gaia Research, the practice she founded in 1996, and the Royal Academy of Engineering Visiting Professor in Engineering Design for Sustainable Development in the School of Architecture, University of Strathclyde.

She was educated in Engineering Design and Appropriate Technology in the early 1980s at Warwick University. It was an inspired course and a privileged learning opportunity at a time when the environment and development were largely considered to be luxury issues by those with no motivation to improve global equity and life quality.

Sandy seeks to improve the built environment through research, education and consultancy. In particular, she tries to promote construction ecology through advocacy, informed project management, interdisciplinary design and community engagement as a means of delivering quality buildings that spare other species, are efficient, healthy, affordable, and fit for individuals and communities now and in the future.

Sandy considers heartening the increasing understanding of appropriate development and design quality as fundamental aspects of social justice. She had humble beginnings. But she finds the widening gap between rhetoric and action takes the edge off any urgency for celebration.

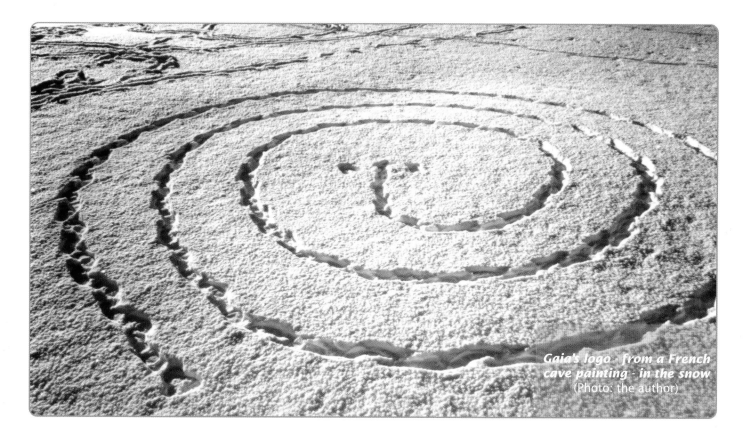

Gaia's logo - from a French cave painting - in the snow
(Photo: the author)

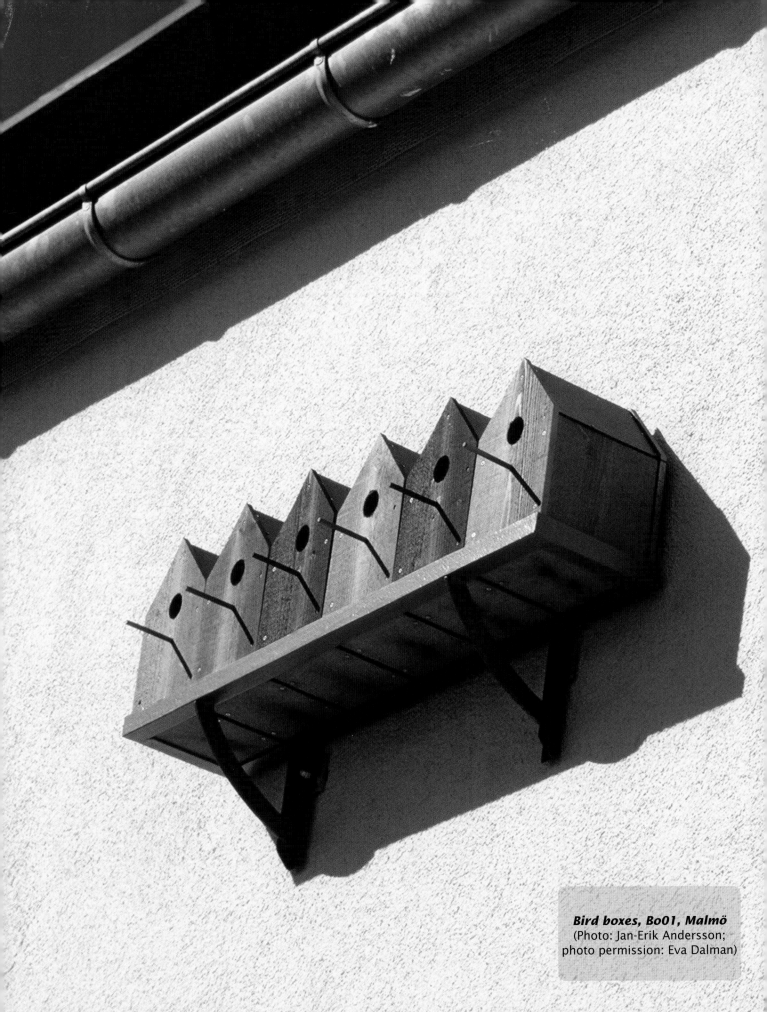

Bird boxes, Bo01, Malmö
(Photo: Jan-Erik Andersson;
photo permission: Eva Dalman)

Acknowledgements

Many people have contributed to bringing this publication to print.

Friends at Gaia Research over the last few years – Cat Button, Sarah Worrall, Steven Downie, Janice May, Paul Jones, Gill Pemberton – have been terrific, always sharp, funny, kind, loyal and dedicated. I wish them every success and happiness in their diverse futures.

A close working relationship with past and present staff at Gaia Architects has been a bridge to sanity. Special thanks to John Kelly, Barbara Chapman, Leanne Campbell, Elaine Rainey, Sam Foster, Steve Malone, Robin Baker, Matt Fox, Kathryn Robinson, Henrietta Temple and Paul Woodville.

I am privileged to be part of the family of Gaia International, a federation of professionals who work internationally in pursuit of the ecological design of buildings and the built environment. In particular, my thanks for their help, inspiration and good company go to: Drew and Carole Mackie, Chris Butters and family, Kimmo and Maritta Kuismaanen, Joachim and Barbara Eble, Margrit and Declan Kennedy, Eva Dalman, Frederica Miller and Julio Perez, Varis Bokalders, Paul Leech and Sally Starbuck, Bjorn Berge, Rolf Jacobson and Marianne Leisner, Dag Roalkvam and Wenche Ellingson, Bruno and Eva Erat, Herbert Dreiseitl, Peter Schmidt and Gabriella Pal-Schmidt.

This book evolved from a training course part funded by the Department of Trade and Industry and the Ecology Building Society, to whom I owe enormous thanks. It aimed to bring together contemporary knowledge for architects, clients, engineers and cost professionals seeking to deal with the challenges and opportunities of designing a sustainable built environment. The modular training packages were a response to the evolving discourse that it was 'all holistic'. Whilst I am totally in agreement with this, there seemed a need for the parts to inform the greater sum that could result, and that became my resolve.

The course involved short summary notes which form the basis of this book, supplemented by lecture, workshop and masterclass sessions with contributions from many of my friends and contemporaries. In particular, I owe huge thanks to Bill Bordass for always being willing to talk, share and play out, to Nick Grant (who co-authored what has become Chapter 12), Clive Beggs (who helped with what has become Chapter 8), Adrian Leaman (who contributed much on post-occupancy evaluation), Roger Venables (who assisted on what has become Chapter 2), and Michiel Haas, Chris Weedon, Cath Hassell, Brian Darcy, Ben Gunn, Koen Steemers, Paul Littlefair, Phil Jones, Paul Jennings, John Gilbert, Fionn Stevenson, Gokay Devici, Max Fordham, David Loe and Tom Morton. I am immensely grateful for the support that they provided. I own the mistakes, errors and omissions.

It is my experience that many in the construction profession have treated sustainable design with cynicism, and even contempt, but that this is changing as increasing understanding leads to respect. So, in 1999, in parallel to the creation of the training programme, I pursued development of an evidence-based accreditation scheme in sustainable building design. I hoped to encourage recognition of the additional skills of those with the dedication to see the many barriers to sustainable design as a challenge to be overcome rather than an excuse for failure. My aim was to help clients, policy-makers and the profession to recognise the clear distinction between aspiration and delivery in sustainable design, in order to find the mechanisms to speed the latter.

With support from Sebastian Tombs at the Royal Incorporation of Architects in Scotland, a steering group chaired by Lord Willie Prosser, and an assessment panel chaired by Raymond Young, the world's first Accreditation Scheme in Sustainable Design was launched in 2005. It is a significant achievement, and one that should now be opened up to other professions and other countries. I am very grateful to all those who assisted in making it happen, but most particularly the dedication of the applicants to delivering sustainable design that made it possible.

Unlimited thanks are reserved for Howard Liddell, the Principal of Gaia Architects, a founder member of Gaia International, an ongoing contributor to the CPD throughout its development and delivery, a guardian of excellence and the only architect yet accredited A* in sustainable design. All of that would be enough, but in addition he has broad shoulders, genius, passion, wit and seemingly boundless capacity for love and unflinching support.

Introduction

Achieving sustainability requires us to live within the limits of the earth's capacity to provide the materials for our activities and to absorb the waste and pollution that our activities generate.

The built environment presents us with a major challenge. The construction, fit-out, operation and ultimate demolition of buildings is a huge factor in human impact on the environment both directly (through material and energy consumption and the consequent pollution and waste) and indirectly (through the pressures on often inefficient infrastructure). The built environment also has a crucial impact on the physical and economic health and well-being of individuals, communities and organisations. A good building is a delight and will enhance a community or organisation, enhance our ability to learn or increase our productivity. A poor building will do the opposite. Where buildings and built environments contribute to ill-health and alienation, undermine community and create excessive financial liability, they are undesirable and unsustainable.

Sustainable development is now the stated policy of local, national and international governments, and of much industry and commerce. More than three decades on from a recognisable start of the environmental movement – the establishment of World Environment Day by the United Nations General Assembly in 1972 – there appears at last to be a growing commitment to reverse unsustainable trends in development.

To meet the challenge we have to enhance quality of life for all by designing healthy buildings and environments fit for individuals and communities both now and in the future. We need to minimise resource throughputs, waste and pollution, and to fulfil our responsibility to protect other species and environments. Buildings and the built environment will therefore increasingly be required to satisfy a number of criteria, including that they should:

- **Enhance biodiversity** – not use materials from threatened species or environments and improve natural habitats where possible through appropriate planting and water use.

- **Support communities** – identify and meet the real needs, requirements and aspirations of communities and stakeholders and involve them in key decisions.

- **Use resources effectively** – not consume a disproportionate amount of resources, including money and land during material sourcing, construction, use or disposal; not cause unnecessary waste of energy, water or materials due to short

life, poor design, inefficiency, or less than ideal construction and manufacturing procedures. Buildings have to be affordable, manageable and maintainable in use.

- **Minimise pollution** – create minimum dependence on polluting products and materials, management practices, energy, power and forms of transport.

- **Create healthy environments** – enhance living, leisure and work environments; and not endanger the health of the builders or occupants, or any other parties, through exposure to pollutants, the use of toxic materials or providing host environments to harmful organisms.

- **Manage the process** – stewardship of projects is a vital and overarching aspect in delivering sustainable projects, both in the first instance and also in ensuring their performance over time. Too many aspirations are undermined by failure to manage the design process, particularly at crucial handover points where responsibilities change. This requires us to identify appropriate targets, tools and benchmarks, and manage their delivery.

There is already a significant amount of information available to all professions on how to design buildings that are attentive to the needs of sustainable construction, but most practice still falls far short of applying even the most easily applicable principles in most projects.

Opportunities that could bring real advantage are being missed every day. The result is that buildings and the industries that supply building designers with products, materials and services are less efficient, less economical and more polluting than they might otherwise be. The positive impact on the environment and on quality of life from addressing these issues could be immense.

This book aims to summarise the existing sources of best practice guidance on the design of sustainable buildings and built environments. Each chapter provides information on critical aspects of a particular topic and sources of further guidance by way of an annotated bibliography. The case studies highlight experiences to date to improve understanding and encourage implementation. They are not all best practice solutions. It is intended that this will help the reader to access the guidance, tools and techniques available for staying abreast of choices and issues and to make informed 'holistic' decisions to assist in designing healthy, affordable, resource-efficient buildings fit for individuals and communities.

Chapter 1
Sustainability drivers

In which we put forward something of the history of ideas that has brought about a shared understanding that it is necessary to implement checks and balances in pursuit of sustained genuine progress for all.

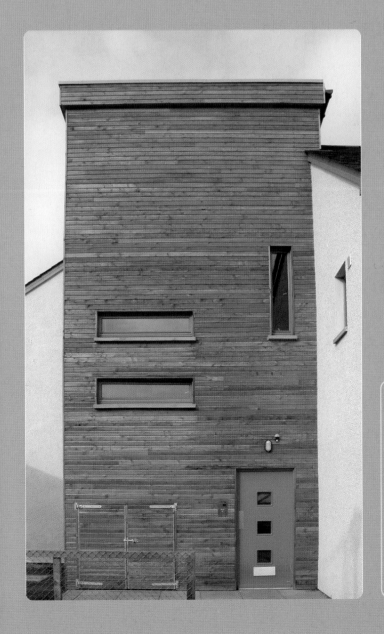

'The choice is simple, sustainable development, unsustainable development or no development at all.'

Sandy Halliday, Build Green (1990)

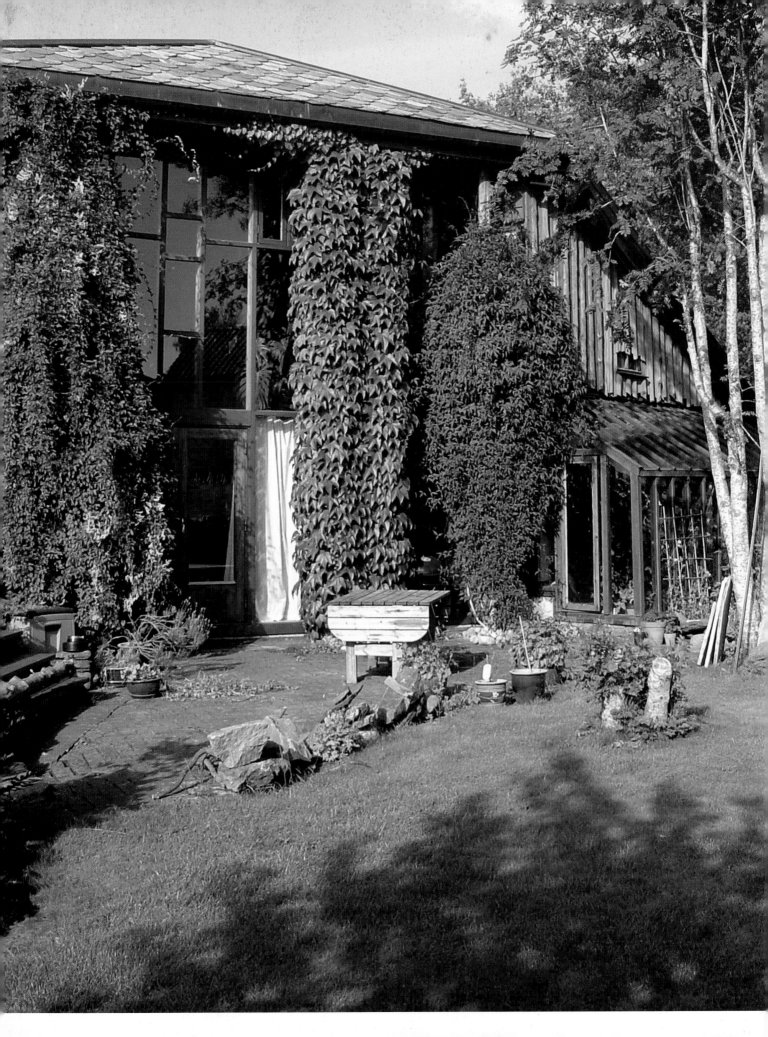

Contents

(Facing page)
Andersen House, Stavanger
The first modern building designed
to be moisture transfusive
(Architects and builders:
Dag Roalkvam and Rolf Jacobsen;
photo: Dag Roalkvam)

(Previous page)
Toll House Gardens
(Architects: Gaia Architects;
photo: Michael Wolshover)

Sustainability drivers

Introduction

There can be few within the professions involved in the built environment for whom sustainability is a new idea. Recently, government policies, international politics and architectural responses mean that it is an issue rarely out of the press and the office. It is an increasingly important aspect of client briefs. Yet, for an issue this ubiquitous it remains poorly understood, and the source of much debate and disagreement.

There is a fundamental misconception that sustainability and the environment are one and the same issue. Whilst there is a lot of evidence that the natural environmental is a powerful driver of human creativity, the concept of sustainability is different. It evolved from a debate about how we develop.

The EcoCity project
A community consultation tool, developed by Gaia Planning and the TASC Agency, in which 10-year-old children plan the development of their community. It has been used to engage children, their teachers, their parents and their communities in sustainable urban design issues in Edinburgh, Glasgow, Halifax, Belfast, Johannesburg and Thessaloniki
(Photo: Gaia Architects)

It is not wholly surprising that the concept of sustainable development is difficult to communicate. Sustainability involves big issues and their complex interaction: the division of wealth and opportunity between the world's rich and poor, health, welfare, safety, security and useful work as basic needs of societies, and rights of individuals. Much is predicated on the rights of the young and future generations and of other species – a concept unimaginable a few generations ago – and much also on the rights of those in society least capable of looking after themselves. The state of the environment is a fundamental aspect because the unintended consequences of our activities impact directly on our current quality of life, impose burdens on others, and threaten other species both now and in the future.

The global, social and cultural issues with which sustainability is concerned are mostly a far cry from the sketchpad, design team meeting and post-tender cost review. We spend relatively little time thinking about what people really need.

As the values of equity and interdependence on the natural environment have rarely been integrated into education and training, they can be difficult to translate into the practicalities of

what building design and cost professionals do on a daily basis. Appropriate and meaningful responses are genuinely hard to identify and we still know little about what responses are adequate.

With evidence of massive environmental damage going on in the developing nations it can seem pointless to try to do anything about it, unless we appreciate that sustainable design is about delivering real benefits. We don't need to look any further than pedestrianisation to see that rules and guidelines on environmental impact reap instant rewards.

Sustainability as vested self-interest has driven the international debate to date, more so than in individual countries, and will do so in the future. Alongside the environmental destruction in developing countries there are exemplar ecological towns being developed in South America, Taiwan, India and the USA. They will challenge people to think about what is appropriate development. Their ambitions and success or failure will probably determine life quality for the majority in this millennium.

The case studies in this chapter intend to highlight some early initiatives and exploration in sustainable design.

Development

'Sustainable development' has suffered from an image problem. It requires us to act in a sensitive manner towards natural systems and has been seen by those who would do otherwise as a restraint on 'development' per se. Astonishingly it has taken a very long time for sustainable development to be recognised as a justified restraint on 'inappropriate' development and a primary driver of improving quality of life for all.

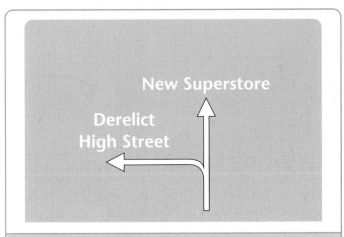

Difficult decisions
Achieving sustainable development requires us to prevent inappropriate development

Many developing countries are adopting styles and scales of development that are now recognised as inappropriate and unsustainable. Only a few are making serious attempts to combine tradition with modernity.

There is ever increasing demand on the earth's limited resources, escalating pollution and growing awareness of moral responsibility favouring greater equity. It is increasingly attractive to some to put in place long-term policies that can reliably deliver social, environmental and economic improvements. It is equally threatening to others, but need not be so.

Human skills have transformed the environment. For the developed world and the wealthy in the developing world, access to sanitation, vaccination, health awareness and treatment, food hygiene and good diet have vastly extended the quality and quantity of life in recent decades. However, the extent to which our activities are unsustainable has become clearer over the same period. There has been an increasing realisation that changes in pursuit of progress can, and often are, accompanied by inadvertent consequences, such as inequity and

hazards, that need to be recognised and avoided. A large proportion of the world still lives with the ever-present threat of drought, pestilence and starvation, often exacerbated by wars. Further billions are subject to scarcity, poor hygiene and unsanitary conditions, often within close proximity of abundance and pristine cleanliness. Some of this is in our nature and some of it is simply inadequate attention to appropriate development.

Humankind faces an awesome challenge to reverse unsustainable trends. Pollution of air, land, water and food that results from our activities threatens to crucially undermine the security, health and quality of life that humankind has pursued and sought to protect. There is now overwhelming acceptance that we face major global problems of climate change, ozone depletion, over-fishing, soil erosion, noise, resource distribution, chemical and electromagnetic pollution, deforestation, desertification, species loss and congestion. We also now know enough of history to appreciate that civilisations fail through abuse of resources.

With rising expectation and industrialisation, questions must at some time surface: can we maintain and improve life quality whilst radically improving the effectiveness in how we use all our resources, and reducing pollution and waste? Evidence suggests we can. It is a very positive agenda.

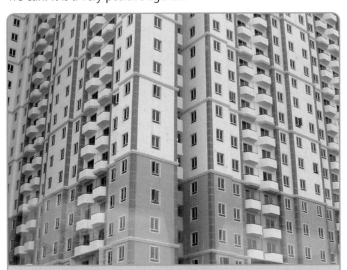

Penang – 2003
It has taken more than three decades for the sustainability agenda to be recognised not as a restraint on development but as a restraint on 'inappropriate' development. We do now have the basis of a common understanding from which to make progress
(Photo: the author)

Case Study 1.1:

Solar Hemicycle, Middleton, Wisconsin

Architect: Frank Lloyd Wright, 1945

The building was designed in 1945 by Frank Lloyd Wright on a hemicycle plan and is an early example of modern passive solar design. Earth is piled up against the northern wall for insulation.

The southern wall has two-storey glass windows and doors to maximise solar gain in winter and to take advantage of the elliptical solar path. An overhang on the southern façade is designed to provide shade from high-level summer sun.

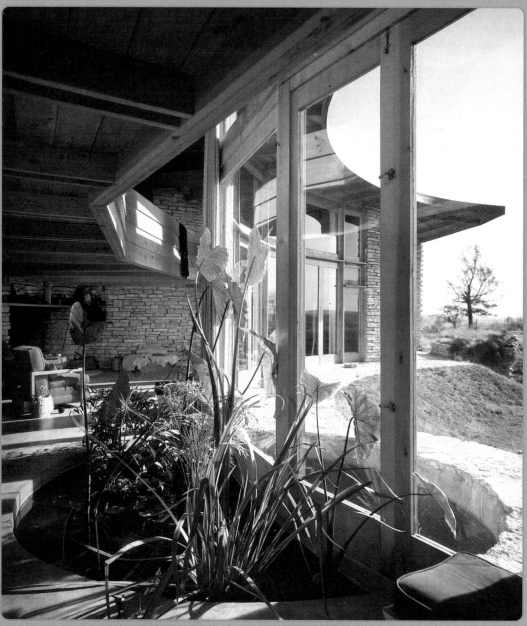

Photo: Ezra Stoller

Optimism versus pessimism

Until recently, environmental concerns were often seen as scaremongering, more so in the UK than many other places in Europe, especially when the demands for urgent action preceded positive proof that the concerns were fully justified. The culture of technological optimism, particularly strong in the 1950s and 1960s, invited confidence in the ability of the earth to provide for human needs in perpetuity. Until quite recently it was widely believed that any action in the face of uncertainty was wasteful, expensive and obstructive to innovation. However, increasing awareness of the costs of postponing action – for instance, the potential costs imposed by global warming and escalating crime and disaffection – have moved opinion to favour precautionary and preventative actions. This precautionary approach is now enshrined in sustainable development principles, albeit scarcely applied.

	State of the World	
	Optimists Right	Pessimists Right
Optimistic Policy	High	Disaster
Pessimistic Policy	Moderate	Tolerable

Optimism–pessimism table

This matrix, which dates back to the 1970s, suggests that within any risk scenario if the optimists are right and there is little to worry about, and if we pursue a policy of optimism, then the potential gains are high. However, if the pessimistic scenario is accurate, following an optimistic policy leads to disaster. Prudent policies based on precautionary action are most sensible

Precautionary principle

A principle adopted by the UN Conference on Environment and Development (UNCED) 1992 that in order to protect the environment a precautionary approach should be widely applied. The Rio declaration interpreted this as:

'where there are threats of serious or irreversible damage to the environment, lack of scientific certainty should not be used as a reason for postponing cost-effective measures to prevent environmental degradation.'

Oversimplification

Too often the scope of concerns and complexity of issues regarding sustainability are over-simplified. Many so-called sustainability arguments equate it with climate change in particular, to the detriment of other considerations. Vitally important as carbon management is, we need action on many fronts. No amount of energy efficiency, nor any other single-issue campaign, will deliver sustainable development, although it will help. Oversimplification encourages one-dimensional solutions, short cuts, shallow questions and potentially bad laws. Oversimplification diverts attention from broader understanding and excludes people who need to be engaged. In terms of the built environment, single issues alienate designers, who are often more comfortable with the resolution of complex problems than with single issues. Hence an attempt in this book to introduce the broad picture of the problems that designers face.

Perhaps most importantly, we need to move from the present rhetoric that sustainability involves environmental, economic and social aspects to actively making and demonstrating those links. It is the lack of real belief in, and evidence of, the linkages that prevents politicians and others from providing long-term solutions to our most basic development problems.

An important aspect of the development of new affordable low-allergy housing in Perth was to look to research on the economic value of improvements in health. Research by Howieson on improvements to existing properties in Scotland indicated that the cost of providing an allergy-resistant environment could be paid back in 23 months from savings in medication. Projects now exist where patients with breathing disabilities are being prescribed housing improvements on the NHS.

Case Study 1.2:

St. George's School, Wallasey, Cheshire

Architect: Emslie Morgan, 1961

St. George's School at Wallasey, 1961, was designed by Emslie Morgan to provide each classroom with natural daylight and sunlight. A long, narrow-plan, two-storey building, it has large south-facing, double-glazed windows deriving maximum benefit from solar gain.

Diffusing glass was used to reduce glare and clear-glazed, openable windows, positioned at intervals, give the occupants control over the internal environment.

The heavyweight structural mass – concrete floors and ceilings – was intended to balance out fluctuations in heat demand, which was first reduced by high levels of insulation and low ventilation rates.

The remainder of the heating was to be met by a combination of the heat produced by the occupants, the solar wall and the heat output of the electric lighting. Conventional heating in the form of a single radiator beneath each of the openable windows was installed as a precaution against the failure of the passive approach.

The auxiliary system was rarely used. Using electrical inefficiency for heating was part of a now outdated approach to design, but the debate on whether well-designed schools need any heating continues.

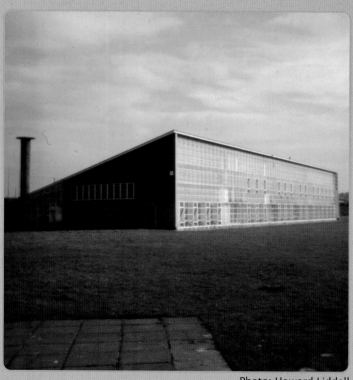

Photo: Howard Liddell

Inertia

A contributing element to the shift in attitude is the recognition of the significant time lag between initial concerns and coordinated action on issues as diverse as desertification, climate change, ozone depletion, acid rain and asbestosis. These man-made disasters have all taken place with prior warning and very slow response. This generation is being starkly confronted by the failure to act of previous generations.

There is an increasing tendency to consider how our environment might be if, instead of foot dragging and talking down concerns, we had committed resources to respond to these threats when they were first identified. In many cases responses are still hugely inadequate.

> **'If we suspect a problem we should talk it up, not talk it down.'**
>
> Bill Bordass

The construction industry, its designers and its suppliers are central to the issues. The construction industry did not start to implement controls on chlorofluorocarbons (CFCs) until the mid-1990s despite significant evidence of the adverse effects. The industry continues to design resource-inefficient buildings, utilises polluting materials, overspecifies inefficient equipment and undertakes developments highly dependent on polluting forms of transport, with poor attention to the long-term communities. The majority of construction activity transforms natural habitats into environments where species other than humans struggle to exist. None of this is necessary. It is just bad design.

In 1974, two independent scientific papers suggested that chlorine atoms were ozone destroyers and that CFCs were breaking up in the stratosphere, releasing chlorine. The devastating consequences were clear. In 1978, a campaign in the USA led to a ban on CFCs for their primary use as propellants. By the mid-1980s, CFC production was surpassing its previous peak as manufacturers sought alternative markets and found uses in the construction industry as cheap refrigerants and blowing agents for insulation materials.

In 1984, a 40% drop in stratospheric ozone was measured in the Antarctic and the ozone hole in the Southern Hemisphere was identified. In 1987, stratospheric chlorine was eventually confirmed as the problem and the Montreal Protocol was signed. Major manufacturers Du Pont agreed to phase out CFCs in 1988. The northern ozone hole was identified in 1991.

If the international agreement was fully applied, CFCs would be gone from the atmosphere in 100 years – but currently the illegal trade in CFCs from South to North America exceeds in cash value the trade in cocaine. North America, it seems, is addicted to air-conditioning and it seems incapable of processing the consequences.

Current predictions for global temperature change as a result of greenhouse gases are not very different from those predicted 40 years ago.

The Swedish chemist Arrhenius is credited with first recognising, and quantifying, that increases in CO_2 would lead to global warming. Scientific papers appeared from the 1930s, but there was little real interest until the 1970s and no consensus until the late 1990s.

esis, and the burning of fossil fuels. Since that time ge cities has risen 10 per cent. is too   Some scientists predict that the amount oxygen carbon dioxide in the air will almost doub r when by the year 2020. Carbon dioxide concentr 119.) tions, through complex reactions, could pr ats and vent the normal escape of radiated heat fro ght also the earth. Therefore, the temperature mig ut these rise about 5° F (2.8° C). This would have fa reaching effects on other aspects of climat up, the such as cloud cover and rainfall. It is al a critical believed that warming of the ocean wate

Impact of greenhouse gases
(Ecology, Basic Biology in Colour, Vol. V, 1972)

Internationally the issue is now very high on the political agenda, but intransigence from the major polluters undermines the will and effectiveness of actions by the global majority. Improved effectiveness in the use of resources sadly remains an unattractive proposition and instead proposed solutions currently include carbon sequestration (not sensibly in tree growth but in underground caverns!) and nuclear power (despite the fact that the lack of a waste management resolution makes it a fundamentally unsustainable solution).

History of international action

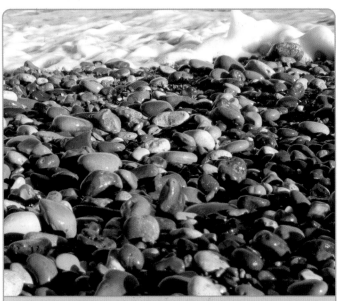

'Beginnings are apt to be shadowy'
Rachel Carson, opening sentence of *The Sea Around Us* (1951)
This classic work remains a source of inspiration for anyone
interested in the combination of the technical and the beautiful
in the natural environment
(Photo: the author)

Much visual art, religion and poetry would indicate that concerns
for the natural environment are deep rooted in the human psyche.
Yet it was very recently in human history that environmental
protection became a respectable concern. It was the early part of
the twentieth century before it formed the basis of international
agreements, with the International Maritime Organisation taking a
leading position. For years the approach to environmental
problems was largely dispersal – build higher chimney stacks – and
there was little thought given to efficiency or health.

In the post-World War 2 period, Western nations experienced
unprecedented economic development, and environmental
concerns were largely perceived as the preserve of the elite and the
politically subversive left wing – strange bedfellows in other times!

The recent positioning of the environment as a central political
issue indicates a fundamental change in attitudes that began in
the 1960s with concerns, mainly in developed countries, about
local and regional issues such as air and water pollution. In 1968,
two significant events established a basis for change.

The Club of Rome – Limits to Growth 1968

In 1968, 30 influential people from 10 countries – scientists,
educators, economists, humanists, industrialists and civil servants
– met in Rome. They shared a common concern that the major
problems faced by humankind were too complex to be dealt
with by traditional institutions and policies. This became 'The
Club of Rome', which set as its objectives to cultivate
understanding of the global system and to promote new policy
initiatives and action in response.

The first meeting led to the commissioning of a project to
examine problems that the group considered common to all
societies but beyond the ability of individual nations and political
structures to resolve independently. These included: wealth
imbalances leading to poverty alongside prosperity;
environmental degradation; loss of faith in existing institutions;
urban spread; insecurity of employment; alienation of youth;
rejection of traditional values; and economic disruptions
including inflation. These problems, which remain fundamental
issues today, were seen to involve the interaction of technical,
social, economic and political aspects.

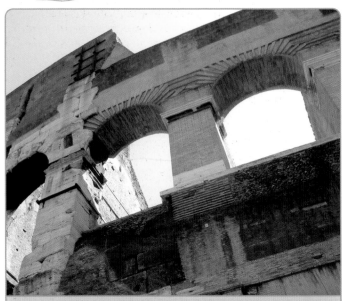

The Club of Rome held its first meeting in the late 1960s
It remains an influential supporter of original thought and action
in respect of sustainable development
(Photo: the author)

> **'Infinite growth on a finite planet is an impossibility.'**
>
> E. F. Schumacher (1973)

The outcome of the first meeting of the Club of Rome, published in 1972 as *Limits to Growth*, included a model of five basic factors thought to determine and limit growth.

These were:

- Population
- Food production
- Natural resources
- Industrial production
- Pollution

The *Limits to Growth* report drew attention to the exponential growth of all these elements. It led to serious concerns that we were using many of the Earth's assets at rates beyond their ability to regenerate and that inevitably we would outstrip the world's ability to support further growth. It predicted that if trends in these factors continue the limits to growth would be reached within 100 years, probably followed by a sudden decline. However, it also indicated that it was possible to establish sustainable ecological and economic stability, and meet the material needs and potential of all people, if we decided to make the effort. The sooner we begin work the better the chance of success.

Food production

To achieve a 34% increase in world food production from 1951 to 1961, investment in nitrates increased by 146%, expenditure on equipment by 63% and pesticide use by 300%.

The *Limits to Growth* report was based on a systems theory that became known as the Meadows–Meadows model. It stated two important principles: that all systems rely upon input of resources

and emit waste; and that the constraints on any finite system, including the Earth, are the ability to supply the required resources and to absorb the wastes emitted. Simply put, it is not the number of babies, cars or refrigerators that put stress on an environment, but the efficiency with which we use resources and minimise pollution and net waste.

It identified many sources utilised by human and economic systems as receding. The conclusion of the Meadows–Meadows scenario is that if you have to invest increasing amounts of a resource such as energy to get more energy, then ultimately overall gains are reduced. Inevitably, more capital and energy will be needed to obtain future supplies.

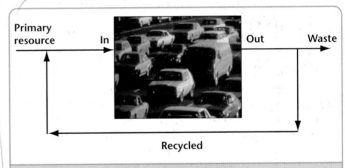

Sources and sinks
Simply put, it is not the number of babies, cars or refrigerators that puts stress on an environment, but the efficiency with which we use resources and minimise pollution and net waste

At the same time, the treatment and storage of waste was identified as becoming more difficult, contentious and expensive as the existing sites (or sinks) became overburdened (such as the atmospheric concentrations of greenhouse gases) and new sites (such as for landfill) become harder to find. Much current policy development is still based around these core principles.

Alternative population models – after the model in *Limits to Growth*.

The model describes the ways in which a system responds to pressures. The solid lines show population, the dashed line shows the carrying capacity.

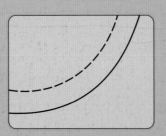

Continuous
A population can grow without interruption as long as the limits (carrying capacity) are far away or growing at the same rate or faster. This is the optimistic scenario, where, for example, a rise in food production matches a rise in population. In reality, it can rarely be sustained without drawing on other additional resources.

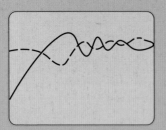

Overshoot
Overshoot occurs because of failure of control, faulty data or slow response. Natural oscillation is typical of populations and occurs when there is opportunity for the system to recover. Examples include fish stocks that are often capable of repair within limits.

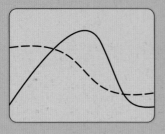

Collapse
Going too far beyond a limit will lead to a crash and a permanently impoverished environment, from which recovery is impossible. This is particularly likely when the limits are unknown or when there are positive feedback loops, such as in the case of greenhouse gas emissions, warming seas or depleting forests, which are a CO_2 sink.

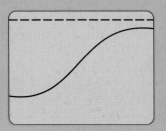

Sigmoid
A growing population takes resources from and emits pollution to a finite space, and puts pressure on that environment. Negative feedback such as scarcity, pollution and ill-health slows down growth if the feedback and the response are rapid and accurate. Growth levels off and the population gradually and stably approaches the carrying capacity.

Case Study 1.3:

Street Farm House, London

Architects: "Street Farmers" – Graham Caine, Bruce Haggart, 1974

An experimental temporary structure constructed in 1974 by Graham Caine and Bruce Haggart, on a sports field in Eltham owned by Thames Polytechnic. The aim was to provide integrated shelter, heat, food, water, cooking facilities and an ecologically sound waste disposal system for a small family in an urban context.

The structure was timber frame and insulated with wood wool. An integral attached semicircular south-facing greenhouse was used to live in, grow food, collect rain and act as a heat source. It incorporated hydroponic beds and a fishpond fertilised with effluent from a methane digester. Warm, oxygenated air from the greenhouse could be vented to the first-floor living space and an openable flap could vent excessively hot air to the outside. Auxiliary heating was provided by a paraffin heater. Domestic hot water was provided by black painted panel radiators with a total surface area of 8.4 m², glazed with two layers of polythene. This thermosiphoned directly to an insulated 225-litre water cylinder.

Rainwater was collected off the greenhouse roof, passed through a sand filter and used, with excess diverted to the fishpond. The design was relatively cheap.

Graham Caine and family lived in the building for 18 months before it was dismantled.

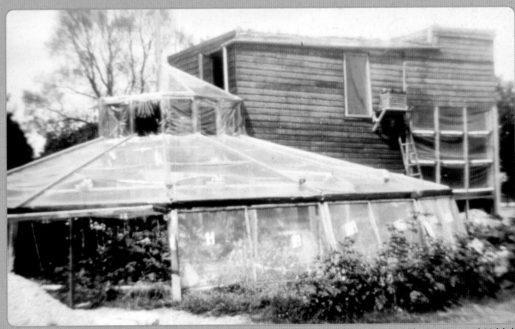

Photo: Howard Liddell

Case Study 1.4:

Wates House, Centre for Alternative Technology

Architect: Peter Bond Associates, 1976

The Centre for Alternative Technology has been a leading proponent of sustainable building, beginning in the 1970s with experiments specifically aimed at reducing energy demand. Completed in 1976, by Peter Bond Associates, Richmond, Surrey, this two-storey 100 m² house was designed with a conventional appearance and emphasis on very-low-energy passive design combined with alternative energy sources. The 700 mm thick walls consist of a rendered 100 mm outer brick skin, 450 mm of glass fibre insulation and an inner skin of 150 mm thick Thermalite concrete block.

The U-value is 0.075 W/m²K and the thermal time lag of 13–14 hours. Other energy-saving measures include a 275-litre waste water heat recovery tank coupled to the 180-litre hot water cylinder by a 0.18 kW heat pump, a cooking stove surrounded with 150 mm of insulation, a single entrance lobby with double doors, and low wattage fluorescent lights. The building consumed about one-fifth of the energy of a similarly sized conventional house built at the same time.

The evaporator of a 0.15 kW air/air heat pump is placed in a stream of outside air (the heat source) and the condenser placed in the stream of recirculating room air (the heat sink). Fresh air is introduced at a rate of one-quarter of an air change per hour, and stale air is extracted from the kitchen and expelled over the evaporator to help prevent icing up in cold weather. The system can be reversed for summer cooling.

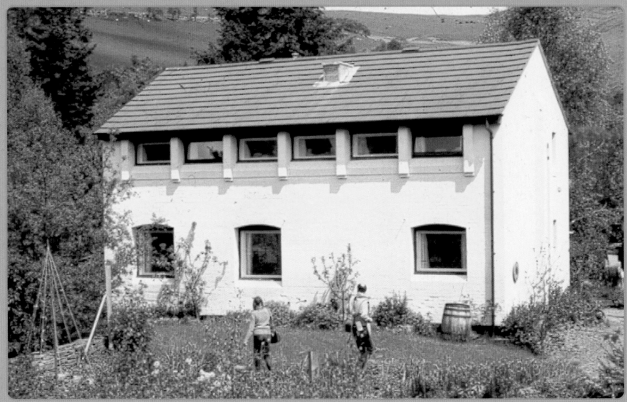

Photo: Pat Borer

UNCHE – 1972

In 1968, motivated primarily by the acidification of Scandinavian lakes and forests, the UN's economic and social council called for a meeting. The meeting eventually took place in 1972 and has since been known as the UN Conference on the Human Environment (UNCHE) or the Stockholm Conference. One hundred and thirteen countries were represented. It was responsible for transforming the environment into a political issue of international importance and made the division of wealth between the Northern and Southern Hemispheres a critical aspect of international policy.

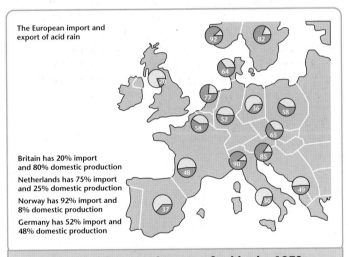

The European import and export of acid rain

Britain has 20% import and 80% domestic production

Netherlands has 75% import and 25% domestic production

Norway has 92% import and 8% domestic production

Germany has 52% import and 48% domestic production

European import and export of acid rain, 1970s
The UK's decision to build higher and higher chimney stacks and to rely on a predominantly westerly wind to take the pollution away led directly to international action on the environment. Ultimately, with global development, everyone catches a westerly (Data: Friends of the Earth, 1970s)

The relationship between environment and development was central to intensive negotiations prior to the meeting. Initially, the calls for environmental protection were thought to be elitist and a form of political and economic restraint. Not surprisingly, developing nations were reluctant to be lectured to about environmental constraints by countries that had grown rich on ignoring these same constraints. Interestingly, the debate and arguments eventually resulted in a very significant agreement that development and the environment were inextricably linked and that 'no one could go it alone'. This understanding, documented in the seminal publication *Only One Earth*, has taken more than 35 years to become widespread. The environment was, for the first time, identified 'as a critical dimension of successful development', and efforts began to resolve the dilemmas of growth, development and environment.

Following from the meeting, many countries established environment agencies and ministries. Legislation followed. The United Nations Environment Programme (UNEP) was created to promote awareness and action within the UN. A number of international and regional agreements were signed related to marine pollution, dumping and trans-boundary movement of waste, and it was at this point that protection of the ozone layer became an international issue, eventually leading to the Montreal Protocol.

> *'Humanity has the ability to make development sustainable – to ensure that it meets the needs of the present without compromising the ability of future generations to meet their own needs.'*
>
> Our Common Future

WCED – The Brundtland Commission 1981

The World Conservation Union (1981) is generally considered the originator of the term 'sustainable development' and it became the focal point of the Brundtland Commission – The World Commission on Environment and Development (WCED) – report Our Common Future published in 1987.

The WCED report was undertaken with an emphasis on social equity, stewardship and responsibility for all members of this generation and the next. Many of the sustainability principles now embodied in national and international agreements and policy stem from this report, including:

- the precautionary principle
- intergenerational equity
- intragenerational equity
- conservation of biodiversity
- internalised environmental costs.

Sustainable development was firmly established as a matter of self-interest for individuals and society, at an international policy level, by 1987.

Case Study 1.5:

The Ark, Prince Edward Island, Canada

The New Alchemy Institute and Solsearch Architects, 1976

The New Alchemy Institute was founded in 1971 by biologists John Todd, Nancy Jack Todd and Bill McLarney in Massachusetts. They later moved to Vermont, where they built a series of buildings to house their experiments. They had a strong academic knowledge of ecology and wanted to develop this by implementing solutions to problems of pollution. Where alchemy is the turning of base metals into gold, so new alchemy, it was proposed, was about turning pollution and toxic sludge into clear air and clean water.

'We asked ourselves the question: is it possible to grow the food needs of a small group of people in a small space without harming the environment and without enormous recourse to external sources of energy and materials on a continuing basis?

The whole idea was: could we design a system that is self-sustainable and capable of functioning as a system?'

John Todd, Design Outlaws on the Ecological Frontier (2000)

The New Alchemy Institute developed 'living machines', where they grew plants and farmed fish, usually housed in great glass domes. These machines replicated various ecosystems to treat sewage and water and to grow vegetables and fish.

A number of bioshelters were built, including the one shown here for extreme northern climates.

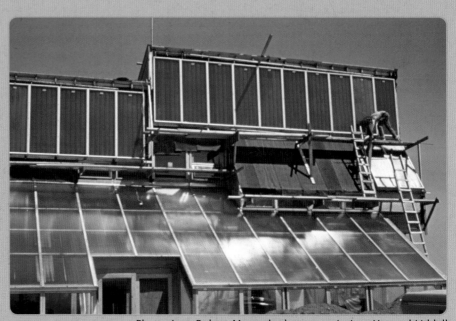

Photo: Jean-Robert Mazaud; photo permission: Howard Liddell

Case Study 1.6:

Granada House, Macclesfield, Cheshire

Architect: Don Wilson, 1976

Experimental passive and active heating technology was implanted in this 125 m² four-bedroom house, which was the subject of Granada Television's House for the Future series in 1976.

A conservatory attached to the south-west elevation provided solar heat, which was delivered to the ground floor by opening the connecting doors and the first-floor bedrooms through flaps at the base of each bedroom window. Excess heat could be stored in the 12 m³ insulated rock store located beneath the conservatory floor.

A trickle-type flat plate collector (42 m²) was installed on the south-west-facing roof at a pitch of 34° to the horizontal. Thermal storage was provided by water tanks containing a total of 5400 litres. A 1.5 kW heat pump transferred low-grade heat from a 2000-litre tank (at below 25°C) to a 3000-litre space heating tank (at 25–45°C). Legionella legislation would not now allow this. The heat was distributed by oversized thermostatically controlled radiators operating at 25–30°C. A 3.5 kW solid fuel boiler provided auxiliary heat.

After a year-long monitoring programme, it was estimated that the passive heating provided 21% of the heat required, the heat pump another 7% and the flat plate collector a further 2%, totalling 30%.

The vast majority of the benefits were due to the insulation. It is interesting to note that there is a contemporary enthusiasm for repeating similar experiments.

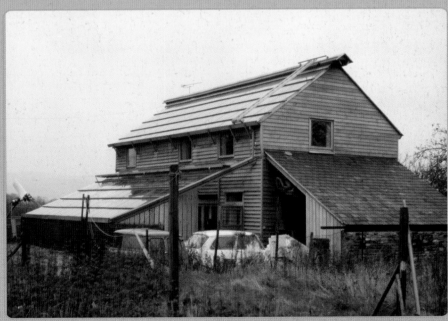

Photo: Howard Liddell

UNCED – 1992

By the early 1990s there was a huge groundswell of opinion that concerted international action on environment and development was needed. In 1992, the UN Conference on Environment and Development (UNCED) or Rio Earth Summit brought together 170 heads of state and government. It aimed to determine the requirements of achieving sustainable development and to agree a worldwide response. One of its biggest challenges proved to be the 'only one earth' approach. By proposing a unified international response it was perceived as threatening the sovereignty of national states. Perhaps inevitably, many were disappointed by the outcomes, including a lack of clarity, but with hindsight it is clear that a significant amount was achieved compared to subsequent events. There were five documents produced for Rio, known as the UNCED Agreements.

The Framework Convention on Climate Change is one of two 'International Agreements' signed by most governments at Rio. It established the principle that climate change was potentially a serious problem; that action could not wait for the resolution of scientific uncertainties; that developed countries should take the lead in mitigation; and that they should compensate developing countries for any additional costs they incurred in meeting the measures. It established a process of government reporting on policies, projections and progress, but no binding commitments were agreed beyond a first step to return GHG emissions to 1990 levels by 2000.

The Convention on Biological Diversity was the second of the 'International Agreements' signed by most governments. It aimed to preserve the biological diversity of the planet through the protection of species and ecosystems, and to establish terms for the uses of biological resources and technology. It affirmed that states have 'sovereign rights' over biological resources on their territory and that benefits should be shared equitably. Countries were required to develop plans to protect biodiversity.

The Rio Declaration was one of two 'Statements of Principles'. It comprises 27 principles for guiding action on environment and development. They stress the right to, and need for, development and poverty alleviation, and the rights and roles of special groups. They are often ambiguous on principles of trade and environment.

The Forest Principles was the second of the 'Statements of Principles'. It is generally agreed to be a failed Convention on Forests. It emphasises the sovereign right to exploit forest resources but does include principles that are intended to guide their management, conservation and sustainable development.

Agenda 21– an agenda for action – is a massive document that was intended as the blueprint for socially, economically and environmentally sustainable development. *Agenda 21* was intended to form the key intergovernmental guide and reference document up to the millennium. It is widely recognised for putting 'bottom-up', participatory and community-based approaches into the forefront of policy-making in many areas, including population policy. A summary document by Michael Keating makes easier reading than the original.

All of these agreements indicate a strong move to manage pollution in all its forms, which does indicate a very real political concern resulting from the evidence of research into chemical dispersal, including climate change. The climate change gases (methane, CO_2, N_2O, CFCs, tropospheric ozone) have continued to be the source of much controversy. It was 2001 before 164 countries were able to agree a methodology for applying the Kyoto agreement – the USA and Australia declined and only in 2003 did Russia ratify the Kyoto Protocol and enable agreements to come into force. It is very interesting that the other countries have gone ahead despite the refusal of major polluters – Australia and the USA – to comply with clear international will.

Rio to Johannesburg – 2002

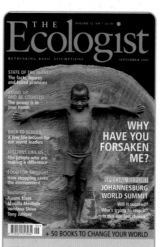

This image first appeared in the September 2002 issue of *The Ecologist* Volume 32, No. 7 (www.theecologist.org)

Following UNCED, a number of international meetings were convened and agreements were reached on a variety of environmental issues of international relevance. The next major world convention, the World Summit for Sustainable Development (WSSD) in Johannesburg in 2002, is generally considered as a failure, with few commitments made.

Whilst it is true in many respects that Rio had limited success and Johannesburg even less, a factual account of what was actually agreed in 2002 makes interesting reading (see *Rio plus Ten* by Middleton and O'Keefe – it covers the ground and is extremely well written).

Case Study 1.7:

The Machynlleth House, CAT

Self-build under the guidance of Jon Broome, Architype, 1993

The development of post and beam timber-frame building owes a great deal to the architect Walter Segal. He refined the building process to make it accessible to all and today his Segal Method is popular with selfbuilders. The Machynlleth House at the Centre for Alternative Technology demonstrates that a low-cost simple Segal construction can incorporate energy-saving features. The Centre arranged a self-build course for eight participants, who had no prior building knowledge. After 10 days of intensive work – under guidance – the structure was complete, under cover and partly enclosed.

The sandwich forming the walls differs from other Segal houses to give higher insulation.

As well as being exceptionally well insulated, it incorporates a south-facing, passive solar conservatory extending the full width of the house. This acts as a buffer between the inside and outside of the building, and provides pre-heated ventilation air.

The core of the sandwich is 100mm of extruded, expanded polystyrene, which has a closed cell structure and includes a sheet of polythene between the core and the internal plasterboard lining, to reduce the infiltration of cold air. The building also includes solar panels for hot water heating. A woodburning stove provides back-up.

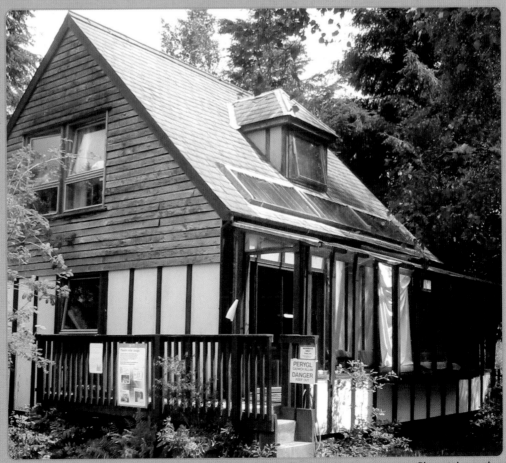

Photo: the author

Case Study 1.8:

Andersen House, Stavanger, Norway

Architects: Dag Roalkvam and Rolf Jacobsen, 1984

This 210 m² wood and stone pentagonal building is the first modern example of the moisture transfusive wall, a construction technique that is now increasing in popularity.

It was designed and built by Dag Roalkvam and Rolf Jacobsen, now of Gaia Norway, in 1984. It was constructed avoiding the use of materials known to contain toxic substances, in keeping with the Gaia architectural philosophy, and was designed with passive air exchange.

It is zoned for temperature with all the warm rooms facing south and cold rooms facing northwest and prevailing wind. A greenhouse on one side of the house provides pre-warmed air.

It has a double skin – or raincoat – hanging 600mm away from the walls on the weather facing sides. This sacrificial wall keeps wind away from the main walls. This wooden skin is broken by gaps to admit light to the windows.

On the south-west aspect a double-height, central room with a glazed external wall acts as an intermediate space, providing light and solar heat to the adjoining rooms through internal windows.

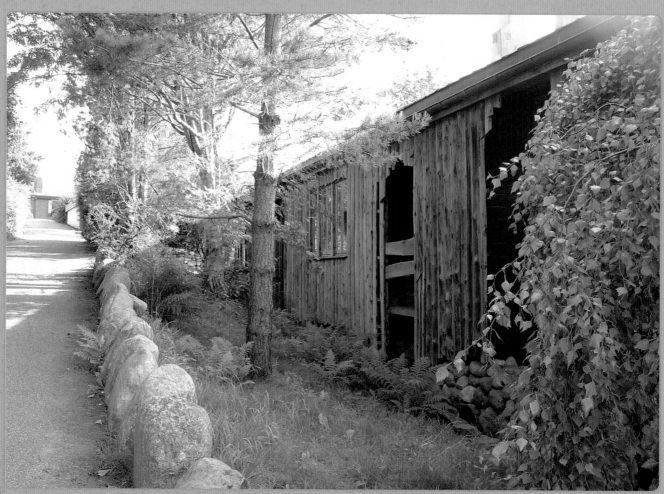

Photo: Dag Roalkvam

Recent progress?

Many gloomy predictions are contradicted by experience. In resource terms we appear to have more than ever, and in developed countries warnings have begun to be heeded. Widespread concern is being translated into policy. Regulations and taxation are slowly taming polluters. The air and rivers are getting cleaner, and many people remain optimistically wedded to the idea that humankind will find solutions to any problems that arise.

> *'Nineteenth and twentieth century models of development are being exported by nineteenth and twentieth century thinkers, ahead of twenty-first century knowledge.*
>
> Sandy Halliday

In many developing countries resource consumption and pollution are escalating in justifiable pursuit of economic development, but the understanding of the fundamental link between development and the environment, forged in the 1970s, is being left behind. A population of 4 million in Finland has discovered the bicycle, whilst a population of a billion in China is trying to consign it to history.

In developing countries environmental problems are immense and increasing. And everywhere, pervasive toxicity remains an immense problem. Global warming and ozone depletion are reminders of unheeded warnings and the construction industry, along with others, continues to ignore them. The onus is on wealthier nations to bear the brunt of the expense and remedial action. It is also a responsibility to set an example of real quality in sustainable buildings and to support native sustainable building techniques where they exist rather than to export inappropriate technologies and techniques. However, the signs are not good.

All the best possible scenarios seem likely to be frustrated unless we actively start to reverse unsustainable trends and support sustainable ones.

Arguments become polarised. In respect of agriculture, those promoting genetically modified crops claim the moral high ground of feeding the world's hungry. Those against invoke the precautionary principle and promote sustainable methods of increasing food production without the risks implicit in genetic modification. The same is true in built environments. A need for housing is used to override any argument for such housing to be affordable, healthy, resource efficient and in the right place. Yet it could be all these things.

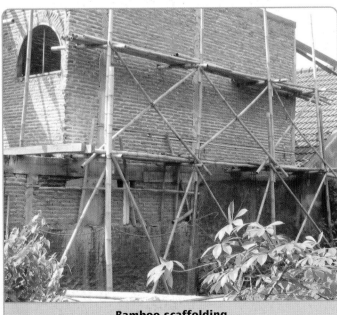

Bamboo scaffolding
Bamboo might reasonably be expected to be used in developing nations for scaffolding, even in large constructions,...
(Photo: the author)

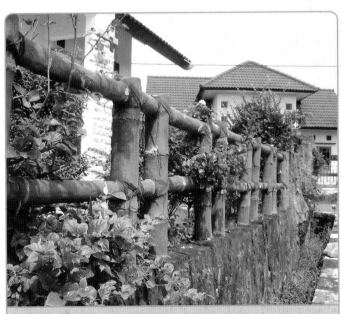

Concrete fenceposts
...but only 50 yards away, traditional bamboo fencing had been replaced by a lookalike concrete substitute
(Photo: the author)

Case Study 1.9:

Rocky Mountain Institute, Colorado

Designers: Lovins and Lovins, 1984

Situated at 2200 m above sea level, outdoor temperatures during the winter can fall as low as minus 44°C. One per cent of the heating needs of the building are provided by two small wood-burning stoves and 99% from passive solar.

The heavy thermal mass curved building stores heat and a large glazed south-facing façade allows three-quarters of the light and half of the solar energy to enter the building and then retains it.

The walls, made from two leaves of 150 mm-thick masonry faced with local stone inside and out, achieve a U-value of 0.14 W/m²K. The highly insulated, earth-covered roof has a U-value of 0.09 W/m²K.

Incoming air is pre-heated by outgoing air through air-to-air heat exchangers. Hot water for the building is provided by a bank of solar collectors connected to a 7000-litre super-insulated water storage tank. Low-energy appliances are used throughout, including a purpose-built super-insulated fridge and freezer and compact fluorescent luminaires.

This results in a 90% saving in household electricity over the norm. The extra cost of installing the passive and active systems in the house was repaid after 10 months, at 1984 prices, and the energy savings will pay for the house in about 40 years.

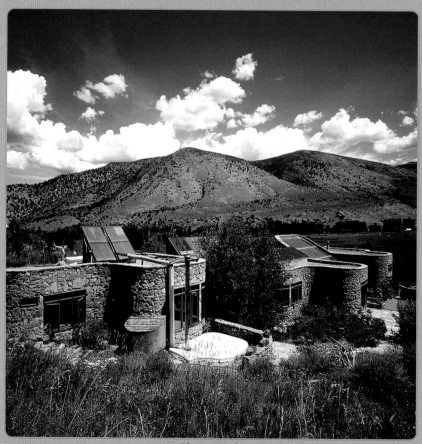

Photo: Rocky Mountain Institute (www.rmi.org)

Case Study 1.10:

NMB Bank, The Netherlands

Architect: Ton Alberts, 1991

Located south-east of Amsterdam, the NMB (now ING) HQ was the largest bank in the Netherlands. This unique building (48 600 m²) was designed by Ton Alberts. It consists of a series of 10 towers strung together by an internal street forming an 'S' shape. Along the street are conference rooms, a lecture theatre, a winter garden, restaurants and eating places. Different coloured towers create distinct identities for each department.

An integrated approach was adopted at the outset of the building project, looking at the overall operation of the organisation and allowing architects, engineers and landscapers to contribute their ideas. Energy efficiency was given a high priority. The building was designed to operate without air-conditioning, and a passive system controls all the heating, cooling and ventilation needs. Located at the top of each tower is a solar collector and a heat recovery unit. The windows are designed to provide an average 500 lux, whilst excluding external traffic noise and preventing excessive heat loss and unwanted gains.

Integration of good insulation levels and careful use of passive heating and ventilation backed up by well-controlled mechanical services mean that it has an energy consumption of 96 kWh/m² per annum, approximately 90% less energy than a typical 1970s office block. Compared to the consumption of the previous HQ building erected 10 years earlier, it gives savings in fuel bills of over a £1 m/year.

Enclosing the south-facing aspect captures passive solar energy and provides a bright circulation space. Its reflective windows reject solar energy from high angles. This plus heat recovery from the printing works provides the heating needs. The heat is distributed via air circulation and through a low-temperature central heating system, fed by a heat pump to a back-up condensing boiler. It uses two conservatories, one to the north and one to the south, which are connected to either pre-heat or cool incoming air to the building as required. The facilities manager reported the heat consumption as 70–80 kWh/m²/year and 25% of normal mains water consumption.

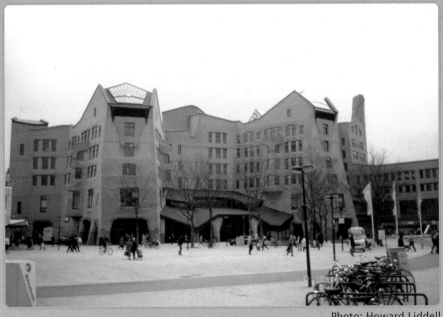

Photo: Howard Liddell

Conclusion

Throughout the 1960s and 1970s the concept of sustainability evolved in the international arena. It was however largely marginalised as a restraint on development. Only in the last few years has there been an evolution of awareness such that sustainability is now recognised as a restraint on inappropriate development and a principal driver of increasing quality of life for all. Even 30 years on, these are still young concepts. There is no longer any excuse for not addressing these issues seriously.

The built environment offers plenty of evidence that there are links between the economy, the environment and society, and plenty of opportunity to reinforce the positive links that generate net benefit. The construction sector has a significant role to play. There is much to do. Many are trying to move in the appropriate direction, but unsustainable building clearly dominates. Indeed, sustainable construction is still marginalised and unsustainable building lauded. In the UK, government policy based on presumptions about economic behaviour of developers is proving to be misguided. As a result we are burdened by unsustainable schools and housing, where ample knowledge exists to do otherwise.

If, as all the international agreements claim, we aim to promote environmental quality, precaution, equity and biodiversity as fundamental aspects of development, then strenuous efforts and constant vigilance are required. Developing countries have to show commitment and responsibility. It is happening slowly but only at a pace that vested interests will tolerate, based on short-termism, not at the rate required or possible.

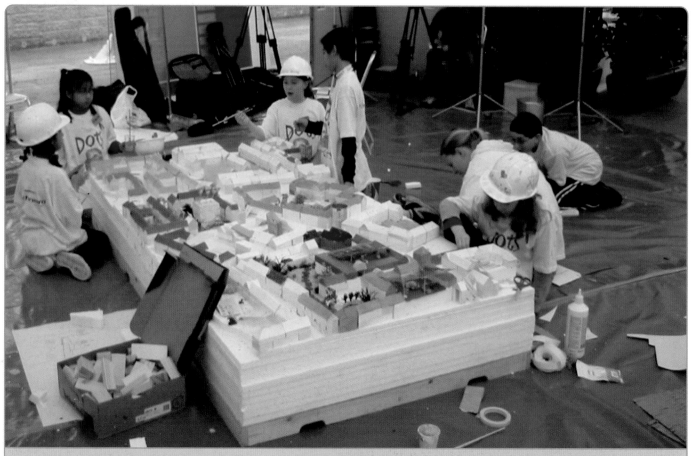

Children's ecocity, Dumbydykes, Edinburgh
(Photo: TASC Agency)

Bibliography

Texts

Jacks, G. V. and Whyte, R. O. (1939) *The Rape of the Earth*. Faber. World survey of soil erosion.

Carson, R. (1951) *The Sea Around Us*. Oxford University Press.

Carson, R. (1962) *Silent Spring*. Haughton Mifflin. Also worth a read is the biography of Rachel Carson, *Witness for Nature*, by Lear.

Brand, S. (ed.) (1971) *The Whole Earth Catalogue*. Penguin Books.

Papanek, V. (1971) *Design for the Real World – Human Ecology and Social Change*. Granada.

Meadows, D., Meadows, D., Randers, J. and Behrens, W. W. (1972) *The Limits to Growth*. Signet.

Ward, B. and Dubois, R. (1972) *Only One Earth*. Norton.

Kolbas, G. H. (1972) *Basic Biology in Colour Vol. V. Ecology – Cycle and Recycle*. Sterling Publishing Co.

Schumacher, E. F. (1973) *Small is Beautiful: A study of economics as if people mattered*. Blond Briggs.

Bacon, J. et al. *Shelter* (1973) Shelter/Random House.

Gorz, A. (1980) *Ecology as Politics*. Pluto Press.

Myers, M. (ed.) (1985) *The Gaia Atlas of Planet Management*. Pan Books.

WCED (1987) *Our Common Future*. Oxford.

Pearson, D. (1989) *The Natural House Book*. Gaia Books.

Kemp, D. D. (1990) *Global Environmental Issues – A Climatological Approach*. Routledge. Physics doesn't change – good coverage of all the major environmental problems for any-one who wants to know how chlorine depletes the ozone layer, acid rain is formed and other such details.

Vale, R and Vale, B. (1991) *Green Architecture: Design for a Sustainable Future*. Thames & Hudson.

Meadows, D., Meadows, D. and Randers, J. (1992). *Beyond the Limits*. Earthscan.

Grubb, M. et al. (1993) *The Earth Summit Agreements – A Guide and Assessment*. RIIA.

Keating, M. (1993) *Agenda for Change. Centre for Our Common Future*. A really useful summary of the Rio agreements, including Agenda 21.

Brenton, T. (1994) *The Greening of Machiavelli*. Earthscan/RIIA. Best title award and a really good summary of the way international agreements have evolved.

von Weizsacker, E., Lovins, A. B. and Lovins, L. H. (1995) *Factor Four – Doubling Wealth, Halving Resource Use*. Earthscan. Upbeat, optimistic, JFDI classic.

Gilpin, A. (1996) *Dictionary of Environment and Sustainable Development*. Wiley.

Tenner, E. (1996) *Why Things Bite Back – Predicting the problems of progress*. Fourth Estate.

Zelov, C. (ed.) (1997) *Design Outlaws on the Ecological Frontier*. The Knossos Project.

McNeil, J. (2000) *Something New Under the Sun – An environmental history of the 20th Century*. Penguin.

Morrison, C. and Halliday, S. P. (2000) *Working with Participation No. 5: EcoCity – A model for children's participation in the planning and regeneration of their local environment*. Children in Scotland.

Zelov C. (ed.) (2000) *Design Outlaws at the Ecological Frontier*. Knossus Publishers

Meadows, D., Meadows, D. and Randers, J. (2002) *Limits to Growth – The Thirty Year Update*. Earthscan.

Middleton, N. and O'Keefe, P. (2003) *Rio plus Ten – Politics, Poverty and the Environment*. Pluto Press.

Stephen, W. (ed.) (2004) *Think Global, Act Local – The Life and Legacy of Patrick Geddes*. Luath Press.

Sacquet, A.-M. (2005) *World Atlas of Sustainable Development – Economic, Social and Environmental Data*. Anthem Press.

Diamond, J. (2006) *Collapse – How Societies Choose to Fail or Survive*. Penguin.

Architecture for Humanity (ed.) (2006) *Design Like You Give a Damn* Thames & Hudson

Sustainable development networks

The Ecologist – www.theecologist.org

Environment Business – www.environment-now.co.uk

Ethical Consumer – www.ethicalconsumer.org

New Internationalist – www.newint.org

Resurgence – www.resurgence.gn.apc.uk

The Club of Rome – www.clubofrome.org

Chapter 2
Policy and legislation

(with thanks to Roger Venables of Crane Environmental for his input to the original)

In which we highlight the key policy drivers for the creation of more sustainable construction, the legislative requirements that the promoters, designers and constructors of built development need to meet, and some pro-active policy initiatives on the part of those really striving to adopt a sustainable approach.

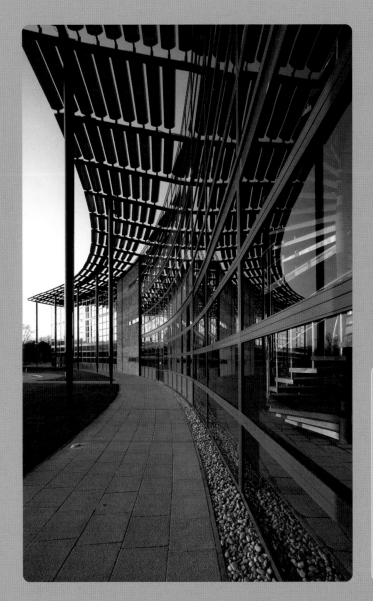

'The construction industry has a huge contribution to make to our quality of life. It provides the delivery mechanism for many aspects of government policy aimed at the provision and modernisation of the nation's built environment ... The economic, social and environmental benefits which can flow from more efficient and sustainable construction are potentially immense.'

Building a Better Quality of Life: a strategy for more sustainable construction in the UK, April 2000

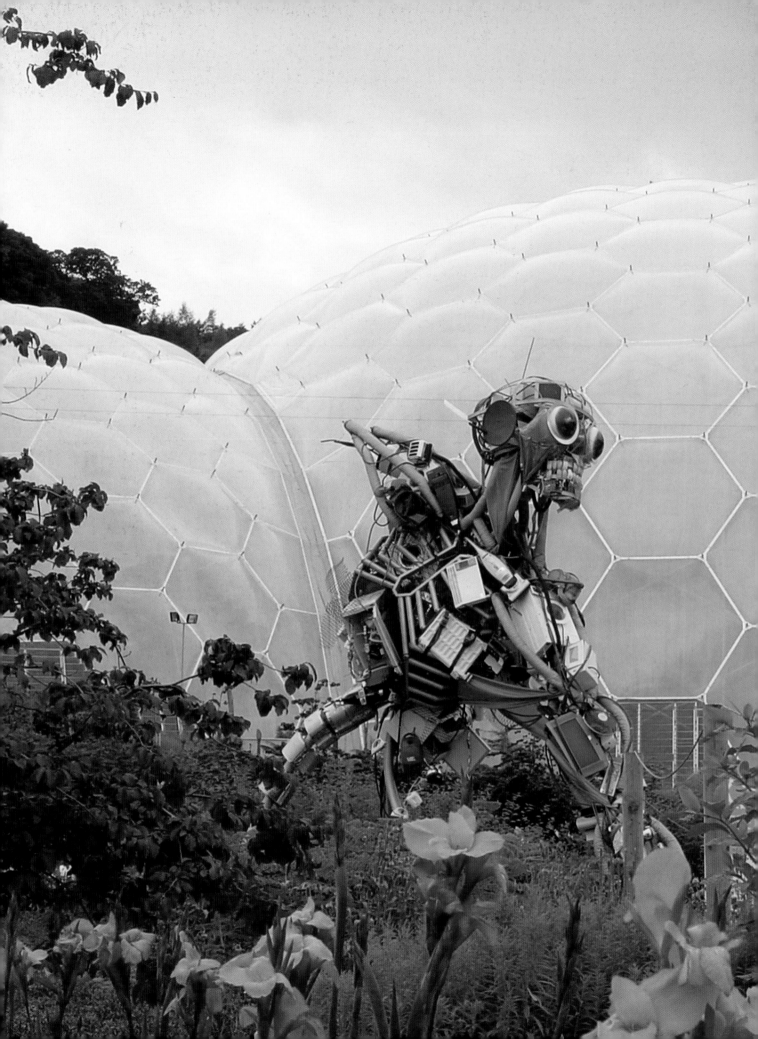

Contents

(Facing page)
WEEE Man at the Eden Project, Cornwall
Sculpted from waste electrical and electronic goods
(Photo: Bill Bordass, William Bordass Associates)

(Previous page)
Red Kite House
(Architects: Scott Brownrigg, photo: Martin Cleveland, www.mc-photostudio.com)

Policy and legislation

Introduction

Significant changes in attitudes towards the environmental and social impact of construction have been taking place in recent years.

Pressures on the industry involving the three strands of sustainability – economics, social equity and environmental enhancement – have led to activity in development of appropriate policies throughout the sector, and to more stringent legislation. This is in part a response to increasing use of economic intervention, which is dealt with in Chapter 3.

As a consequence, the construction industry, along with other industries, is developing policies and practices that are environmentally and socially more responsible. This emergence of 'business with a conscience' is a very significant recent trend.

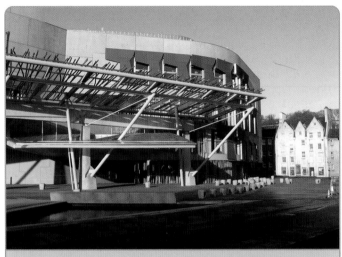

Scottish Parliament building, Edinburgh
Scottish Executive now has power to make building regulations
that support sustainable development
(Photo: Howard Liddell)

Emerging policies are leading to mainstreaming of community and environmentally responsible building and design practices, which until recently were largely marginalised.

This trend has the potential to lead to many more built development projects that are simultaneously more efficient and profitable, much more socially accountable, and much less damaging to the environment than before. This is called sustainable construction. Understanding and adoption of sustainable construction are rapidly increasing. However, the practices that can deliver sustainable construction are being adopted by a very small minority of organisations involved in built development, and on only a tiny percentage of construction projects.

Legislation is inadequate. It could, and should, be more pro-active in moving to eliminate unsustainable practices, so that

benefits in health and well-being would flow. Much more is required. However, legislation can only ever be a lowest common denominator. It is the actions of industry leaders, responsive to and seeking out contemporary knowledge, that are at the forefront of change. Businesses and individuals are driving improvements in the sustainability performance of mainstream construction practice, not the other way around.

This is gradually being translated into policies issued by governments, industry bodies, professional institutions and individual companies, and ultimately setting the guidelines for changing legislation. Recent experience indicates that it is central European practice that is delivering the appropriate tools, products and materials to drive change in sustainable construction within Europe.

Impact

The UK construction industry provides a tenth of the UK's gross domestic product and employs 1.4 million people. It is responsible for over 25% of all industry-related pollution incidents. Construction and demolition waste represent 19% of UK waste. The energy used in constructing, occupying and operating buildings is responsible for about 50% of the UK's greenhouse gas emissions. Our buildings are less healthy, less efficient, generate more waste, and are more polluting and more costly to run than those in many European countries.

There is an intention to significantly expand the house building target, but there are concerns about the impact on individuals, and on the wider environment, of many of the materials in common use. There is strong evidence that building performance is not achieving building standards. Houses are getting bigger, so improving energy efficiency standards on a per m^2 basis is unlikely to keep pace with real consumption. Water is a particular concern in some places. Improvements in performance are therefore necessary even to maintain a level playing field, to protect biodiversity, to ensure built quality and to keep within available resource limits. Providing improvements

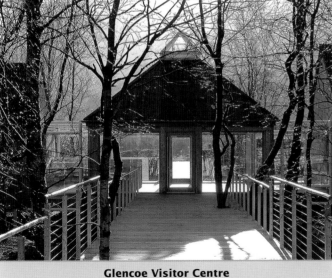

Glencoe Visitor Centre
(Architects: Gaia Architects; photo: Michael Wolshover)

that can deliver the health, environmental and economic benefits is a major challenge.

Changes in attitude

The changes in attitudes, and consequential changes in policies and legislation, have been prompted by a range of factors, including:

- the disturbing results of research into climate change, depletion of the ozone layer and widespread chemical pollution of the environment
- the increased awareness of these and other environmental issues and their increasing presence and importance on the political agenda – locally, nationally and internationally – especially since the *UN Conference on Environment and Development* in Rio, 1992 and its *Agenda 21* declaration
- increasing concern about the adverse impact of typical construction activity on neighbours and on the environment
- the action of individuals and environmental groups in challenging norms about consumption of resources, generation of waste and damage to biodiversity
- increasing concern about poor indoor air quality and other adverse factors within buildings
- increasing concerns about the type of developments that are being permitted and the imposition of development projects on communities, resulting in disaffection, rather than development that meets the identified needs of communities
- increasing recognition that achieving a high-quality built environment can be a major contribution to improvements in our quality of life, as well as delivering productivity and health and financial benefits
- challenges to conventional arguments about the cost of construction and embracing the cost of externalities, leading to better understanding of the inter-relationship between a high-quality environment, productivity, education and health, in turn leading to financial benefits and improvements in quality of life and business performance
- increasing focus on the corporate responsibilities of businesses, leading to greater emphasis on good business practice and fair trade.

Whilst there is uncertainty about the extent of the action required, it is clear that in recent years legislation and policy, including economic policy, has been moving to reverse unsustainable trends.

Policy integration

The holistic nature of the sustainable construction agenda and the fact that the built environment affects the quality of our lives so fundamentally, and in so many diverse ways, means that the built environment has the potential to be a focus for a wide range of policy. This increasingly appears to be the case.

Policy on architectural quality, planning and community participation, pollution prevention, biodiversity and animal habitats, transport infrastructure, the relationship between town and hinterland, health at home, crime in communities, energy use and generation, and developing appropriate new jobs and skills are all intrinsically connected to the environments in which we live and work. The integrative aspects are increasingly apparent and interesting, and the development of overarching indicators of sustainable development have much to do with the quality of construction per se.

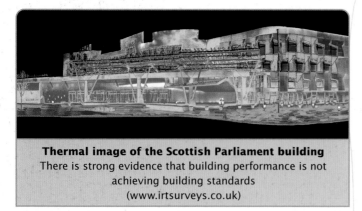

Thermal image of the Scottish Parliament building
There is strong evidence that building performance is not achieving building standards
(www.irtsurveys.co.uk)

Policy responses

Sustainability policies represent the stated priorities, aims, aspirations and objectives of international bodies, national governments, professions and companies. They are increasingly used by a wide range of players in the construction scene as a means of communicating commitment to improving practice beyond the regulatory standard and to show evidence of improving their sustainability performance. They are fast becoming a requirement on construction projects and are increasingly used to raise standards beyond a legislative requirement.

There is now a lot of knowledge and great opportunity to develop improved buildings and built environments. In order to move forward the industry needs to commit to firm deliverables, but also requires education on product and process issues. Clients have the opportunity to look at models of best practice and to recognise the benefits that can accrue from it. Governments need to take a more forthright role in raising the policy commitments and the legislative requirements, linking policy and legislation to the available knowledge at an ambitious pace commensurate with delivering much needed changes.

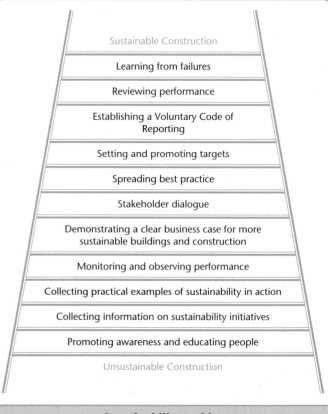

Sustainable Construction

Learning from failures

Reviewing performance

Establishing a Voluntary Code of Reporting

Setting and promoting targets

Spreading best practice

Stakeholder dialogue

Demonstrating a clear business case for more sustainable buildings and construction

Monitoring and observing performance

Collecting practical examples of sustainability in action

Collecting information on sustainability initiatives

Promoting awareness and educating people

Unsustainable Construction

Sustainability Ladder
(from Sustainable Action Group of the Construction Federation (2000), *Towards Sustainability*, CIP Ltd)

Case Study 2.1:

Municipal Building Department, Tübingen

Architects: Various

When the city of Tübingen in south Germany decided to undertake the development of a derelict French barracks into a new city quarter in the 1990s, they developed a number of innovative strategies for procurement and for environmental protection. Rather than selling the land to a developer, they determined to set the guidelines and to oversee the development themselves. In this way they have been able to maintain control and to recycle the profits into the infrastructure, including transport and landscape. They decided to go beyond the regulatory framework in setting environmental guidelines for the development. Overleaf is the contractual agreement that forms the basis for environmental protection.

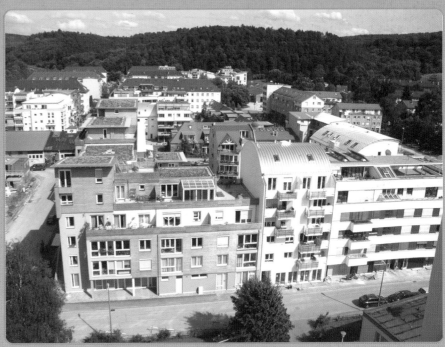

Photo: Joachim Eble Architects

Case Study 2.1 (Continued):

Municipal Building Department, Tübingen

Regarding compliance with the conditions for environmental protection

The architect/engineer commits:
- to include the following regulations in planning and tendering, and
- guarantee the compliance of the following regulations in the submission as well as in the project monitoring.

This commitment is part of the contract.

1 *Protection of wood*

On principle the use of wood preserver is not allowed. If the construction necessitates wood preserver (see examples in DIN 68 800 Part 3, April 1990), the following products are allowed: inside the building only pure boris salt products and outside the building beech distillates or CKB salts (chromate/potassium/boric acid).

2 *Paint, varnish, adhesives* (for carpets, coverings, etc.)

Only non-solvent materials signed with RAL-UZ 12 (Blue Angel, Environmental Label No. 12) are allowed.

3 *Halogen-free materials*

Exceptions are admitted in the field of electric cables as well as tubes for the sewage system. In the last case the tender must include the following sentence: 'The contractor is committed to recycle PVC waste from the building site separately.'

4 *Materials containing CFCs*

The use of materials containing totally halogenated chlorofluorocarbons (for example, R11 and R12) is not permitted. The use of partly halogenated chlorofluorocarbons is exceptionally not allowed, but reasons must be given for each individual case.

5 *Tropical timber*

The use of tropical timber is not allowed.

6 *Mineral fibrous insulating material*

Only mineral fibrous insulating material with carcinogenic index lower than 40 is allowed.

(Carcinogenic index in the meaning of technical guideline for hazardous materials 905.)

7 *Resolution of the City Council to the use of grey water*

8 *Resolution of the City Council to the low-energy standard*

9 *Consideration of the accident prevention regulations*

Sometimes the architect or engineer may think it unavoidable to use a material not in accordance with according to numbers 1–5. In this case the deviation must be explained in detail and the municipality must agree before tendering. The valid alternatives must be nominated precisely in the tender.

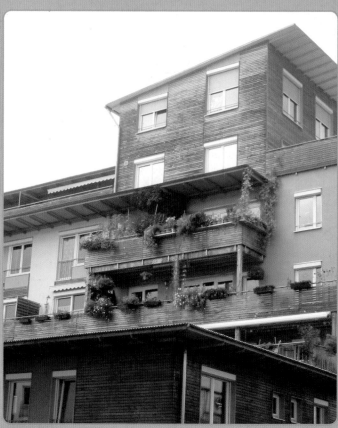

Architects: Joachim Eble Architects
Photo: the author

Key players

Leading-edge organisations and designers have been at the forefront of change, applying their knowledge to address problems of unsustainable patterns of development for decades, well in advance of governments, clients or the professional bodies. Taking a wide perspective of the role of construction, and linking this to contemporary issues, they have pushed the forefront of building design in relation to communities, materials, health and resource effectiveness, and by highlighting the positive benefits of sustainable design through the delivery of good quality, healthy, efficient, value-for-money buildings. It is notable that they may be the least likely to have formal policies, instead operating from a base understanding.

Government, government agencies and local authorities have been addressing the issue seriously since the early 1990s, and are gradually cascading requirements. As part of the implementation strategy for the policy, the RIAS has also spearheaded an accreditation scheme to acknowledge the contribution of accomplished sustainable building designers. The scheme was launched in February 2005. Thirteen architects gained a personal accreditation award down the supply chain of construction clients, through much needed formal policies and the guidance that underpins them, and through legislation passed by parliaments.

The *European Union* is very actively supporting sustainable development through directives and guidance. It consolidates and disseminates best practice from leading-edge countries and uses this to drive up standards and the regulatory benchmark. It enables individuals and governments in other countries to use this as a precedent.

Local authorities became more proactive across a wide range of issues, including construction, in response to the *Agenda 21* commitments made in Rio in 1992. As well as developing local environmental and community plans, many drew up checklists and began developing policies for sustainable construction and the natural environment. The advent of partnership as the principal means of delivering public sector buildings such as hospitals and schools – prior to the development of best practice guidance – has presented barriers to delivery. Although in principle financial partners would be expected to take a long-term interest in resource issues, health and potential legal responsibilities, the majority have largely pursued policies of short-term financial gain.

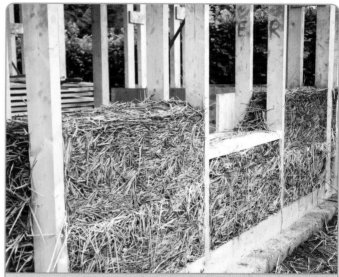

European precedents
European practice was cited in addressing building regulations issues for this light earth construction in the Scottish Borders
(Photo: Steven Downie)

Leading-edge contractors, developers, suppliers and constructors are beginning to use sustainability policies to bring about change in the way they carry out their operations. Expectations, rising costs and legal precautions have significantly changed behaviour in site operations and these have been formalised, particularly in larger companies.

Clients, conventional businesses, designers and developers are increasingly aware of consumer power and trends to ensure that business impacts on the environment and society are positive. There is curiosity and concern about how this will impact on bottom-line profits. Indeed, the triple bottom line – meeting social, environmental and economic obligations to consumers and shareholders – is increasingly the boardroom agenda. Understanding and adoption of sustainable construction is evolving. Few businesses now seem to openly commit to unsustainable building, although there is much confusion about what it means in practice. As a consequence, increasing numbers of developers and designers are prepared to indicate sustainable design amongst their services, although the claims are often in advance of the evidence and results can be disappointing.

Industry and professional bodies are developing policies and action plans to be adopted by their members, including introducing sustainability as a fundamental requirement in undergraduate education, leading to a professional qualification. They are also bringing demonstration projects to the fore through seminars, professional development opportunities and award schemes in order to help to disseminate good practice.

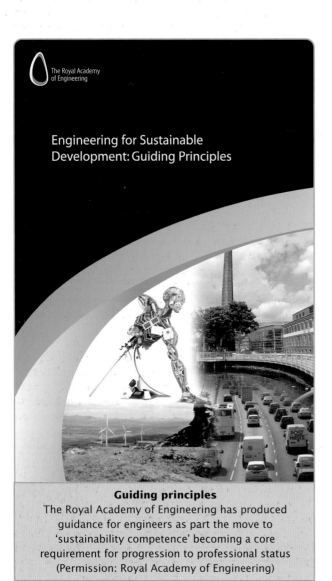

Guiding principles
The Royal Academy of Engineering has produced guidance for engineers as part the move to 'sustainability competence' becoming a core requirement for progression to professional status
(Permission: Royal Academy of Engineering)

How does sustainable development challenge us?

Sustainability challenges us to ensure that we do not cause harm whilst maintaining a non-declining stock of capital assets, including environmental assets, to meet the needs of society in the future. Success relies on action at different levels. Consider the actions required on transport:

- At product design and manufacturing level, eco-efficiency and innovation are needed to reduce unnecessary resource consumption and to generate products and services that minimise waste and pollution.
- At industry level, joined-up thinking and action are needed to provide a joined-up local, regional and national transport infrastructure (i.e. trains, buses, safe cycle and walk routes). This already happens very effectively in many European countries and successful policies have been implemented, but it is not helped by privatisations that do not make it a requirement.
- At national and international levels, policies and actions to motivate usage of alternative modes of transport are vital.
- At business and societal levels, much could be done in terms of mixed use development and IT infrastructure to reduce the need or desire to travel.
- At the societal level, people and communities need to be better served by local facilities and designed environments, so that they can alter their travel habits and expectations in ways compatible with improving their health and life quality.

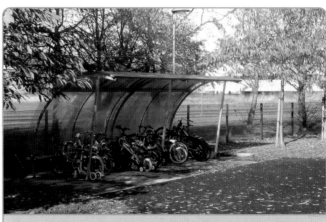

Cycles at Westmoor School. Tyne and Wear
Children and parents can be provided with the opportunity to alter their travel habits to reduce pollution and improve their health and life quality
(Photo: the author)

Development of UK policy for sustainable development

1990

The UK government formally set out its environmental aims in the White Paper *This Common Inheritance*. It suggested four principles of sustainability:

1 Decisions should be based on the best scientific information and analysis of risks.
2 Where there is uncertainty and potentially serious risks exist, precautionary action may be necessary.
3 Ecological impacts must be considered, particularly where resources are non-renewable or effects may be irreversible.
4 Cost implications should be brought home directly to the people responsible – 'polluter pays'.

1994

The UK strategy was published subsequent to the 1992 Rio de Janeiro UN Conference on the Environment and Development. It identified a number of sectors of the economy that are significant to sustainable development. Amongst these were:

- Minerals extraction
- Energy
- Transport
- Manufacturing and services
- Development and construction
- Waste.

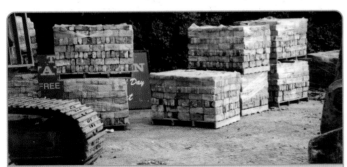

Brick recycling
The construction industry has significantly changed its behaviour and become increasingly resource efficient and less wasteful as a response to policy and legislation
(Photo: Crane Environmental)

A Better Quality of Life – A strategy for sustainable development in the UK

1999

After extensive consultation, through 'Sustainable Development: Opportunities for Change', the UK government published the policy paper *A Better Quality of Life – A strategy for sustainable development in the UK*. This emphasised that 'one of the fundamental principles of sustainable development is that it is a process with economic, social and ethical, as well as environmental dimensions'. The publication was reviewed and a progress report published in 2002.

Four tenets of sustainable development were included in the consultation paper that led to *A Better Quality of Life*:

1 *Social progress which recognises the needs of everyone.* Everyone should share in the benefits of increased prosperity and a clean and safe environment. We have to improve access to services, tackle social exclusion, and reduce the harm to health caused by poverty, poor housing, unemployment and pollution. Our needs must not be met by treating others, including future generations and people elsewhere in the world, unfairly.
2 *Effective protection of the environment.* We must act to limit global environmental threats, such as climate change; to protect human health and safety from hazards, such as poor air quality and toxic chemicals; and to protect things which people need or value, such as wildlife, landscapes and historic buildings.
3 *Prudent use of natural resources.* This does not mean denying ourselves the use of non-renewable resources like oil and gas, but we do need to make sure that we use them efficiently and that alternatives are developed to replace them in due course. Renewable resources, such as water, should be used in ways that do not endanger the resource or cause serious damage or pollution.
4 *Maintenance of high and stable levels of economic growth and employment.* Everyone can then share in high living standards and greater job opportunities. The UK is a trading nation in a rapidly changing world. For our country to prosper, our businesses must produce the high-quality goods and services that consumers throughout the world want, at prices they are prepared to pay. To achieve that, we need a workforce that is equipped with the education and skills for the twenty-first century. We need businesses ready to invest and an infrastructure to support them.

Case Study 2.2:

Glencoe Visitor Centre, Argyll

Architects: Gaia Architects, 2002

Reconciling access and conservation

Architects committed to sustainable design have argued that quantitative assessment methods often and indicators are irreconcilable with the qualitative nature of the design process. Quantitative indicators can lead to reductionism, sometimes to a single digit and reward the measurable at the expense of the important. Few respond to context, so urban, suburban and rural projects are subject to similar rules. Instead, indicators and guidance must encourage and excite design professionals to creative problem-solving.

In 2001, the Sustainable Construction Strategy Group set out 13 such measures. Here they form the backdrop to a case study.

1 *Reuse and improve existing built assets.* Resolving the dilemma of providing access whilst preserving nature and heritage – was the driver of the brief when a decision was made to replace the outdated Glencoe Visitor Centre. The former centre was badly situated in the heart of the Glen. It had altered the mood and was facilitating the destruction of one of Scotland's most treasured environments. To renovate or develop in this place would have compounded an earlier error. A decision was made to seek another site and to return the existing one to its former ecology. The old centre has since been dismantled, and the materials recycled locally.

2 *Locate appropriately.* Gaia responded with a low-lying, modern building on a brownfield site close to Glencoe village and adjacent to the campsite. The Centre now forms a link between these places. It is designed as a clachan which reflects the massing, proportions and scale of local low-lying, polyglot villages. The building (1500m^2) comprises a café, exhibition area, viewing platform, shop, toilets, education centre, offices and a warden's house. The building and parking was fitted into the existing matured Sylvia Crowe landscape. Careful siting avoided the loss of healthy trees and strict site boundaries avoided contractor damage. Pad foundations minimise disruption to roots and groundwater. All topsoil was retained for reuse.

3 *Relate land-use planning to transport infrastructure.* The aim was to allow visitors to experience a uniquely beautiful and evocative place, whilst avoiding or mitigating any damage. Locating the building next to the campsite and a safe pathway to the local village has opened up access that otherwise required transport. Visitors can now take advantage of local services and business. There was a tradition of fly-parking, which is hazardous and deleterious to the local fauna. Off-road parking facilities have been enhanced and walkers are encouraged to begin and end walks at the Centre, which is also more secure.

4 *Design for effective resource use.* All the timber – bolted and demountable portal frames, larch cladding and roofing, oak windows and doors, nail-free oak and sycamore floors, and birch ceiling finishes – is Scottish and untreated. Non-galvanised, tin roofing was sourced from the mining industry. Now rusted, it reflects the west coast vernacular. After a failed attempt to reopen the Ballachullish quarry, Gaia resorted to recycled Ballachullish and Cumbrian slate.

5 *Design for life.* The clachan form allows for future expansion or contraction. All the materials are easy to dismantle, separate and identify for repair, reuse or recycling. Few materials used are polymeric or bonded and all but sacrificial elements of the construction are nail free, so that they are removable, for maintenance or replacement.

6 *Aim for lean construction.* The project delivers value for money and high environmental quality with a cost yardstick level at, or below, equivalent buildings.

7 *Minimise energy use.* Cellulose fibre super-insulated breathing walls (250mm), floors and roofs are airtight construction. Windows and doors are sealed with sheep's wool, which provides permanently flexible airtight detail, unlike toxic hard-setting sprays that are inflexible. Ventilation is through designed fanlights. Daylighting is extensive with energy efficient fittings. Heating is simple with domestic style thermostats and manual controls.

8 *Utilise renewable energy sources.* Hot water from wood-CHP district heating serves the building and caravan site.

9 *Do not pollute the wider environment.* The building has 100% untreated timber, uses carbon-neutral fuel, is PVC and glue free, uses only natural paints and stains, and has on-site water gathering and treatment.

10 *Preserve/enhance biodiversity.* Significant flora from the building footprint were relocated. The interplay between buildings, stream and new planting was balanced to optimise diverse ecologies, including sunlight and shade. Existing healthy, mature trees were supplemented with new growth. All planting was sourced from the bio-region.

11 *Conserve water resources.* Water off the hill serves the Centre and caravan site. It is collected, filtered, conserved, recycled and treated on site, and delivered pure to the River Coe.

12 *Respect people and local environment.* Consultation took place to ensure that the project benefited the local community. Attention was given to the size of restaurant, its opening hours and contents of the shop to ensure it complements the local economy. A path to the village opens up access to local business.

13 *Set targets.* Gaia had a two-year involvement beyond handover, to ensure that the operation and maintenance is in sympathy with the design intentions. Environmental, social and economic indicators will be established by consensus with local people, clients and users, as will care regimes.

Conclusion. As a context of what is possible within an existing project, the 13 measures can be shown to have an extremely valuable role in explaining to an audience that seeks qualitative information the benefits and opportunities offered by a sustainable approach. Assessing projects on the basis of these qualitative aspects should be encouraged.

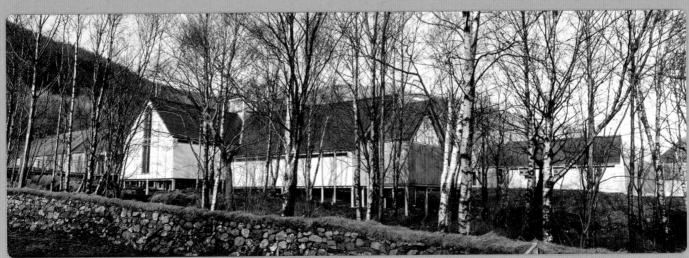

Photo: Michael Wolshover

For sustainable construction – Building a Better Quality of Life: A strategy for more sustainable construction in the UK

April 2000

In parallel with the sustainable development consultation, five further consultation papers were issued covering issues that the government felt they needed to consult on in greater depth due to the effects they have on society and the environment: business, tourism, forestry, biodiversity and construction. This resulted in a policy paper on construction, *Building a Better Quality of Life: A strategy for more sustainable construction in the UK*. It highlighted priorities from the sustainable development review, of particular relevance to construction, including:

- more investment in people and equipment for a competitive economy
- achieving higher growth whilst reducing pollution and use of resources
- sharing the benefits of growth more widely and more fairly
- improving our towns and cities, and protecting the quality of the countryside
- contributing to sustainable development internationally.

The policy paper indicates that a sustainable construction approach involves all the following actions:

- delivering buildings and structures that provide greater satisfaction, well-being and value to customers and users
- respecting and treating its stakeholders more fairly
- enhancing and better protecting the natural environment
- minimising its impact on the consumption of energy (especially carbon-based energy) and natural resources
- being more profitable and more competitive.

Achieving Sustainability in Construction Procurement

June 2000

The UK Government Construction Clients' Panel published a Sustainability Action Plan, *Achieving Sustainability in Construction Procurement*. This represented the first indication of a commitment to implementation. The Panel comprised representatives of Defence Estates; the Department for Education and Employment; the Department for Food, Environment and Rural Affairs; the Department of Transport; Local Government and the Regions; the Department of Trade and Industry; English Heritage; Environment Agency, Health and Safety Executive; Highways Agency; NHS Estates; Office of Government Commerce; and the Prison Service. The plan sets out how government clients of construction will take forward the sustainable development agenda through better procurement of new works, maintenance and refurbishment. This plan is already changing the way that government procures construction, leading to the purchase of better built development.

An example of the targets set down is that from March 2003 all new projects should achieve an excellent rating under BREEAM or equivalent. They didn't.

Industry and Professional Bodies' Policies

The Royal Incorporation of Architects in Scotland has an Environmental Statement and Implementation Strategy, including the Mission Statement: -

'Maximum Architectural Value – Minimum Environmental Harm'.

Under 'Policy', it states:

'The RIAS promotes a life-cycle approach to the design and construction of buildings and their components, which does not endanger environmental or personal health, and which respects biodiversity, inter-generational responsibility and social equity.'

As part of the implementation strategy for the policy, the RIAS has also spearheaded an accreditation scheme to acknowledge the contribution of accomplished sustainable building designers. The scheme was launched in February 2005. Thirteen architects gained a personal accreditation award.

The current position

Building a Better Quality of Life: A strategy for more sustainable construction was published in 2001. There have been a number of publications in the intervening period looking at, for example, the business case for sustainable construction (*Reputation, Risk and Reward – business case for more sustainable construction*, 2002) and the forthcoming legislative environment. The strategy for sustainable development was updated in 2005 and indicated that the UK Government wished to be amongst the leaders in the EU on sustainable procurement by 2009. The Sustainable Procurement Task Force (SPTF) was set up and delivered its findings and recommendations *Procuring the Future* in 2006. The Office of Government Commerce (OGC) now provides guidance on construction procurement and sustainability.

> ### Significant changes since publication of Building a Better Quality of Life
>
> - UK Climate Change Programme
> - The Energy Efficiency Commitment (EEC; an obligation on energy suppliers to encourage household energy efficiency)
> - The UK and EU Emissions Trading Schemes
> - Aggregates levy and landfill tax
> - Formation of sector skills councils
> - Launch of Respect for People Code of Good Working Health and Safety Practices
> - Formation of Constructing Excellence
> - Revision to *Part L of the Building Regulations* leading to tighter Building Regulations
> - *Code for Sustainable Homes*
> - Site Waste Management Plans
> - Planning policy developments
> - *The Sustainable and Secure Buildings Act*
> - Design for manufacture
> - The introduction of minimum standards for products and product labelling.

In early 2006 a consultation was launched in recognition of the significant changes in practice and policy since 2001 and *to provide a framework to identify* what progress has been made and to *guide future progress within the construction industry.*

The *Sustainable Construction Strategy Report 2006* provides a good overview of recent policy action with respect to people, the environment and sector initiatives to support more sustainable construction, including the crucial area of skills development, and links to more information. This is part of the emerging picture of the integrative aspect of the built environment.

The regulatory framework has changed, with an extensive consultation in England leading to new building regulations brought into effect on 6 April 2006 aimed at delivering significant improvements in energy efficiency in both new and existing buildings. There is also a move to develop voluntary guidelines which take the sector beyond current legislative requirements and there is consultation on a code for sustainable homes. The standards are still significantly below what is required and possible and affordable.

Sustainable Communities

The Office of the Deputy Prime Minster (ODPM) has also widened its perspective on the construction industry to address sustainable communities, which they define as:

'... places where people want to live and work, now and in the future. They meet the diverse needs of existing and future residents, are sensitive to their environment, and contribute to a high quality of life. They are safe and inclusive, well planned, built and run, and offer equality of opportunity and good services for all.'

Greater choice and opportunity in housing are aspects of the sustainable communities strategy. It includes the launch of a Sustainable Communities Award in 2003. The award criteria are based on the agreed definition of a sustainable community as published in the Department's two five-year plans – *Homes for All* and *People, Places and Prosperity* (published in January 2005).

The rising price of housing, far in excess of other basic necessities, means that the government has been forced to look to affordability as a key aspect of sustainable communities and a cornerstone of the strategy is to offer everyone the opportunity of a decent home at a price they can afford. As well as environmental protection it includes assistance to first-time buyers, social tenants and key workers, for whom the lack of adequate and affordable provision was leading to shortages in some areas.

Case Study 2.3:

Red Kite House, Wallingford

Architects: Scott Brownrigg, 2005

Red Kite House is a new office for the UK Environment Agency. It aimed to demonstrate the EA's leadership in the design of improved workplaces and to help raise awareness for the potential for businesses, organisations and the public to make positive choices to protect and improve the environment.

Before Red Kite House was built, the area's 250 staff occupied eight inflexible, inefficient buildings. As well as addressing these issues, a new single building was also perceived as aiding effective and efficient teamworking.

The Howbery business/science park site was chosen because of the competitive lease terms, minimal business disruption, a beautiful parkland situation next to the River Thames and the site owners/developers allowing us to influence the design of the building. The Environment Agency worked closely with the design team to construct an office that would meet the operational needs and serve as an example of best practice in sustainable office development.

The three-storey building has an internal floor area of approximately 3000 m². It is naturally ventilated with thoughtful and innovative passive design features to provide the required airflow through the building. Manually operated window openings allow cross-ventilation and high-level exposed concrete ceilings on each floor provide thermal mass, and an overhang to the south prevents solar ingress in summer. Additional air movement to the top floor, the most vulnerable to overheating, is provided by roof-mounted turbines.

Photovoltaic cell and solar thermal panels contribute to the electrical and hot water demand, with a predicted saving of nearly 14 tonnes of CO_2/year and predicted carbon emissions target 26% below that defined as 'good practice'. Rainwater is collected from the roof sufficient to meet about 40% of the building's annual demand for water. Overspill from the tank goes to a reed bed. The car park uses pervious blocks, over a geotextile membrane that traps oil and other pollutants.

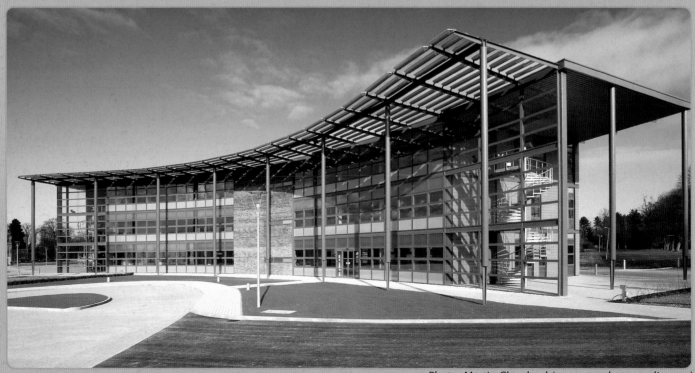

Photo: Martin Cleveland (www.mc-photo-studio.com)

Case Study 2.4:

Springhill, Stroud Co-housing

Architects: Architype, 2005

Stroud Co-housing is the first new-build collaborative housing in the UK. It aims to create a real sense of community. There are 35 private houses and flats with a shared Common House where people can cook and eat together. Cars and parking are kept to the edge of the site, leaving the majority of the area pedestrian only and safe for children and the elderly.

This Common House is the hub, meeting and event space, and also has a workshop, table tennis area and laundry facilities.

Timber construction and cladding give the hill-slope site a distinctive character, and the relatively narrow, pedestrianised 'main street' meanders around the site parallel with the contours, creating a characterful village feel. Walking and cycling are priority modes of transport within the area and beyond. While car ownership remains high, car use is reportedly lower than average, with easy walking access to the town centre.

Recycling, community composting, high-intensity insulation, a Sustainable Urban Drainage System (SUDS) and a car-sharing scheme all contribute to an environmentally sensitive scheme. The project also has the largest array of photovoltaic cells on private housing in the UK; this was achieved with help from a £400,000 government grant for the installation and monitoring of the tiles.

Co-housing aims to promote a strong sense of belonging and encourages friendly, cooperative and helpful behaviour, including self-policing. The residents all became directors of the development company, so were involved in commissioning the construction. Three housing units are subsidised in perpetuity at 15% below market value.

In Denmark, from a standing start in the 1970s, 3–4% of the population now live in co-housing. In Stroud they are already working on schemes for co-flats and actively looking for other sites to develop.

Many of the residents of Springhill work from home and the nature of the community means there is a lot of business support sharing, offering a glimpse of a possible future for home-based enterprise integrated with more sustainable living. Springhill is innovative and practical, and offers a real alternative for future housing.

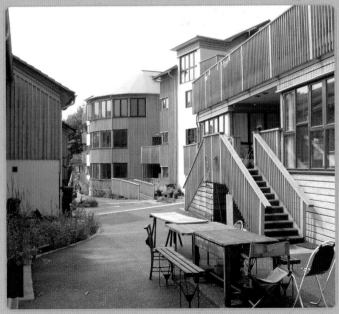

Photo: the author

Limitations of policies

The international community increasingly acknowledges that current legislation is inadequate and that it is ethically reprehensible to do nothing in the face of current threats. Taking a lead through policy commitments represents a real opportunity.

The failure of the UK government to fully implement its commitments is unfortunate, but probably results from a greater malaise, the lack of public engagement in the problems that then empower and support the actions of politicians. The 2005 crisis over costs of oil, resulting in a demonstration by hauliers, and the failure to identify a workable policy solution is the kind of situation politicians wish to avoid.

Published policies exhibit a degree of consensus on sustainability issues but little agreement on the extent of the problems, priorities, the action required, the targets to be achieved or timescales for implementation. As a consequence, many more preach the virtues of sustainability than deliver in practice. In part this may result from lack of real commitment, but there are also knowledge gaps and huge difficulties encountered in practice. The fact that many policies lack targets or timescales is a notable aspect.

Yet, by linking the three strands of sustainability, there is great opportunity to develop improved buildings and built environments. In order to do so, we need to identify carrots to balance the necessary sticks and commit to firm deliverables, including education on product and process issues. We need to link policy commitments to best practice and knowledge. This is a vital aspect in meeting our ethical responsibilities to contribute to a sustainable future. There is at last a serious policy discussion emerging about the need to tax resources and throughputs, rather than people. This accords with the limits to growth systems theory mentioned in Chapter 1.

In parallel to the development of policies, a vast and expanding variety of tools and techniques have emerged to promote, guide and appraise sustainable construction. Chapter 4 considers the scope of tools available and attempts to present them as a hierarchy. It aims to encourage critical engagement in what types of measures can be incorporated into policy to assist delivery of sustainable construction. Ultimately, we need tools and techniques with third-party validation and linked to real measurable environmental limits on the use of resources, minimising pollution, community enhancement and protection of biodiversity to be incorporated as the legislative bottom line.

Legislation in the UK

The previous section concentrated on the shift in attitudes towards the environment, and showed how political statements have, over the last decade, filtered down to a local and practical level of action. This section deals with the established legal framework, which partly goes back to before the 1992 Rio Conference, and partly has come into force as a result of renewed government commitment in response to Rio and the 'Sustainable Development' pledge.

There is no framework of common legislation in the countries that make up the UK. Neither is there any specific Legislation in the UK – Act of Parliament, regulation or by-law – that forces designers, builders, developers or clients of construction to adopt a sustainable approach.

Although there is no legislation that forces a sustainable approach to construction, planning, building control and environmental legislation control and influence three significant aspects of construction – what can be built, where it can be built and how it can or should be built.

There is a considerable body of legislation on issues such as planning, environmental assessment and protection, employment practice, nuisance to neighbours, quality of indoor environments and financial propriety that anyone seeking to adopt a sustainable construction approach must comply with. Primary legislation in Scotland, the *Building (Scotland) Act 2003*, made provision for ministers to make building regulations for the purpose of 'furthering the achievements of sustainable development'. This was an important shift. By going beyond the framework of purely *sustainable construction*, the bill acknowledges the role of buildings and the built environment in responding to social, economic and cultural imperatives.

Until recently the UK's record on building regulations was poor compared to our near neighbours. Energy Advisory Associates compiled a graph to compare our building standards with European practice and show how far behind we are. Whilst the latest regulations are an improvement, many of our neighbours are now developing even better standards and implementing financial and other incentives to move towards *Minergie* and passive housing types.

Anyone involved in the development of schemes and their designs is required to keep up to date with the latest position. The up-to-date simplified reference source that can be consulted for the latest legislative provisions related to sustainable construction is *www.natregs.org*. A number of other online sources of information are listed in the Bibliography. The nature of legislation is that it is continually changing, so the site is for information only and does not constitute legal advice.

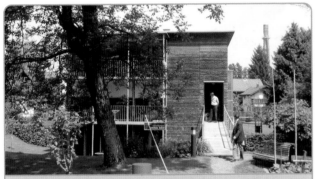

Oelzbundt housing apartment block, Austria
Built to Minergie standard, defined as half the energy consumption of a building regulations dwelling
(Architect: Kaufman; photo: the author)

Legislation controlling or influencing *how* you can build includes:

- Building law and regulations
- *Environmental Protection Act 1990*
- Water pollution control law, especially the *Water Resources Act*
- Waste law
- Contaminated land law
- Noise control law
- Other pollution control law
- Wildlife and countryside law
- Land drainage law
- Dumping at sea provisions
- Enabling acts for individual projects (e.g. *Channel Tunnel Rail Link (CTRL) Act 1996*).

Legislation controlling or influencing *what* and *where* you can build includes:

- Planning law
- Environmental impact assessment regulations
- Pollution control law, especially the *Integrated Pollution Prevention and Control Directive, Water Resources* and *Clean Air Acts*
- Wildlife and countryside law
- Contaminated land law
- Land drainage law
- Highway law
- *Reservoirs Act*
- Enabling acts for individual projects (e.g. *CTRL Act 1996*).

Case Study 2.5:

Examples of contraventions of environmental legislation

Waste offences

Employees of Company A had been taking rubble from building operations and storing it on their site. The waste, containing asbestos, over time built up to over 190 tonnes. The company then paid for the rubble to be removed, but failed to supply the correct information about the nature of the waste.

The contractor removing the waste from the site subsequently used it to construct part of a public amenity. Company A were fined £4000 plus costs (from *Environment Times*, Vol. 7/3, p. 45).

Company B were fined £1000 plus costs for burning waste containing fibreglass at their depot. Fibreglass releases a toxic/irritant smoke when burnt.

The company claimed that they were not the owners of the land in question but were renting it. The material had been deposited on the site by others and they did not know that they were committing an offence by burning it. On fining the defendant, the magistrate ruled that there was no defence in ignorance (from *Environment Times*, Vol. 7/4, p. 44).

Individual C was conditionally discharged for 12 months with costs of £8000 after spreading controlled waste (excavation material) on a site in Leeds without a waste management licence. The material contained wood, plastic and paper.

He did not think he needed a licence because he was spreading the waste. The Environment Agency disagreed and felt he was tipping and using the waste to infill (from *Environment Times*, Vol. 7/3, p. 48).

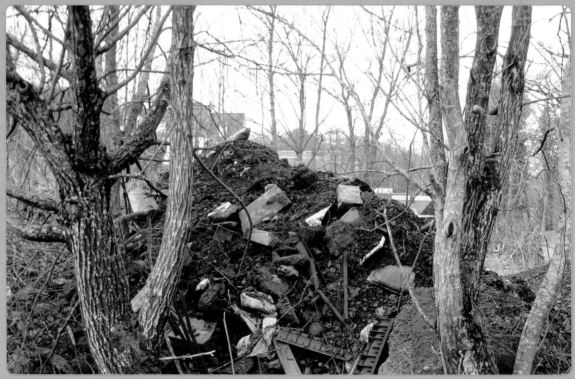

Photo: Howard Liddell

The environmental legal framework

There has been a substantial increase both in the amount and the scope of environmental legislation and regulation in the last decade throughout the world and especially in Europe. As a result of all these new laws and regulations, organisations are beginning to realise that environmental issues are a serious concern that influences their success and potentially survival.

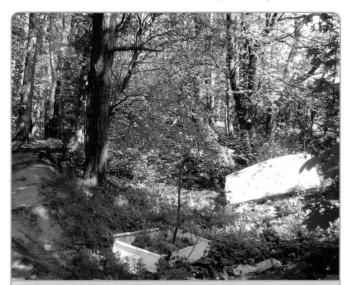

Waste management
Laws have been extended considerably – from preventing fly-tipping such as this, to taking serious control of the construction industry
(Photo: the author)

Directors are more likely to be subject to criminal proceedings. They may be personally liable for crimes committed in the course of running a company's business or where they decide deliberately to commit the company to a criminal course of action. A director's or manager's liability may also arise as a result of giving directions (e.g. to employees) for the offence to be committed, in which case he/she would be an aider, abettor, counsellor or procurer, and thus tried and punished as a principal offender.

Criminal prosecution may be brought by citizens whether or not they have suffered any special harm. However, in practice, regulatory authorities carry out most environmental prosecutions. A criminal offence is followed by a fine or imprisonment, the level of fine under environmental litigation being limited in Magistrates' Court and unlimited in the Crown Court. Criminal courts also have the power to make compensation orders – for example, fish restocking to rivers after a pollution incident.

Environmental liability

Employees have a duty of care for their actions in relation to others and the environment. They can be prosecuted personally in the event of an offence being committed under criminal law (for non-compliance), and can be sued under civil law (for compensation) in the event of their (allegedly) causing damage to persons and/or their property.

Property owners and occupiers, persons who 'cause or knowingly permit' pollution or 'persons responsible' for the pollution may all be held to be liable.

Reducing a company's environmental legal liability

There is a straightforward approach:

- Take a board-level decision to be environmentally responsible and ensure this is recorded.
- Appoint a board-level director or equivalent to be responsible for environmental issues.
- Introduce and implement an environmental management system to help prevent liability being incurred and to provide documented evidence of a defence to a criminal prosecution (e.g. showing that reasonable precautions were taken).
- Implement a training programme to ensure that everyone is aware of the issues.
- Highlight the requirements of due diligence.
- Take reasonable precautions to prevent liability.
- Use best practicable means.
- Use BATNEEC (Best Available Technology Not Entailing Excessive Cost).
- Be able to demonstrate that directors and managers have not consented, connived or been neglectful in respect of environmental performance.

Any person may commit an offence where they perform an act that is specifically prohibited by statute. In general, the crucial factor will be evidence of 'consent', 'connivance' or 'neglect'.

Case Study 2.6:

Examples of contraventions of environmental legislation

Water offences

The Environment Agency received a report about oil pollution to a farm pond and brook in Essex. The Agency traced the source back to Company D's project office. The company was unaware of any problem, but on inspection with the officer conceded that their fuel compound was the source of pollution. The company had installed a bund wall around the oil storage tanks, but later a management decision was made to circumvent these measures by drilling a hole through the bund wall to prevent the accumulation of excessive rainwater. This led to subsequent oil spillages being passed directly into the adjacent watercourse. The company cooperated fully with the Agency and employed oil clean-up contractors to deal with the pollution to the brook and pond, but nevertheless was fined £8000 plus costs (from *Environment Times*, Vol. 7/3, p. 45).

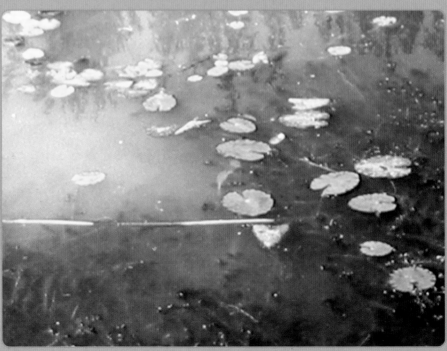

Photo: the author

EU legislation

The EU (European Union) has been responsible for a significant raft of environmental legislation that has impacted directly on the construction industry. UK governments are obliged to incorporate this legislation into their own frameworks within a given period of time. EU legislation is following the best practice lead of regulations established locally by member states and it is these policies that are slowly finding their way into UK legislation. Issues arising under policy by leading-edge organisations are finding their way into European legislation, but the responses of the individual countries are not always rapid.

Construction Products Directive (CPD)

This Construction Products Directive (CPD) was introduced in order to harmonise and reduce barriers to free trade in construction products. It requires member states to replace their national standards for construction products (British Standards, in the case of the UK) with European Technical Assessments (ETA) leading to European Certification (CEN). Products covered by the directive are those incorporated within building and civil engineering construction works.

At present the CPD does not address many environmental requirements, but it is inevitable that these will be integrated in the harmonised specifications (ETA and CEN) in the longer term. For example:

- the life-cycle costs of products in relation to disposal and reuse
- energy over the complete life cycle of the construction
- risk assessment to ensure compliance with the EU obligation to address the precautionary principle.

Energy Performance of Buildings Directive

The *European Commission's Action Plan on Energy Efficiency (2000)* indicated the need for specific measures to address the performance of buildings and to help the EU to meet its climate change objectives under the Kyoto Protocol commitments. In response, the European Commission (EC) proposed the Directive on the *Energy Performance of Buildings*, with a timetable for implementation by 2006. The aim was to create a common framework for calculating the energy performance of buildings and thereby provide a level playing field for judging the efforts of member states in achieving energy savings. It would also facilitate transparency for prospective building owners and tenants across Europe, although each EU country could set minimum performance levels at its own discretion. The directive applies to new buildings, large existing buildings facing major renovation, energy certification of buildings at point of sale or transfer, and involves mandatory inspections of boilers and air-conditioning systems. It will put pressure on energy requirements to be applied to existing buildings, as is now the case in a number of European countries.

At the time of going to press the Government had not announced how it would put in place UK requirements.

Environmental Impact Assessment

In certain cases an application for planning permission will be required to be accompanied by an environmental statement prepared through the process of Environmental Impact Assessment (EIA). This is a process by which information about the positive and negative environmental effects of a new development, and of alternative schemes, are collected by the developer and taken into account by the local planning authority in deciding whether or not to grant planning permission. The 1997 EC Directive on environmental assessment was amended to include a broadening of the categories of development to which it applies, resulting in the 1999 regulations on EIAs, which involve local authorities in deciding whether an environmental statement is required and what its scope should be. Even if an EIA is not required, many developers are finding that applications for planning permission are more effectively dealt with if accompanied by a (voluntary) environmental commentary on the proposed development.

Waste Electrical and Electronic Equipment (WEEE) Directive

The Waste Electrical and Electronic Equipment (WEEE) Directive was agreed on 13 February 2003, along with the related Directive on Restrictions of the use of certain Hazardous Substances in electrical and electronic equipment (RoHS).

The Waste Electrical and Electronic Equipment Directive aims to minimise the impacts of electrical and electronic equipment on the environment during their lifetimes and when they become waste. It applies to a huge spectrum of products. It encourages and sets criteria for the collection, treatment, recycling and recovery of waste electrical and electronic equipment. It makes producers responsible for financing most of these activities (producer responsibility). Private householders are to be able to return WEEE without charge.

RoHS (Restrictions of the use of certain Hazardous Substances)

The RoHS Directive bans the placing on the EU market of new electrical and electronic equipment containing more than agreed levels of lead, cadmium, mercury, hexavalent chromium, polybrominated biphenyl (PBB) and polybrominated diphenyl ether (PBDE) flame retardants. There are a number of exempted applications for these substances. The RoHS takes its scope broadly from the WEEE Directive. Manufacturers have to ensure that their products – and their components – comply. This directive introduces the concept of cradle-to-grave environmental considerations for products.

> **'Manufacturers ... will provide information on the material composition and the consumption of energy and/or resources of their components ... and, where available, the results of environmental assessments and/or case reference studies which concern the use and end-of-life management of the components ...'**
>
> (Article 11.2)

The aim is to reduce hazardous waste from the industry and encourage an increase in recycling and sustainable production. Some of the most hazardous products when landfilled are electronic and electrical. The directive states that manufacturers must retain responsibility for their products throughout their life cycles. It came into force in 2006 and encourages manufacturers to look at more benign materials and processes if their long-term management is ultimately their responsibility. Take-back and collection schemes for obsolete products will be more commonplace, as companies recycle their branded goods.

Potential barriers and how to deal with them

It must be recognised that some current legal provisions do not help moves towards more sustainable construction.

A recent Scottish Executive Report (*Scottish House: A review of recent experience in building individual and small groups of houses with a view to sustainability, the use of traditional and new materials and innovative design*, 2001) demonstrates that planning and building control provisions can sometimes be used or very strictly interpreted, not necessarily deliberately to stifle

innovation and more sustainable construction, but nevertheless having the same effect. For example, Scottish building regulations specify that a toilet shall be a 'water closet', thus precluding the use of composting toilets because they self-evidently do not use water. A special dispensation was required from the authorities to allow the first use of such toilets in 2001.

Other examples of issues affected by barriers include the use of rain downpipes – despite their being common and proven elsewhere; new materials – such as unfired earth, which is now gaining increased acceptance; solar-orientated layouts; density of dwellings and alternative traffic arrangements. The stance of a client, designer or developer who wishes to adopt innovative techniques that appear to be precluded by regulation often needs to be focused on the aim of the regulatory regime and the outcome that the regulation seeks to achieve. Demonstrating how the alternative provides an equal or better outcome can lead to a change of heart on the part of the regulators.

On the environmental front, the definitions of waste can sometimes militate against a creative approach to solving resource-use issues. For example, it may become clear during the construction phase of a project that it would be possible and advantageous (to the environment as well as the developer) to use more of the excavation arisings on site than the original design had included, for example to create noise bunds. Very careful steps must be taken in conjunction with the regulatory authorities to ensure that such bunds are not designated as waste disposal sites, thus requiring licensing and active management long into the future.

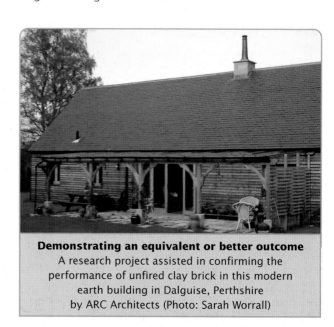

Demonstrating an equivalent or better outcome
A research project assisted in confirming the performance of unfired clay brick in this modern earth building in Dalguise, Perthshire by ARC Architects (Photo: Sarah Worrall)

Case Study 2.7:

Examples of contraventions of environmental legislation

Wildlife offence

Japanese knotweed is a highly invasive plant, which the *Wildlife and Countryside Act 1981* makes it illegal to plant or otherwise introduce into the wild.

The recommendations are that soil up to 7m diameter around each plant and up to 3.5 m in depth has to be removed and buried at a minimum of 5 m depth. That is roughly 75 m^3 of fill to be removed and buried for each plant! The other way of treating Japanese knotweed is to spray it with herbicide for a minimum of three years until sure that the plants are dead.

However, on most construction sites this form of treatment is not practical. A contractor in Kent knew that they had Japanese knotweed on their site, but ignored warnings about how to handle the soil it was growing in. They transferred a small amount of knotweed-contaminated soil to a stockpile within the construction site and before long the majority of the stockpile had been colonised by Japanese knotweed. As a result they had to treat far more material than they would have done if they had dealt with it more carefully in the first place. This cost the contractor in excess of £50,000.

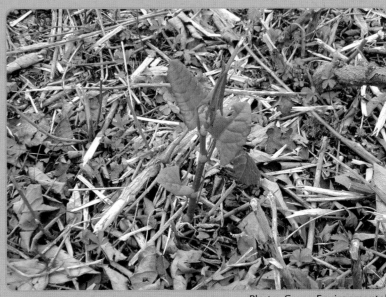

Photo: Crane Environmental

Conclusion

Ultimately, the responsibilities lie with national governments to legislate against unsustainable practices and to penalise failure. The rules are changing and enforcement in Europe is a reality but progress is slow. Some countries resist change. At least in the short term, it is dependent on the industry, its clients and its professional bodies to take appropriate action to eliminate unsustainable practices and to seek continual environmental enhancement strategies. If the construction industry is to be accountable then it must develop its policies such that it is in a position to adequately respond to current threats and reverse unsustainable trends.

Increasing numbers of international bodies, national governments, professions, clients, builders and designers are embracing the need for improving their construction performance and that of the resulting buildings. Many governments and organisations have responded to the public and/or contractual requirements with sustainable construction polices, but the resulting outcomes are disappointing – with little delivered.

Whilst the aspirations they contain are often laudable, they also fail to adequately promote effective change in so far as they fail to acknowledge the extent of action required, to identify tools and techniques by which to implement change and therefore to provide for adequate and decisive action.

Company, professional and government policies must embrace serious commitment to education on design and process, and to meeting targets that will deliver the much needed change. The best policies would properly reward best practice, have firm targets based on real limits, and have an integrative, overarching aspect to link business, economic, social and environmental policies. The use of tools is a fundamental part of this process, but the tools adopted must be appropriate.

There is a need to better understand what is really required (checklists) and to develop the skills to deliver (critical path tools). In addition, we need to radically improve current third-party-approved label and certification schemes so that they relate to real limits and hence targets that must be achieved for action to be meaningful (targeting tools). Labelling schemes can then act as proper auditing mechanisms to ensure that we are adequately responding to threats.

It is likely that the EU will continue to pursue ecological considerations for products. There is a draft directive on Eco-Design for End-Use Products, which aims to bring construction more closely in line with environmental objectives.

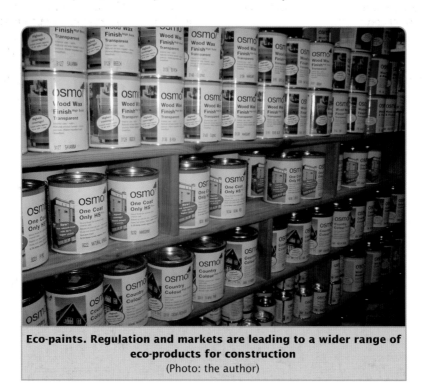

Eco-paints. Regulation and markets are leading to a wider range of eco-products for construction
(Photo: the author)

Handy hints and tips

The principal requirements on water pollution, waste and wildlife, especially during construction, are as follows:

- Do not pollute inland waters, groundwater/aquifers or the sea.
- Do not discharge specified substances into a foul sewer without a licence.
- Do not disturb birds or their nests during the breeding season.
- Do not disturb or handle certain species of mammals, invertebrates or birds specified in an Appendix to the *Wildlife and Countryside Act* – for example, badgers, bats or great-crested newts.
- Do not uproot any wild flower without the landowner's permission.
- Respect and avoid damaging special habitats such as those designated as Sites of Special Scientific Interest (SSSIs), Sites of Nature Conservation Importance (SNCIs) or similar.
- Know that construction waste is always 'controlled waste' and that some (e.g. oil and fluorescent tubes) is 'special waste'.
- Exercise the duty of care for waste, including subcontractors' waste if you are the principal contractor.
- Ensure that appropriately licensed waste carriers are used, and that all waste has correctly completed waste transfer notes.
- Know when a Waste Management Licence is required.

- Know that some exemptions are possible – for example, when waste is kept for less than three months before it is used for construction or as a planned part of a development such as noise bunds. But a material can still be regarded as waste in law even if someone else can use it as a primary material – it stops being waste when received by the transferee.
- Keep records of waste disposal and transfers for at least two years.
- Keep waste in appropriate, labelled containers.
- Prevent and report:
  - corrosion or damage to containers
  - accidental spillages or leaks
  - waste escaping or blowing away
  - scavenging
  - vandalism.
- Do not store waste or allow it to accumulate in such a way that it could harm the environment or be prejudicial to human health – a statutory nuisance.
- Plan for waste management.
- Know the cost of Landfill Tax.

It is important that reclaimed and recycled products are traceable, with an available product history, so that dangerous products are not reintroduced into buildings. The lack of traceability and hence variable risk entailed in reusing construction products has hampered attempts to gain greater acceptance. Also, there is a strong suggestion that efforts to move to a solution have been hampered because reuse is seen by many as diminishing market share for new products. Consequently, many resist increasing the acceptance of reuse.

Bibliography

DETR (1999) *A Better Quality of Life: A Strategy for Sustainable Development for the UK.* The Stationery Office, London.

CIRIA (2000) *Environmental Handbooks for Building and Civil Engineering Projects.* CIRIA, London.

DEFRA (2000) *Foundation For Our Future.* The Stationery Office, London.

DETR (2000) *Building a Better Quality of Life: A Strategy for More Sustainable Construction in the UK.* The Stationery Office, London.

Sustainability Action Group of the Government Construction Clients' Panel (2000) *Achieving Sustainability in Construction Procurement.* Centre for Sustainable Construction, BRE, Watford.

Sustainable Construction Focus Group of the Construction Confederation (2000) *Towards Sustainability – A Strategy for the Construction Industry.* CIP Ltd.

Sustainable Construction Task Force (2002) *Reputation, Risk and Reward* – the business case for more sustainable construction This research report demonstrates the business case for more sustainable construction. BRE.

Rethinking Construction (2003) *Demonstrations of Sustainability* This document reviews the Rethinking Construction demonstration projects addressing sustainability. Those featured provide tangible evidence of the construction industry's adoption of more sustainable practices Constructing Excellence. (www.constructingexcellence.org.uk).

Scottish Parliament *Building (Scotland) Bill 2003* (2003). The Stationery Office, Edinburgh (www.scottish.parliament.uk/parl_bus/legis.html).

CIRIA C587 (2004) *Working with Wildlife Resource and Training Pack.* Contains a 20-page table of wildlife law affecting construction projects

Halliday, S. P. and Stevenson, F. (2004) *Sustainable Construction and the Regulatory Framework.* Gaia Research. (www.gaiagroup.org/Research/IDS/Suc-con-reg/index.html)

UK Strategy for Sustainable Development (2005) www.sustainabledevelopment.gov.uk/publications/uk-strategy/uk-strategy-2005.htm

DEFRA (2006) *The National Action Plan*, 'Procuring the Future' www.sustainable-development.gov.uk/publications/procurement-action-plan/index.htm.

Websites

Construction Products Directive – www.dti.gov.uk/construction/sustain/EA_Sustainable_Report_41564_2.pdf

Croner's Environmental Management – www.croner.co.uk

Croner's Environmental Policy and Procedures – www.croner.co.uk

DEFRA's site for environmental legislation and forthcoming EU directives, affecting sustainability – www.dti.gov.uk/construction/sustain/scb.pdf

Environment Agency (http://www.environment-agency.gov.uk/), including Netregs (http://www.netregs.gov.uk/)

EU Directive on the Energy Performance of Buildings – www.defra.gov.uk/ENVIRONMENT/energy/internat/ecbuildings.htm

Office of the Government Commerce – www.ogc.gov.uk

SEPA (Scottish Environmental Protection Agency) – www.sepa.gov.uk

Thomson/Gee Environmental Compliance Manual – www.gee.co.uk

Waste and Resources Action Programme – www.wrap.org.uk/materials/plasterboard/useful_links.html

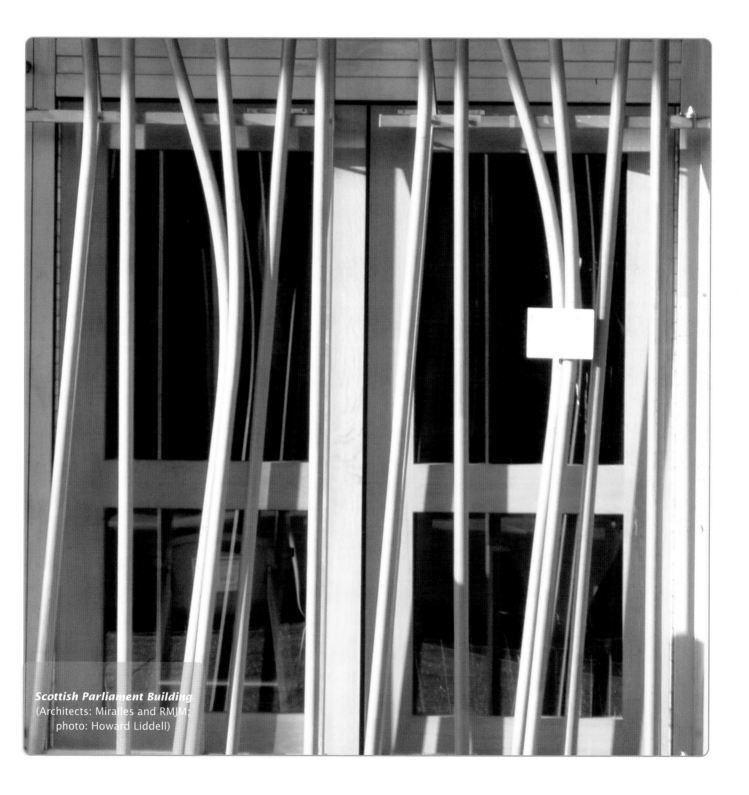

Scottish Parliament Building
(Architects: Miralles and RMJM;
photo: Howard Liddell)

Chapter 3
Cost issues

In which we address the recurring themes concerned with costs of sustainable construction and highlight some advanced class thinking to challenge the conventional approaches to money, cost, value and price that drive most projects.

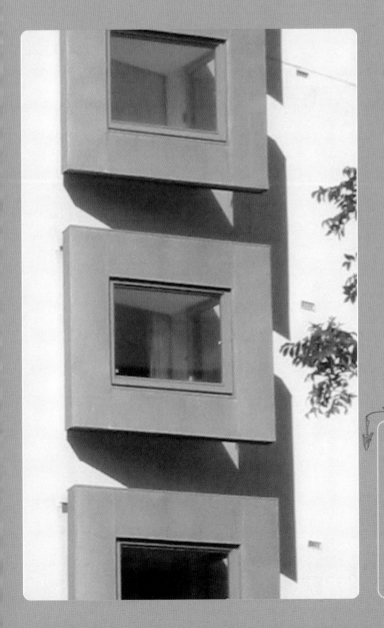

'It is unwise to pay too much, but it's worse to pay too little. When you pay too much, you lose a little money – that is all. When you pay too little, you sometimes lose everything, because the thing you bought is incapable of doing the thing it was bought to do. The common law of business balance prohibits paying a little and getting a lot.'

John Ruskin (1860), as quoted in Accelerating Change (2002)

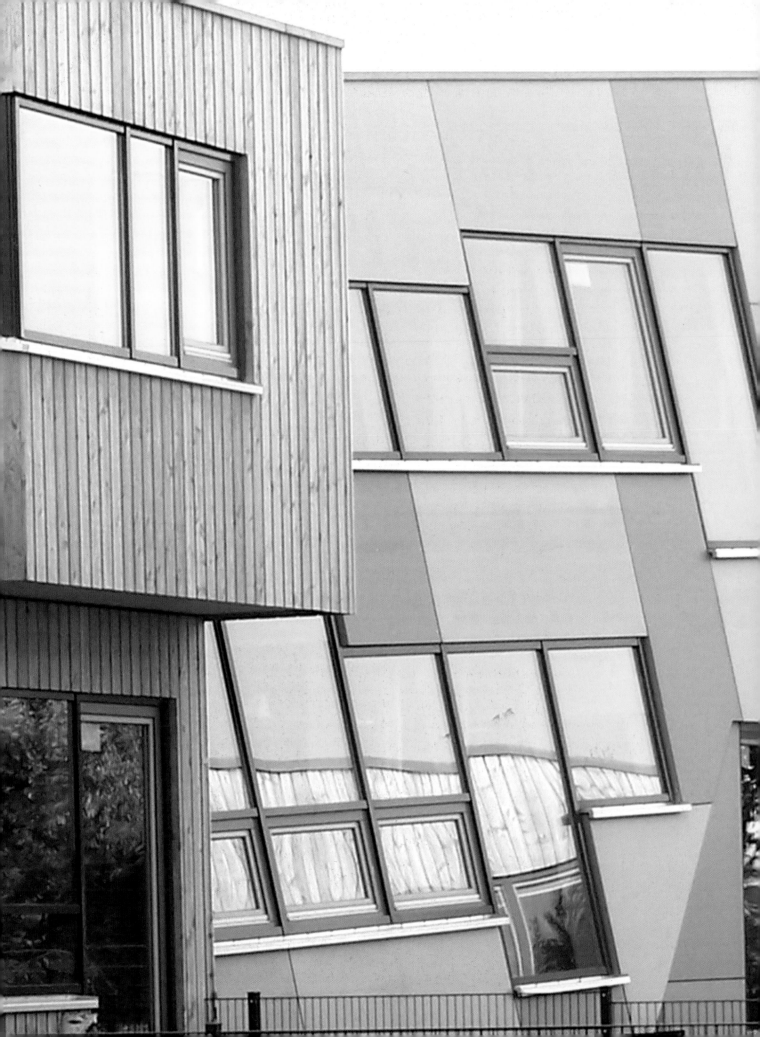

Contents

(Facing page)
Gelsenkirchen School
The impact on users was a principal driver of the design of this school in Gelsenkirchen (Architects: Peter Hübner Architects; photo: Ian Cameron)

(Previous page)
Crown St, Gorbals, Glasgow
(Photo: the author)

Cost issues

Introduction

Cost is the primary aspect of discussion on sustainable building. The perceived additional cost of sustainable building and the low perceived value of environmental and social quality have largely prevented positive action except by the most committed. Much current thinking on this issue is unbearably banal. Even the newest convert to 'sustainability' can present the tripolar diagram representing the links between society, environment and economy, but few resources have been committed to the proof, from which real benefits in all three areas could follow.

Pollution avoidance and costed benefits
We have to prove the links between the environment, society and the economy in order that we can encourage better decision-making and reverse unsustainable trends

The construction industry is constantly making financial decisions that have wide-ranging environmental and social impacts, driven largely from a viewpoint that we cannot afford to build in a sustainable manner. Until recently there was very little information on how much more sustainable building costs are. Any amount of 'more' is seemingly just too much. Given purchasing trends in other sectors, it is not credible that clients and consumers want leaky, inefficient and polluting buildings. More likely the problem is that with limited choice and little information on best value alternatives they are powerless and that opportunities are significantly lagging behind consumer preferences in many regions.

Cost information is now beginning to emerge, and with it questions about impacts on infrastructure and people, running costs, the quality of an environment or workplace, and maintaining the value of long-term investments.

This chapter looks at costs of sustainable buildings and introduces the background to evolving attitudes to environmental and social costs. There is underlying criticism of traditional economic systems, which put the financial bottom line before environmental protection or quality of life, and there are emerging policy responses, including alternative indicators.

It draws on national and international evidence to highlight the significant trends in policy, consumerism and investment which impact on our built environment, and draws on a number of sources and built projects to explain why we need to get smarter about cost. This chapter does not seek to revisit the traditional approaches to construction cost evaluation covered in most textbooks.

All the information available only tells us the additional cost of our best-practice assessed buildings. Without an indication of what the real limits of our activity are, we are still not in a position to determine whether it really does cost more to build in a genuinely sustainable manner.

> *'How long can we go on pretending that the environment is not the economy, is not health, is not the prerequisite to development, is not recreation... '*
>
> C. Caccia, WCED, Ottawa, 1986

The role of construction

The construction industry plays an enormous role in our lives. It provides for one of our most basic needs and is also an immense factor in the economy. The built environment also has a financial impact through its influence on the physical and economic health and well-being of individuals, communities and organisations. Poorly designed buildings and built environments contribute directly to ill-health, crime and disaffection, undermine community and create excessive financial liability in the long term. If they are well designed they can do the opposite.

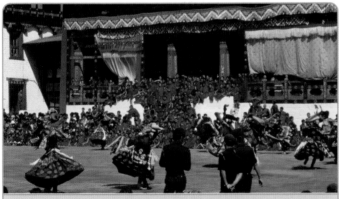

Thimpu Tschechu celebrations
In Bhutan the king has identified Gross National Happiness as more important than Gross National Product
(Photo: Ingun B. Amundsen)

Can we afford sustainable buildings?

The overriding assumption is that sustainable building inevitably costs more or is less profitable. It appears self-evident. If it were cheaper or more profitable, then in market-driven economies surely everyone would be doing it. It is also reasonable to assume that the innovation required has a cost implication of time, planning, risk and enhanced information requirements, so inevitably innovators will be penalised and their profit margins reduced when put in direct competition with unsustainable practices. For the same reason fossil fuel energy is unrealistically cheap because we ultimately pay the price of global warming and the potentially extraordinary cost of remediation. Current funding means that, at best, some additional resources might assist to level the playing field in some areas, but we are far from

creating a positive flow towards more sustainable practice in any sector. As a consequence the perceived additional cost of sustainable building largely prevents action by all but the most committed and well-informed. So lack of innovation and unsustainable building is the norm. This is within a culture where environmental concern has largely been perceived as a luxury and even now is often vilified or derided as 'moralising'.

> **Public opinion**
>
> Fifty-five per cent of householders in the UK are willing to pay a premium for green electricity. Around 30% of them indicated a willingness to pay up to 10% extra. Enthusiasm is greatest for suppliers of 100% green energy.

Interestingly, cost assumptions are increasingly challenged by joined-up approaches to development, health and well-being, long-term thinking and actual cost data. There is change afoot as clients, managers and designers better understand the business case (responsibilities and benefits) of engagement with sustainability initiatives, and to a lesser degree the risks associated with non-compliance with regulation.

There is pressure on everyone concerned to work towards a more sustainable construction industry with a better process and product. Environmental concerns are at last being viewed as socially and economically responsible. Clients are more aware of the political and fiscal trends, and are looking to life-cycle implications of design choices. Waste minimisation and energy efficiency are increasingly seen as good sense, while healthy

> **Reasons for resource efficiency**
> - **1960s:** resource limits
> - **1970s:** security
> - **1980s:** economy
> - **1990s:** environment
> - **2000s:** all the above.

housing, affordable warmth and clean air are recognised as aspects of social justice that should be available to all.

Case Study 3.1:

Mass timber for CO_2 sequestration

Ludesch Village Centre, Austria. Architect: Herman Kaufmann, 2003

Mass timber construction is increasingly common in Austria for offices, housing and even this passive standard village centre in Ludesch.

A study undertaken by Gaia Architects into savings in CO_2 emissions compared a mass timber construction house with a house of standard construction using photovoltaic (PV) cells.

The timber house of a nominal 160m² on two floors was conceived as constructed using 200 mm timber of 170 kg/m², resulting in 100 tonnes of timber material. The additional cost was £20 000 with a net sequestration of 180 tonnes of CO_2 or 3.6 tonnes/year assuming a modest 50-year life. This was compared with a known three-storey, 250 m² detached dwelling with a roof-integrated, grid-connected PV system generating 4 kW peak of electricity. It powers the house and an electric car and saves 90 tonnes of CO_2 over the lifetime of the active PV cells.

The cost of the solar roof was £22 000, with a predicted payback of around 68 years. Changes to net metering in the intervening period may have changed the economic case. The government is currently offering grants to encourage take-up of PV technology. A Carbon Tax, based upon whole-life greenhouse gas impact of products, could encourage innovation in a range of passive solutions and promote long-term ecological approaches.

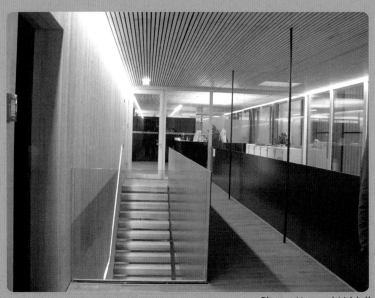

Photo: Howard Liddell

Policy trends

Most of the information throughout the 1960s, 1970s and 1980s on the potential cost benefits of resource conservation and environmental improvement was generated by the voluntary sector. The benefits were not widely appreciated or exploited. Changing attitudes have led to more mainstream pursuit of economic, social and environmental benefits, with some surprising results. Policy has become increasingly proactive in looking to such direct financial benefits, but also in using economic policy to meet social and environmental goals.

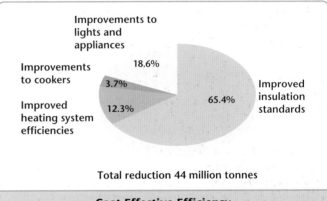

Improvements to lights and appliances 18.6%

Improvements to cookers 3.7%

Improved heating system efficiencies 12.3%

Improved insulation standards 65.4%

Total reduction 44 million tonnes

Cost Effective Efficiency

Research by BRE produced in 1990 showed that 25% of energy could be saved through cost-effective measures, begging the question why the economic benefits were not being reaped and indeed still aren't. (From Shorrock and Henderson 1990)

A note on products and materials

Awareness of issues, responsibilities, liabilities and mitigation strategies in materials, products and component manufacture is presently low in the UK. Frequently, only imports are available with an appropriate performance specification – for example, non-toxic, super-efficient, no/low pollution and recyclable. Many of these lack competitors and so they are unreasonably perceived as specialist. They are invariably more expensive than less benign alternatives. This presents real challenges to delivery of competitive sustainable buildings.

Whilst there is increasing consensus on the market-driven approach, and a large number of initiatives to promote the business case, there is still little real debate on what to do when the best option really does cost more! This will change as manufacturers and suppliers become motivated by loss of markets, increasing costs associated with energy and waste issues, and end-of-life liabilities. Present responses to pressures are not always constructive, with common perceptions that such costs are an unfair burden. There is real failure at all levels to grasp the opportunities for long-term manufacturing and employment and the downstream benefits.

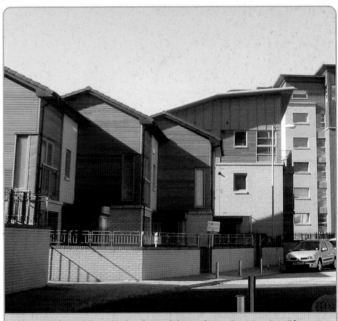

Affordable and well-designed housing, Crown St, Glasgow
(Photo: the author)

Old idealism versus modern realism

Old idealism

- In order to promote its use, clean electricity would be cheaper than dirty electricity, which has 'external costs' – that is, it requires society to repair social and environmental damage.

- Business, clients and designers of inefficient and polluting buildings would be penalised for the impacts of their decisions, including the contribution to global warming, poor productivity and ill-health of employees.

- Manufacturers of products that cause pollution in manufacture, in use or at the end of their life, would be responsible for control, management and remediation of that pollution throughout the product life and beyond.

- Looking at investment over a building's life would make more sense than cheapest capital cost. Whole-life cost and revenue budgets would be a vital aspect of publicly funded projects.

- Designers would be rewarded on the basis of designing out long-term costs.

- Investors would seek clients and buildings that minimise the risk of incurring future penalties.

Modern realism

- A combination of financial incentives, taxation and regulation, are creating a more level playing field between clean and dirty technology to help meet stringent targets.

- There is evidence of business benefits of sustainable building, not just energy and maintenance, but health, productivity and performance. Responsible clients are being rewarded, perhaps one day designers too.

- Polluters are being expected to pay. This is likely to become more apparent as environmental controls inevitably tighten towards European practice and we set more and more stringent regulatory requirements.

- Many of today's buildings will be unfit for tomorrow's business, economic and societal demands.

- There is increasing evidence that even small investments in design time can deliver major capital and running cost benefits.

- Whole-life costing is an increasingly common aspect of building design approaches, as a host of Millennium projects with inadequate revenue forecasts are being found out.

Negawatts and negalitres

Replacing a 100W bulb with a 20W bulb providing the same light output (lumens level) means that the required power has been reduced by 80W. This has become known colloquially as the production of negawatts. Similarly, water conservation measures result in negalitres. Traditionally known as demand-side management, these are useful concepts to promote change.

The concept may have been first established when Scandinavian utilities recognised that the increasing costs and liabilities associated with building new generating plants meant there was potentially more profit available from energy conservation. They distributed free energy-efficient bulbs and thereby enabled the available generating capacity to do more. With the current endemic waste of energy, negawatts are attractive and, at least as a starting point, invariably cheaper than watts. Resource conservation has suffered from poor image and public relations. It is widely interpreted as meaning that we should expect less quality/heating/cooling or space. Communicating the importance of doing *'more with less'* by focusing on using resources more effectively and reducing waste is vitally important. The 1995 report to the Club of Rome *Factor Four* documents a wide range of examples to demonstrate 'resource productivity' – the case for a fourfold increase in wealth by using resources more effectively and by a shift in our approach to progress from increasing labour productivity to resource productivity.

The concept is also now being adopted as part of *'ecominimalist'* design strategies (see Liddell, 2006) that focus on reducing loads and unnecessary losses rather than promoting the add-on ecoclichés of sustainable technology.

Case Study 3.2:

Demolition of an office block

IBM, Hursley, 1991

This demolition project was undertaken in the early 1990s. The building at IBM's former offices at Hursley was an eight-storey, concrete framed office block that because of the building programme was enclosed between new occupied buildings. Due to the constraints of the tight demolition site a decision was made to seek to minimise the disruption of the process by dismantling. Safety and lack of disruption were principal concerns, and once it was determined that the building would need to be dismantled it became possible to consider the recovery of as much material as possible.

The tendering process was viewed by all involved as crucial to the success or failure. Hence the clients drafted a profile of the contractor sought, which included turnover, experience, health and safety record, and availability of plant and personnel to ensure minimum disruption. This enabled a shortlist to be drawn up. These were all subjected to a pre-tender site visit with minimum notice and as a consequence only two were invited to tender. A further interview covered disruption and recycling.

The contractor proposing separation of materials at the workface was successful and they brought with them experience of recycling. Markets for most of the materials were identified prior to the start of demolition. This relied in part on existing knowledge, but also on new information gathering.

The demolition contract resulted in cost efficiencies, despite being slightly longer in duration than a conventional process. It achieved a 27% reduction in cost due to landfill avoidance. A total of 3999 tonnes of material was recycled (99% of the construction waste), saving £39 990 in landfill duty.

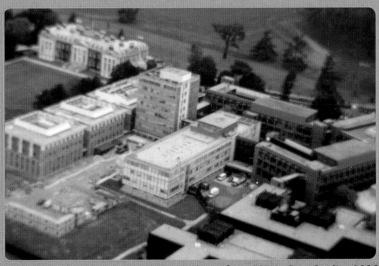

Photo: from BSRIA, Case Studies 1996

What do sustainable buildings cost?

The industry is notoriously shy in revealing information on cost and what is and isn't included. Information on the cost of sustainable building is therefore only slowly beginning to emerge. At best it can be said to give an indication of current knowledge, but it is far from being robust or reliable.

We know that many beneficial features have little or no additional capital cost, but deliver cost benefits in use – for example, site selection, attention to layout, form and window orientation, eliminating oversizing and pre-thinking staffing and security issues. On the other hand, additional costs can accrue from high-performance products, some benign materials such as paints and from extra design time.

Some requirements that were in the past assumed to increase costs are currently proving to be cost neutral or better. An example of this is sustainable urban drainage schemes (SuDs), where savings are evident from the reduced costs of pipes and hard drainage.

Transfer of expenditure to fabric and design time and away from mechanical services equipment, which is taking an increasingly large share of the cost of buildings, is one means of balancing budgets. High insulation levels and passive moisture management can cost more elementally, but require smaller heating and ventilation systems, giving both capital and running cost benefits.

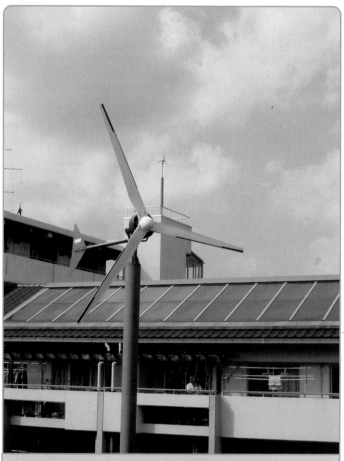

Modern Realism
A combination of instruments including financial incentives, taxation and regulation are creating a more level playing field between clean and dirty technology to help meet stringent targets, but are still difficult to justify against many simpler, cheaper and more effective measures
(Photo: the author)

Savings accrue from:

- Simplicity
- Orientation
- Lighting efficiency
- Design for flexibility
- Energy conservation
- Avoiding oversizing
- Waste management
- Good-quality air
- Passive design
- Native landscaping
- Attention to power
- Water conservation
- Reduction of emissions
- Design for operation and maintenance
- Materials efficiency
- Design for recycling.

Case Study 3.3:

Lighting replacement

Lighting is a major factor in determining the way in which people experience the internal environment and how they are able to respond to certain tasks. Good lighting design takes account of the quality and quantity of light, including natural daylight, in a space.

The qualitative and performance benefits have been well documented. However, this is still an area where significant money is wasted and where attention could save on power demand and energy, with capital and running cost benefits for homes, schools and offices.

There is an ever increasing range of energy-efficient lamps and luminaires on the market to assist good lighting design. Compact fluorescent lamps (CFLs) have a low electrical consumption, long life and good colour-rendering properties, which make them a good alternative to other lamp types in many situations. Over recent years they have under gone many improvements and the price has fallen dramatically. CFLs are available in many shapes and sizes, use 75–80% less energy and last 8–10 times longer than a conventional incandescent lamp (Table 3.1).

	Incandescent	CFL
	75 Watts	15 Watts
Purchase price	£0.40	£1.50
Lifetime	1000 hours	7000 hours
Cost of bulbs for 7000 hours of use	£2.80	£1.50
Cost of electricity for 7000 hours of use*	£36.75	£7.35
Total cost for 7000 hours	£39.55	£8.85

Total saving using CFL = £30.70
*at £0.07 per kWh

Table 3.1 Comparison of Lifetime Cost Benefit of Compact Fluorescent Lamps (CFL) versus Incandescent Bulbs

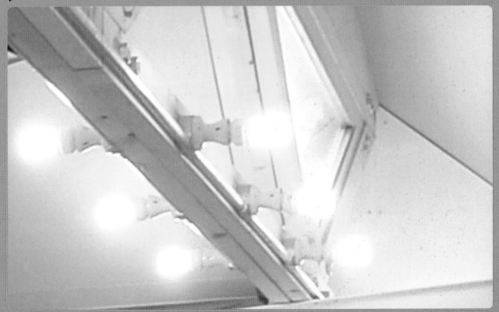

Photo: Bill Bordass, William Bordass Associates

Case Study 3.4:

Window replacement

Morley, Leeds, 2003

This conversation took place in Leeds in 2003:

Architect: **How much would it cost to replace the bottom sill on this timber window?**

Joiner: **It's not worth it – just take the whole window out and replace it with uPVC. Timber windows are virtually obsolete.**

Architect: **How much would that cost?**

Joiner: **About £600.**

Architect: **How much of that do you get?**

Joiner: **£80 per window – and we can usually fit them in an hour, so it's good money.**

Architect: **Okay, just humour me. Let us say for a moment I really insist on having this bottom sill replaced. How long would it take to strip out the bottom panes of glass, refit the bottom astragals and the sill, and then put the glass back in?**

Joiner: **About three to four hours.**

Architect: **So if we were to use the same rate of £80 an hour you could do it for, say, £300 including materials.**

Joiner: **Yes.**

Architect: **Doesn't that mean that you get all the benefit – at least three times more to yourself and you are not having to pay for the uPVC window – but just a small amount of timber.**

Joiner: **[Pause] Tell you what – I'll do it for £200 a window.**

Architect: **Would you give a 30-year guarantee on that?**

Joiner: **Yes.**

Architect: **And what kind of guarantee would you give on uPVC windows?**

Joiner: **I wouldn't.**

(With thanks to Howard Liddell, Joyce Heaton and the joiner.)

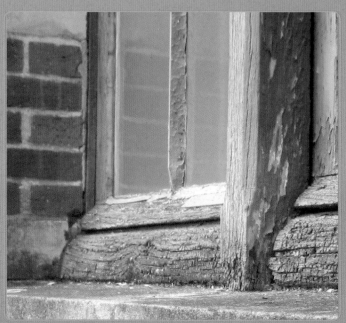

Photo: the author

Case Study 3.5:

Fabric not services

Arup Campus, Solihull. Architects: Arup Associates, 2001

The brief called for a well-equipped, socially cohesive and productive environment for 350 staff of diverse design and engineering disciplines. The distinctive feature of the development is a brief stating that it should fully satisfy developer requirements for market acceptability – that is, be cost-effective, flexible and commercially viable.

In the early stages of the design development (1998), cost benchmarking was established. A typical Midlands-based commercial office of similar scale (with air-conditioning) was identified, against which the cost-effectiveness of the design was to be monitored. A tender target of £89/sq. ft was used for the alternative naturally ventilated building (Table 3.2).

Phase 1 of the development was completed in February 2001. It consists of two pavilions that accommodate design studios. The pavilions are large, long, single volumes with interconnections between floors to encourage social cohesiveness through visual and actual linkages.

The central facilities (café, fitness room, library and a 150-seat auditorium) link the two pavilions. The 24 metre-deep building is naturally ventilated via roof openings, with passive climate control assisted by the use of thermal mass. The option to retrofit air-conditioning has been maintained by defined service areas and plant room spaces.

Reliance on artificial lighting is minimised, with daylighting from the roof and extensive glazing in the façades. Solar gain and glare are controlled by shutters and louvres, electrically or manually operated depending on their orientation. Automatic lighting controls include daylight linking to dim the direct (down) element of lighting and balance the natural light. Where possible, the design allows for occupant control – for example, manual operation of the windows.

	Midlands Office	Arup Campus
	% of total cost	% of total cost
Roof	4.19	11.57
External Cladding	13.70	26.13
Mechanical Services	22.36	4.82

Table 3.2 *BCO Guide to sustainability 2002* Shell and Core, Cat A Only (Excludes Fit Out)

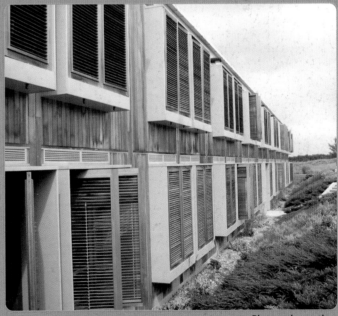

Photo: the author

Cost information

The available information on cost is essentially of four types:

- Elemental costing of sustainable attributes, resulting in figures for the additional costs of buildings accredited through assessment schemes. These give some comfort in that the additional costs are perhaps much lower than people might assume. However, the buildings themselves are not identified and questions must be raised about the priorities, weightings and response to context embodied in such assessment.

- Research data indicating the most and least cost-effective measures.

- Comparisons of overall building costs that have and have not been appraised in terms of their sustainability attributes, which demonstrate no discernible cost associated with sustainability.

- Costed exemplars open to third-party assessment, which demonstrate evidence of costs comparable with less sustainable buildings and additional life-cycle benefits.

Elemental costs

Estimates based on UK projects certified under the Building Research Establishment's Environmental Assessment Method (BREEAM) provide the best source of information available to date in the UK. This indicates less than 1% increase in capital cost to achieve the lower BREEAM ratings, which represent a significant improvement on legislative requirements. To achieve

the highest rating, cost implications are up to 7% for housing and 3.5% for office accommodation.

The figures compare with data from American projects, certified under an equivalent scheme – Leadership in Energy and Environmental Design (LEED) – that identified additional costs of a similar order. This indicates 0–3% increase in capital cost for the lower ratings, and up to 6.5% for the highest rating. However, the samples are small.

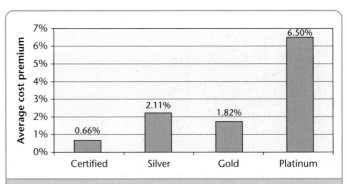

Cost premium of achieving USA's LEED classification
This is a similar scheme to UK's EcoHomes with similar estimates of additional cost based on the costs of specific 'sustainability options'

Discussion

The above data has to be treated with extreme caution. There are so many unknowns and all information on building cost is notoriously unreliable. In the cases where additional costs have been identified under BREEAM and LEED, the samples are small. For instance, the 6.5% cost increase for LEED platinum classification was based on only one building.

As the buildings themselves are not presented, or discussed in detail, it is unclear whether the fundamentals of good design were addressed and therefore whether the costs were additional to essentially good projects or poor ones. In the projects where total costs are compared, it is unclear whether the projects were in the hands of experienced sustainable building designers, which would be likely to have the effect of reducing costs, especially at the crucial procurement stage. The report itself notes that we do not even know whether the 'blue' projects might achieve a LEED classification if they were assessed.

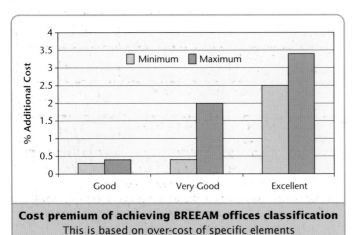

Cost premium of achieving BREEAM offices classification
This is based on over-cost of specific elements

This last issue is important. Experience in Scotland, with the launch of the RIAS Accreditation Scheme for Sustainable Design, suggests that those at the forefront of design might be cognisant of third-party assessment methods but be the least inclined to use them in a formal manner. Whilst such schemes can provide a client with evidence of achievements, in the hands of experienced designers accruing credits through assessment schemes, and paying external assessors, may not always be the best use of limited resources.

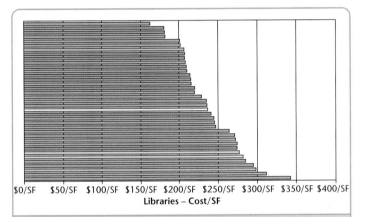

Actual costs of US library buildings in $/sq.ft.
These costs are based on the actual costs of building and the bar colour indicates the LEED classification achieved. Certified, silver and gold correspond to green, silver and gold. The blue ones are unassessed and we do not know how they would rate. There is no statistical basis for the assumption that the better rated buildings were more expensive. There are so many other factors involved

Total costs

These highlighted additional costs appear to contrast with other American data that looked at the overall costs of buildings rather than isolating specific costs. These look at specific building types, some of which had been appraised under LEED. LEED uses a green, silver, gold and platinum (none noted) rating for projects. These are reproduced to indicate the cost/square foot of a range of libraries and academic buildings.

This study found no statistical evidence for increased capital cost of sustainable design. The appraised buildings are distributed through the range of costs and are amongst both the cheapest and the most expensive.

The conclusion of this research was that there is already a vast range of building costs and that the sustainability aspects were simply one aspect 'lost in the noise'. There is no statistical basis for the assumption that the better rated buildings were more expensive.

Cost-effectiveness

There is undoubtedly a tendency for clients and to some extent policymakers to think that sustainable design is primarily concerned with adding on expensive elements such as photovoltaic panels or geothermal heat pumps. Work has been undertaken into developing a matrix of interventions against cost and impact, from low cost/high impact through to high cost/low impact. Table 3.3 is an extract from a table covering factory units (F) and warehouse distribution centres (W).

Measure	Cost £ / Unit
Lighting controls for intermittently used areas – PIRs	1000 (F) – 2000 (W)
4/2 litre dual flush WCs	1200
Modular condensing boilers (F)	1000 (F)
Zoned heating control of individual rooms (F)	1000 (F)
Timer and daylight controls. Average efficacy >100 lumens/watt	500
Shower with a flow rate of less than 9l/min	250 (F) – 500 (W)
Urinals fitted with a time switch or an automatic control device	120

Table 3.3 Low Cost / High Benefit Measures Factory and Warehouse Buildings
Interventions have different cost benefits from low cost with high benefit to high cost low benefit (Data taken from www.sustainableconstruction.org.uk/)

Costed exemplars

The following three projects were submitted with costs to the RIAS accreditation scheme. Each was assessed to be in the top class of sustainable design and each fell within benchmark costs.

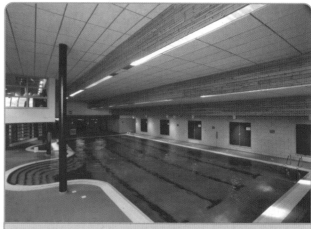

Sports facility
McLaren Community Leisure Facility, Callander is a sports and swimming pool completed in 1998 at £875/m^2, significantly lower than the benchmark costs supplied by Glasgow Council (dry only) project at £1350/m^2. It had an innovative ventilation strategy as part of a Sportscotland policy of Healthy Buildings for Healthy Pursuits. The services content was only 16% of the costs, much lower than on other pools
(Photo: Gaia Architects)

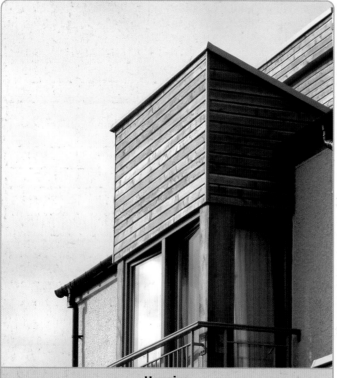

Housing
Toll House Gardens, Perth is a new-build housing completed in 2004 and designed to low-allergy specification at £780/m^2. This was within the standard cost range for housing as set by Communities Scotland
(Photo: Michael Wolshover)

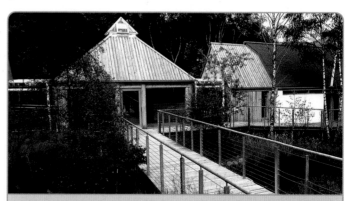

Visitor centre and offices
Glencoe Visitor Management Centre was completed in 2001 @ £980/m^2, lower than the benchmark of £1450/m^2 for an equivalent facility for the same client at the same time. The services content was 9% of the overall building cost
(Photo: Michael Wolshover)

Case Study 3.6:

Costed factory specification

Forfar, Perthshire. Architects: Gaia Architects, 2001

In 2000, Ballindarg Buildings Ltd approached Scottish Enterprise Tayside for advice and assistance in a proposed development of light industrial units as a model example of sustainable development. Gaia Architects were subsequently appointed to undertake a feasibility study.

A visit to the Centre for Alternative Technology provided a balance between practical and educational content, and gave considerable food for thought with regard to the material selection. The Dyfi Eco-park, Machynlleth, was used as a case study. Although the majority of the buildings there are offices rather than industrial units, a feel for green specification was gained. A cost comparison was undertaken by quantity surveyors, Ralph Ogg and Partners, to compare three types of industrial unit: the standard, a light green and a dark green specification.

The latter included consideration of reclaimed, hygroscopic and very-low-impact materials, improved daylighting, carbon-neutral heating, and low-carbon transport strategy, water conservation and management. Costs of the standard industrial units were based on six units in a single block, whereas the costs for the light and dark green industrial units were based on seven units in two blocks. Opportunities for trade offs that can often be readily achieved proved difficult to find from such a low cost base.

Element	Standard	Light green	Dark green
Substructure	28,025	19,298	37,343
Superstructure	86,915	109,434	127,602
Internal finishes	1,830	22,588	37,328
Services	8,310	9,590	11,340
External works	54,785	61,743	69,757
Preliminaries	17,985	22,265	28,337
Contingencies	9,895	12,246	15,525
Total costs	207,745	257,164	327,232
Cost/m^2	£617.62	£655.29	£835.5

Table 3.4 Comparative Costs (GBP) of Specifications

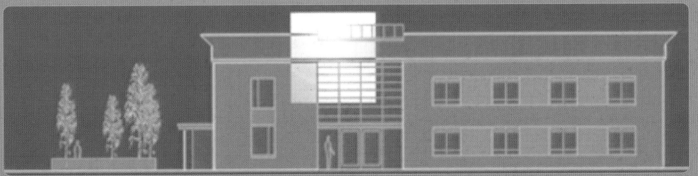

(Image: Lona Architects)

Adding value through design

The design fees and construction costs of a typical office building are a tiny proportion of the total costs of a building. Operations, maintenance, finance and employees often account for as much as 99%. Arguments for increased investment at the design stage are persuasive. It makes excellent business sense to seek a design and construction process that minimises capital cost, maximises those attributes that contribute to better business operation and minimises those elements that will be a financial drain over the building's life.

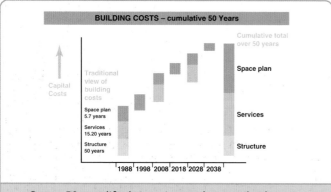

Over a 50-year life the services and space plan become the most significant costs of a building and it makes sense to design them out as far as possible
(Image after original work by DEGW)

Environmental design

The services and space planning are the most significant aspects of the whole-life costs of most buildings. Mechanical services are an escalating aspect of building costs and typically account for more than 25% of capital costs – 50% has been known. Since the mechanical services have to be replaced frequently within the life of a building, have significant maintenance implications and are responsible for much of the resource consumption, there is keen interest in ensuring that their whole-life costs are well understood and minimised.

Designers are increasingly looking to trade-offs between fabric and services, and this is made easier in an interdisciplinary design team environment. If fabric, services and financial appraisals are undertaken by individuals working independently it does not facilitate the best decision-making.

For example, increasing insulation levels do not produce a pro-rata reduction in energy saving. So traditionally the return on additional insulation beyond a certain – quite low – level is considered so close to zero that it cannot justify the additional energy required to manufacture, transport and install higher levels. Evidently, if sufficient insulation can radically reduce or completely remove the need for a heating system then the benefits in capital and running costs are enormous.

Evidence on these aspects is slowly beginning to emerge, as are cost comparisons between passive and mechanical solutions. There has been discussion for many years about the need to move from a fee basis that rewards expenditure on services equipment to one that rewards a reduction in long-term running and maintenance costs. There is no formal basis for this approach, which requires more design time, although some practices claim to work on this basis.

Evidence suggests that cost savings can be optimised when the issues are addressed at the conceptual design phase by an integrated design team. This ensures that a project is designed as one system rather than a collection of stand-alone components.

Cost and quality benefits

A significant issue for environmental designers is the extent to which good environmental design (e.g. air quality and lighting) contributes to operational efficiency and simultaneously to improving the performance of people and processes within buildings

Lighting is a source of significant energy savings and is amongst the shortest payback of any energy efficiency measure. Design input to lighting and luminaires, window design, reflection and glare can contribute to direct savings – that is, in cooling requirement as well as increased worker satisfaction and productivity. An American study compared daylit and non-daylit schools; energy reductions with daylighting were 22–64% and payback for new daylit schools three years. There was also an increase in student performance.

Case Study 3.7:

Design support

Prisma, Nuremburg. Architects: Joachim Eble Architects, 1996

This German SolarBau funding programme provided support for demonstration projects in energy saving. It consciously did not provide capital funding but instead supported design work.

A review of completed demonstration projects concluded that in most cases the expenditure on energy conservation and environmental aspects was marginal. Another aspect of the review related the demonstration projects to the 'normal' building industry. The costs of construction and services were considered (exclusive of planning/design and the associated SolarBau funding). The buildings had a tendency to show below average costs and indicated that energy-related measures integrated at an early stage do not adversely impact on building costs. If this trend to comparable lower costs continued then it would appear conclusive that:

- **additional design input leads to savings in capital costs, and/or**
- **additional costs are entirely compensated through lower costs elsewhere (shifted priorities) – for example, in fitout standards.**

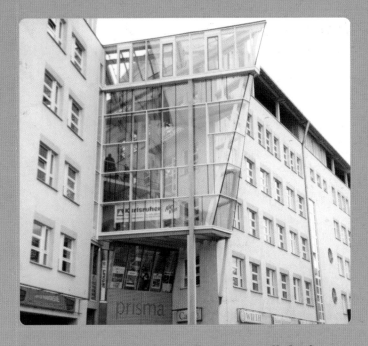

In Germany fee scales are percentage linked to the construction costs. These are strictly controlled within agreed limits and have not fallen into the downward competitive spiral now evident in the UK. These results supported the demand for a reform of the fee structure for architects and engineers in Germany to decouple the design fee from the capital cost. Similar arguments have been made about costs of building services in the UK. Some practices claim to operate on a percentage of building rather than services costs, with incentive bonuses to design out services. However, there has been little movement on the issue on the part of the professional bodies. In the UK there are no incentives currently operating to encourage more design input at the early stages.

Data from www.solarbau.de

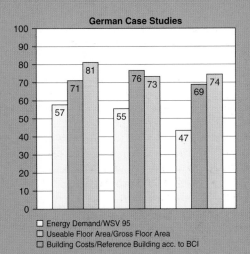

German Case Studies

☐ Energy Demand/WSV 95
☐ Useable Floor Area/Gross Floor Area
☐ Building Costs/Reference Building acc. to BCI

Photo: Joachim Eble Architects

What are the economic benefits of sustainable buildings?

A significant aspect of the growing interest in sustainable building design can be attributed to the recognition, on the part of clients, that there are direct economic benefits from sustainable building: from real savings and by improving the financial performance of a building.

Claims are also made for benefits from public relations, niche marketing and streamlined approvals for more responsible design. Of course, many clients and planners are still largely unmoved by life-cycle considerations and resist rather than encourage innovation.

Reduced operating costs

It is possible to reduce resource use by 30% – from regulatory requirements – within the constraints of most building budgets. Attention to basic details, simplicity, passive solutions and avoiding oversizing should be the first considerations, before add-on technology.

Reduced waste

Construction activity gives rise to the largest quantity of solid waste of any sector in the UK. Reductions are possible with major savings in construction and demolition costs. But efficient use of land, energy and water conservation, native landscaping and solid waste management all have financial benefits. This provides a useful policy fit with the *Limits to Growth* model described in Chapter 1 and provides the basis for many of the case studies in *Factor Four*. Designing buildings for long life and with flexible spaces can significantly reduce waste and disruption during maintenance and refurbishment, and facilitate recycling.

Reduced liability

Legislation is now a vital consideration as environmental bodies show increased willingness to introduce and use the law to prevent poor environmental practice. Future-proofing is important as changes in regulatory requirements can have significant associated costs if they lead to major contract variations.

There is also a clear intention that trends in fiscal policy and in regulatory policy will increasingly tax pollution and inefficiency, and impose increasingly higher targets for environmental performance and social responsibility, in an effort to raise standards. This is reinforcing good practice. Selection of systems that are long-lasting and readily manageable and maintainable, and selection of building materials that are non-polluting in use and at the end of their life, are becoming standard good-practice elements of future-proofing. Attention to the indoor environment reduces the risk of 'building related ill-health', with legal and productivity implications.

Enhanced productivity and learning

Many studies have shown improvements in productivity and in performance when good air quality, personal environmental control, daylight, and a connection to plant features and the outdoors are provided.

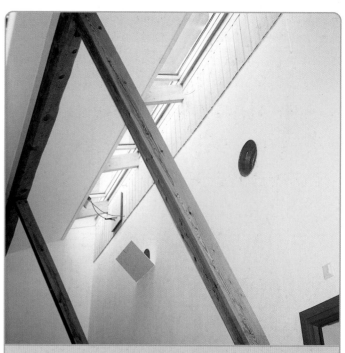

Vanse School, Norway
The health and productivity gains from creating better learning environments has been well documented. It is known that in schools the environment is crucial in promoting opportunities for children, enabling teachers to carry out their tasks and in creating a sense of community
(Architects: Gaia Lista; photo: Fionn Stevenson)

Social costs and the environment

There is a cost associated with ill-health. The National Asthma Campaign statistics indicate that in the UK one in 25 adults and one in seven children have asthma. It accounts for 1500 deaths each year. Seven million lost work days due to asthma result in £350 million in lost productivity and costs of approximately £60 million in sickness benefit. The cost of asthma treatment to the NHS is £850 million a year.

The noticeable rise in asthma/allergy in the UK in recent years provided motivation for research to identify whether the removal of dust mite colonies and their allergens from domestic dwellings has any effect on asthmatic/ allergic symptoms.

Incoming residents of the new 14 house development at Toll House Gardens, Fairfield, were provided with information on the design. Where they were interested in pursuing aspects outside the Housing Association provision, Gaia Architects assisted with flooring finishes, treatments, and low allergy beds and bedding. The dwellings were examined for temperature, damp and dust mites shortly after occupation, and if there was evidence of dust mites brought from elsewhere then the opportunity for steam cleaning was provided.

Case study – female aged 50				
	Before	**After**	**Reduction**	
Salbutamol	700g	520g	31%	
Beclamethasone	875g	650g	31%	
Cost saving in drugs based on Sept 2001 benchmark				£176
No of GP visits Apr 97 – Mar 99 = 17 @ £20				£340
No of GP visits Apr 99 – Mar 01 = 4 @ £20				£80
Total saving on medical costs = £176 + £260 =				£436
Cost of intervention =				£492
Payback period < 27 months				

Table 3.5 Making the link between environment, society and economy
Results of University of Strathclyde study into GP visits and medication taken after interventions to remove dust mites from 45 existing homes. Howieson (2003)

Asthma children 'no better off' in the fume-free country air

By JENNY HOPE
Medical Correspondent

CLAIMS that worsening traffic pollution is to blame for the rising number of children with asthma have been called into doubt by researchers.

They found that youngsters in the country were just as likely to have the condition as those in towns.

A survey of children aged 12 and 13 in the Highlands revealed that 14 per cent had asthma — a proportion similar to the national average — while on Skye it was actually higher at 17 per cent. The busiest road in the areas covered by the study — Skye, Lochaber, Ross and Cromarty and Inverness — was used by an average of 23,000 vehicles a day compared with the 120,000 on the M25 around London each day.

The leader of the survey team, Dr Jane Austin, past chairman of the National Asthma Campaign's Highlands branch, said the results 'certainly contradict popular opinion, which tends to link childhood asthma over the last couple of decades with the huge growth of traffic'. A study in Norway also found no link.

Dr Jon Ayres, the National Asthma Campaign's medical adviser on the environment, said the findings reinforced the view that asthma is 'multi-factorial — you can line up a dozen people with asthma and they will all have different histories and different triggers'.

Experts suspect that, since more time is now spent indoors, the home may hold the key. The Highland team is looking into lifestyles there, including how homes are ventilated, whether they are double-glazed and whether parents smoke.

Daily Mail Article

At a time when car fumes were being targetted for the potential asthma inducing effects, this article reported on research indicating that asthma was as prevalent in remote rural regions as in polluted and congested cities

Every 13 weeks the research team collected data to determine whether there was any change in the dust mite colonies and compared these with results from a study of 45 existing dwellings in Scotland being studied by the University of Strathclyde.

Questionnaires were used to determine whether there had been a reduction in asthmatic symptoms for the occupants. Residents indicated marked improvements in health. The data collected on the different ventilation strategies and impact on moisture regimes is covered in Chapter 10.

Case Study 3.8:

Air leakage – new-build townhouse

A new three-storey mid-terrace townhouse – part of a substantial development by a volume house-builder – was tested as part of a training course. Of masonry construction, it has cavity walls, a suspended concrete ground floor and timber intermediate floors.

Extractor fans from two internal bathrooms and the cooker hood extract were sealed. It achieved an air change rate of 9.8 air changes/hour (ACH) and an air permeability of 9.7 m³/h/m² of total surface area at 50 Pa. This is slightly better than the proposed regulations maximum of 10ACH and substantially worse than the TM23 'best practice' target of 5.0 m³/h/m² at the same pressure. Many of the leakage sites identified occurred in several locations throughout the house:

- beneath the window sill in the groundfloor kitchen
- through a hole in plasterboard drylining in the kitchen
- through holes around water pipes from the gas boiler
- through the room thermostat mounted on an internal partition wall
- through gaps in the panelling around the bath and hand basin
- through spotlights mounted in the ceiling, and around ceiling roses and other light fittings
- around hot and cold water pipes, and waste pipes passing through the backs of kitchen units
- through plumbing and waste pipes in the bathroom on the ground floor
- through wiring to the gas boiler
- through a ceiling-mounted extract vent
- around and through French doors
- along a top edge of skirting board
- around and through electricity sockets and switches, and television connections, in internal and external walls

- at the sides of the internal staircase
- through and around the cooker hood extract.

There was no effective air barrier between the cavity in the external wall and the hollow first and second floors. With plasterboard drylining and hollow partition walls, leakage is to every part of the house and remedial sealing is very difficult.

Despite this, the building would meet the proposed Building Regulations Air Permeability target, at least when new. Yet much more could be achieved with a little more care and attention to detail during the design and construction phases. Good design for low infiltration and controllable ventilation could save 1.2 kW (1200 negawatts) and around £150/annum over a badly designed and constructed building.

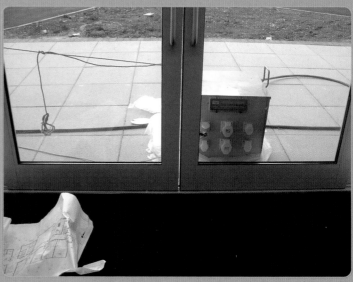

Photo: Paul Jennings

Whole-life costs

Estimates vary, but typical relative figures for buildings' whole-life costs are: for every 1 unit spent on construction, 5 are spent on operation and 200 on salaries. Only 0.1 unit is spent on design.

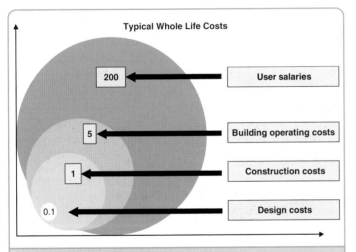

Typical Whole Life Costs

200	←	User salaries
5	←	Building operating costs
1	←	Construction costs
0.1	←	Design costs

Added value of design
An upfront investment of less than 2% of construction costs yields life-cycle savings of over 10 times the initial investment

A 20% reduction in operating costs is negligible compared to salaries, but is equivalent to the construction costs. Designing an environment in which employees are 5% more productive is equivalent to 10 times the construction costs. Interest in whole-life costing has vastly increased with the recognition that first costs are a very small part of the overall cost of buildings.

Clients are increasingly keen to have a realistic indication of the ongoing operational costs to ensure that buildings are affordable in the long term. Potential benefits may include reduced running costs (maintenance, cleaning, energy, water) or because design increases productivity, image and/or business opportunities. Increasing scrutiny of a wide range of issues from the impacts of climate change to built environments which contribute to

deprivation and ill-health are also recognisable as having financial implications and are grabbing the attention of social landlords, property managers, business and investors. Attention to these issues is justified as good business practice.

All the evidence suggests that poor environmental performance will be penalised in future and the benefits of good performance will be increasingly apparent as economic instruments begin to penalise and reward. Treasury as well as other pressures, including the introduction of Public Finance Initiatives (PFIs) and Public–Private Partnerships (PPPs), have an inbuilt incentive to reduce operating costs. However, predicting whole-life costs is still in its infancy and it is very difficult to get data even on relatively simple aspects such as long-term performance, durability and maintenance requirements of components. Even operating costs can be unpredictable, especially those associated with electrical consumption.

Life-cycle assessment (LCA) – sometimes also called life-cycle analysis – is a method to measure and evaluate the environmental burdens associated with a product system or activity, by describing and assessing the energy and materials used and released to the environment over the life cycle. LCA looks at the 'cradle-to-grave' impact of elements, materials and components, and is the basis of most product labelling.

Whole-life cost (WLC) – sometimes also called life-cycle cost (LCC) – is the assessment of all relevant costs and revenues associated with a building over an agreed period, including procurement, operation and sometimes disposal. WLC looks at the life cycle from the start of design and construction, and might include:

- Procurement costs – feasibility, design, construction, purchase/lease, interest, fees
- Operating costs – energy, water/sewage, waste disposal, cleaning, security and management
- Recurring costs – rent, rates, maintenance, repair, refurbishment, replacement/renewal
- End-of-life costs – decommissioning, dismantling or disposal
- Revenue – sales of recycled materials, rental income, asset value accrued.

WLC is still in a formative stage of development, with a variety of techniques still emerging.

Environmental economics – external costs

Environmental economics aims to promote sustainable development through market incentives that reduce conflict between economic growth and environmental protection. By setting a framework of how we grow, it aims to eliminate fears that environmental protection will prevent economic growth. Environmental economics increasingly drives policy. Financial considerations that were once limited to first cost and some rudimentary pay-back or discounting calculation have begun to change dramatically. There is increasing recognition that our natural resources do have an economic value and the impact of unsustainable development – inefficiency, ill-health, community dissatisfaction, pollution, resource depletion, toxicity – do have a cost in quality of life as well as requiring financial remediation.

It is these social and financial implications of unsustainable development (known as external costs) that are now leading to change. There are an increasing number of measures that are aimed at protecting these resources by internalising costs through taxation, legislation, changes in building standards and positive incentives to encourage sustainable development.

Economic instruments

Economic instruments are policies that affect price – for example, to enable clean products and services to compete with unclean alternatives. They are also referred to as 'measures that internalise externalised costs' and take the form of regulatory controls and market-based measures, including pollution charges, user charges, deposit refunds and tradable pollution permits/resource rights. The case for the use of economic instruments to assist in delivering environmental and sustainable development objectives has been made.

> **A report by the UK Round Table on Sustainable Development identified energy, traffic and transport, agriculture, waste management, consumer behaviour, poverty and social exclusion as areas in need of attention to reverse unsustainable trends and where economic instruments could help.**

Fiscal measures include Enhanced Capital Allowances, which incentivise companies to invest in energy-saving equipment; reduced VAT on some energy-saving products; and the Landlord's Energy Saving Allowance. Current policies and measures are projected to save around 12 million tonnes of carbon per year by 2010, saving households and businesses £3 billion per year on their energy bills.

The Marshall Report (1998) investigated their use in energy-related matters and recognised the need for tradable permits and taxation. It advocated a mixed approach of economic instruments alongside regulation, voluntary and negotiated agreements. The review recommended taxation be related to carbon content of fuels and be introduced in a gradual and predictable way to give business time to plan and respond. It was agreed as part of the Kyoto Protocol. By setting caps on emissions the scheme provides incentives for investment in energy efficiency and cleaner technologies.

A voluntary UK pilot scheme is running, and electricity generators and oil refineries are expected to take part in a European scheme. An international scheme will begin in 2008. Attention has been given to ensuring that instruments assist current objectives – such as eliminating fuel poverty – and do not penalise those least advantaged or adversely affect business competitiveness. It was recommended that all tax revenue is recycled into business through awareness, advice and incentives, so as to promote the required change and maintain international competitiveness.

> ### Economic instruments in construction – an international survey (Drouet, D. 2003)
>
> 1 Preferential credit conditions for sustainable buildings.
>
> 2 Reimbursement, rebates and investment aid offered by water or energy utilities, equipment suppliers, and so on.
>
> 3 Preferential insurance conditions for sustainable buildings; new insurance products.
>
> 4 Setting up specialised funds for sustainable construction.
>
> 5 Fiscal bonus for the construction or renovation of green buildings.
>
> 6 Heavier fiscal burden on non-sustainable construction.
>
> 7 Grants, subsidies.
>
> 8 Density bonus and/or accelerated building permit processing for sustainable construction.
>
> 9 Business rating indexes including sustainable building management criteria.
>
> 10 Trade of CO_2 certificates.

Redefining progress

Sustainable development is about ensuring a better quality of life for everyone, now and for future generations. It is important that our economic, social and environmental policies all improve our quality of life, and we need suitable indicators of all three elements to measure progress toward a sustainable economy that meets people's real needs. We should be looking to set policy, indicators and targets that promote those aspects of our economic activity that improve our quality of life.

The principal indicator of well-being and quality of life for the last century has been the gross domestic product (GDP) – the sum of all the money we spend. Increasing GDP is the indicator of progress, but its real value has been challenged for decades.

GDP takes no account of social or environmental issues. Rising oil consumption increases GDP, as do environmental disasters, crime and car crashes, if money has to be spent on remediation. GDP favours cures rather than prevention – good health has no economic value but pills do. Inevitably, therefore, GDP promotes the pursuit of quantity over quality. GDP also fails to reflect the underlying sustainability of any pattern of economic activity. An economy that grows on the basis of depleting oil reserves is spending a non-renewable asset. This ought to be reflected in accounts, but is not.

> '...a new single measure of welfare could play a very useful part in increasing awareness of the different elements that contribute to the well-being of society and to the achievement of sustainable development.. the government should examine this concept with a view to developing and publishing an index of this kind by the year 2000.'
>
> – Parliamentary Committee

With a rise in enlightened attitudes to development economics – and amid concern for resource depletion, environmental quality, social stability and downstream costs – criticism of GDP is ever more justified. There is now a move towards forms of social and environmental costing to provide a framework for sustainable development, and there is real activity to develop indicators that relate economic change to quality of life. The EU 5th Environmental Action Programme committed members to developing pilot systems of 'environmental adjusted national accounts' by 1995, with a view to adopting them by 2000.

A note on VAT and regeneration

EU tax rules are implicated in promoting new build over repair and refurbishment of existing buildings. Demolition and rebuild are zero-rated for VAT against 17.5% for repairs and extensions. This militates against bringing existing buildings back into habitable use. Recent changes may provide member states with an option to establish a flat rate, which would be welcomed as a contribution to sustainability.

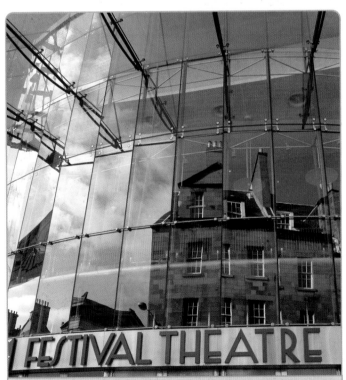

Ecological refurbishment of Nicolson Street, Edinburgh
There are different VAT rules applied to old and new buildings in the same street and this militates against refurbishment
(Architects: Gaia Architects; photo: Michael Wolshover)

Ethical investment

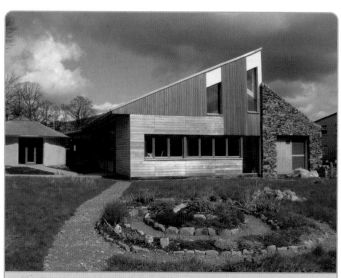

Ecology Building Society HQ, Silsden, Yorkshire
(Architects: Hodson Architects, photo permission: EBS
www.ecology.co.uk)

Ethical investment involves investing surplus money in such a way as to support environmentally and socially responsible activities. Early ethical trusts tended to avoid firms involved in environmental damage, pollution, weapons and the arms trade, nuclear activities and support of oppressive regimes.

An ethical portfolio will normally be tied to a published set of principles that guide investment. These have developed from the formative 'Valdez' principles established following the Alaskan oil pollution disaster. More information can be found from the Ethical Investments Research and Information Service (EIRIS), www.eiris.org/.

Increasingly, there is a strategy to talk up business benefits of a sustainable approach that involves responsibilities, precautionary judgements and use of resources in a sustainable manner. Hence a limited but growing number of opportunities exist for investment in such business. Benefits are increasingly evident because of tax trends, risk assessments and public image, and some ethical investment portfolios are highly competitive. The development of the notion of 'business accountability' has given rise to a number of initiatives to monitor business performance, such as 'sustainability accounting'.

Interestingly, the Pension Act 2000 makes it mandatory for fund managers to disclose to what extent social, environmental and ethical considerations affect their investment strategy.

Money

Money is the measure in which most – but not all – economic concepts are expressed. It was a brilliant invention. Money allows individuals to specialise in a particular area and transcend beyond a basic exchange economy by putting a price on activities.

However, as money has developed an existence in its own right, there is increasing criticism of the way that it is used. Exponential growth, in particular, is a dilemma that makes our economic system less sustainable than one which followed a natural growth curve. For many (see Kennedy, 1988) it is one of the most important issues of today and one that has to be resolved for the long term. Importantly, there are some meaningful proposals for alternatives, which could be better able to deliver sustainable development and prevent centralisation of wealth.

Local Exchange Trading Scheme (LETS) systems have been developed to achieve similar ends to money. A LETS is a system of trading based on agreed barter terms usually, but not exclusively, at a local level. Members receive LET units in return for goods or services and in turn pay for services from others, in the same units. Credits and debits can accrue for anything (childcare/massage) and are recorded in a common, open account. The aim is to keep balances close to zero. The account network enables the barter system to extend trading from a two-person activity to an interdisciplinary one with unlimited access to a wide and varied group of services. There are about 450 LET schemes in the UK.

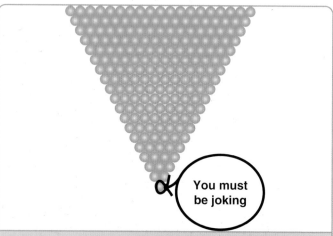

Gold earths
One penny invested at the birth of Jesus Christ at 4% interest would have bought a ball of gold the weight of the earth in 1821, two in 1839 and over 1200 solid gold earths in 2003. At 5% interest it would have bought 260 billion gold earths in 2003
(Cartoon: Howard Liddell)

Conclusion: a discussion on capital

The World Commission on Environment and Development (WCED) – the 'Brundtland Commission' – was seminal in that it gave a precise definition to sustainable development. It also went further than previous international development strategies in that it identified the possibility for the right sort of economic policy to be a positive force in environmental terms. In so doing it pointed out the degrading impact on the environment of the wrong sort of economic policy.

The Brundtland Commission introduced the notion of a non-declining stock of capital assets. This non-declining stock of capital assets, including environmental assets, exists to meet the needs of industry, individual consumers and society in the future.

The Brundtland definition of sustainable development indicated that the assets of each generation combined knowledge, understanding, technology, man-made capital and environmental assets.

They concluded that the sum of a generation's assets should be no less generation on generation, i.e. that each generation should pass on to the next at least the same or equivalent assets. This is at the core of the many interpretations of sustainable development.

David Pearce and colleagues took the theory further in the late 1980s and early 1990s by investigating the concept of economically valuing the environment – that is, placing proper values on the services it provides. The issue that the work highlighted is that as some vital services provided by the environment have no cost directly associated with them – such as the ozone layer – there is no incentive for individuals to protect them. However, as we now know, its depletion has major cost (protection and health treatment) and quality implications. The issue remains unresolved by most commercial activity.

Pearce produced a number of invaluable case studies and a methodology in which man-made and natural capital were largely inter-tradable (except some critical natural capital). This provided the basis for a new pricing structure. Other studies looked at ways of placing value on the environment through assessment of markets known as hedonic pricing, i.e. the value of a lake was estimated from what people were prepared to pay to live next to it.

More recently, a framework for sustainable development has been developed. Five 'Capitals' have been identified to describe what a sustainable society should look like. These are Natural Capital, Human Capital, Social Capital, Manufactured Capital and Financial Capital. It is in many ways a logical expansion on the Brundtland definition of sustainable development. They aim to represent the outcome of a successful capital investment strategy for sustainable development – that is, a sustainable society.

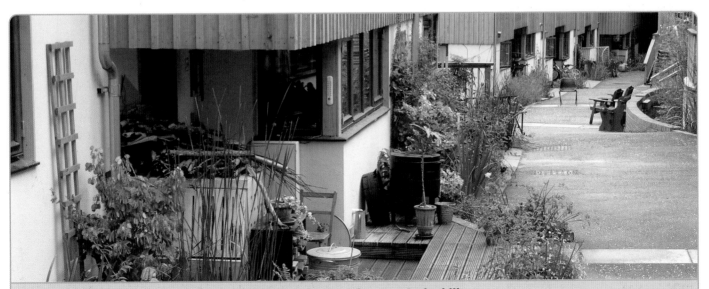

Integrated SuDs Scheme at Springhill
Some requirements that were in the past assumed to increase costs are currently proving to be cost neutral or better. An example of this is sustainable urban drainage schemes, where savings are evident from the reduced costs of pipes and hard drainage
(Architects: Architype, photo: the author)

Bibliography

Mishan, E. J. (1967) *The Costs of Economic Growth*. Pelican. A social sciences classic.

Schumacher, E. F. (1973) *Small is Beautiful: A study of economics as if people mattered*. Blond Briggs.

Hawken, P. (1987) *Growing a Business*. Simon & Schuster.

Kennedy, M. (1988) *Interest and Inflation-Free Money – How to create an exchange mechanism that works for everybody*. Permakultur Publ., ISBN 3 98802184 0 6. This is a look at how money does not work – in particular, the 'invisible wrecking machine' of compound interest.

Pearce, D. et al. (1989) *Blueprint for a Green Economy*. Earthscan.

Shorrock J., and Henderson G (1990) *Greenhouse gas emissions and buildings in the United Kingdom*. BRE

Pearce, D. (ed.) (1991) *Blueprint 2*. Earthscan.

Cairncross, F. (1991) *Costing the Earth*. Economist Books.

Pearce, D. and Barde, J-P. (eds) (1991) *Valuing the Environment*. Earthscan.

Douthwaite, R. (1992) *The Growth Illusion – How economic growth has enriched the few, impoverished the many and endangered the planet*. Green Books.

Elkington, J. and Knight, P. (1992) *The Green Business Guide*. Victor Gollancz.

von Weizsacker, E., Lovins, A. B. and Lovins, L. H. (1995) *Factor Four– Doubling Wealth, Halving Resource Use*. Earthscan.

Halliday S.P. (1996) *Environmental Code of Practice for Buildings and their Services – Case Studies*. BSRIA

Henderson, H. (1996) *Creating Alternative Futures*. Kumarian.

Lord Marshall's Report on Economic Instruments and the Business Use of Energy (1998) http://archive.treasury.gov.uk/pub/html/.

Hawken, P., Lovins, A. B. and Lovins L. H. (1999) *Natural Capitalism*. Earthscan.

Digest 452 (2000) *Whole Life Costing and Life-cycle Assessment for Sustainable Building Design*. BRE.

TemaNord (2002) *The Use of Economic Instruments in Nordic Environmental Policy 1999–2001* (www.norden.org).

DEFRA/DTI (2003) Sustainable Consumption and Production Indicators (www.defra.gov.uk).

Drouet, D. (2003) Economic Instruments for Sustainable Construction, English summary. www.areneidf.com/english/pdf/BLComHQEnglish.pdf.

Energy White Paper (2003) *Our Energy Future – Creating a low carbon economy*. Sets out a long-term strategy to give industry confidence to invest in meeting a truly sustainable energy policy (www.dti.gov.uk/energy/whitepaper/index.shtml).

Fabian Society (2003) *A Better Choice of Choice* (www.fabian-society.org.uk).

Grant, N. (2003) *The Economics of Water Efficient Products in the Household*, EA from 01903-832073.

Howieson, S. G. (2003) *Housing and Health: Are our homes causing the asthma pandemic?* University of Strathclyde.

Jackson, T. and Michaelis, L. (2003) *Policies for Sustainable Consumption*. Sustainable Development Commission.

Kats, G. (2003) *The Costs and Financial Benefits of Green Buildings*. California's Sustainable Building Task Force.

Porritt, J. (2003) *Redefining Prosperity*. Sustainable Development Commission.

Cyril Swett (2005) *Putting a Price on Sustainability* BRE Trust

Liddell, H. L. (2006) *Eco-minimalism, Green Building Bible Vol. 1*, Green Building Press, pp. 98–103.

BRE also produce a number of Good Practice Guides on cost-effectiveness for building managers: search www.energy-efficiency.gov.uk.

CIBSE publications that address WLC issues including ownership, operation and maintenance, durability, replacement intervals, cost benefits of airtightness/insulation and guidance on improving life-cycle performance of systems – search www.cibse.org.uk.

Sustainable development networks

The Ecologist – www.theecologist.org

Environment Business (fortnightly news briefings, listings and occasional supplements on specific topics) – www.environment-now.co.uk

Ethical Consumer – www.ethicalconsumer.org

New Internationalist – www.newint.org

Resurgence – www.resurgence.gn.apc.uk

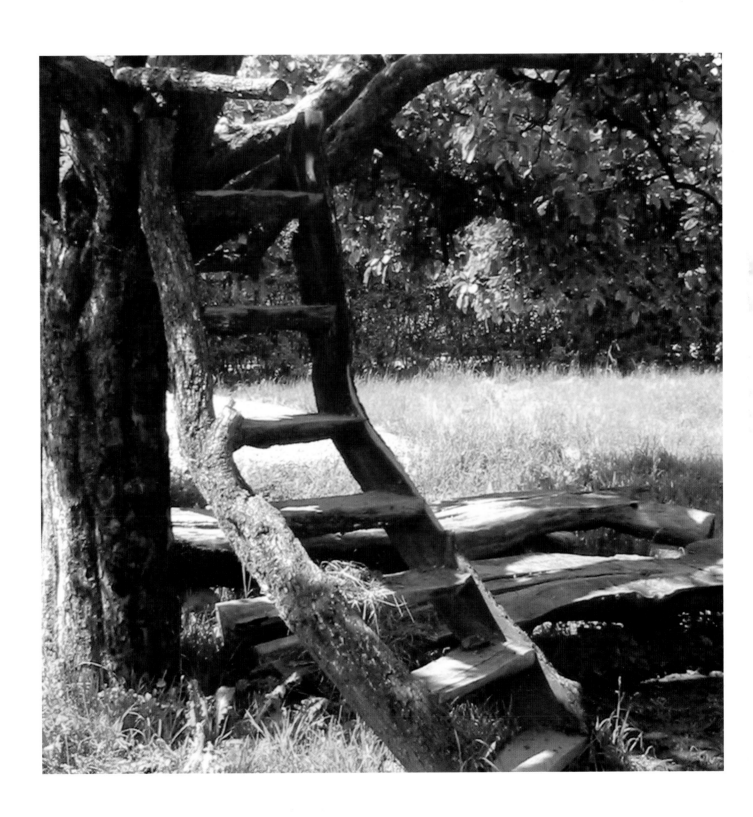

Chapter 4
Appraisal tools and techniques

In which we look at a range of tools and techniques that promote, assist and measure achievements in sustainable construction and attempt to provide a hierarchy. Only those tools and techniques with a degree of objective appraisal and traceability are considered in any depth.

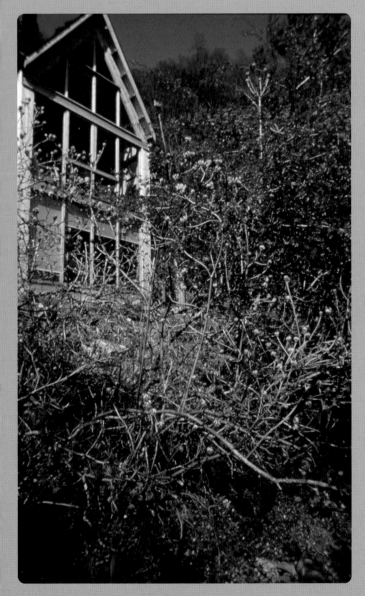

'A great building must begin with the unmeasurable. Must go through measurable means when it is being designed and in the end must be unmeasurable.'

Louis Kahn

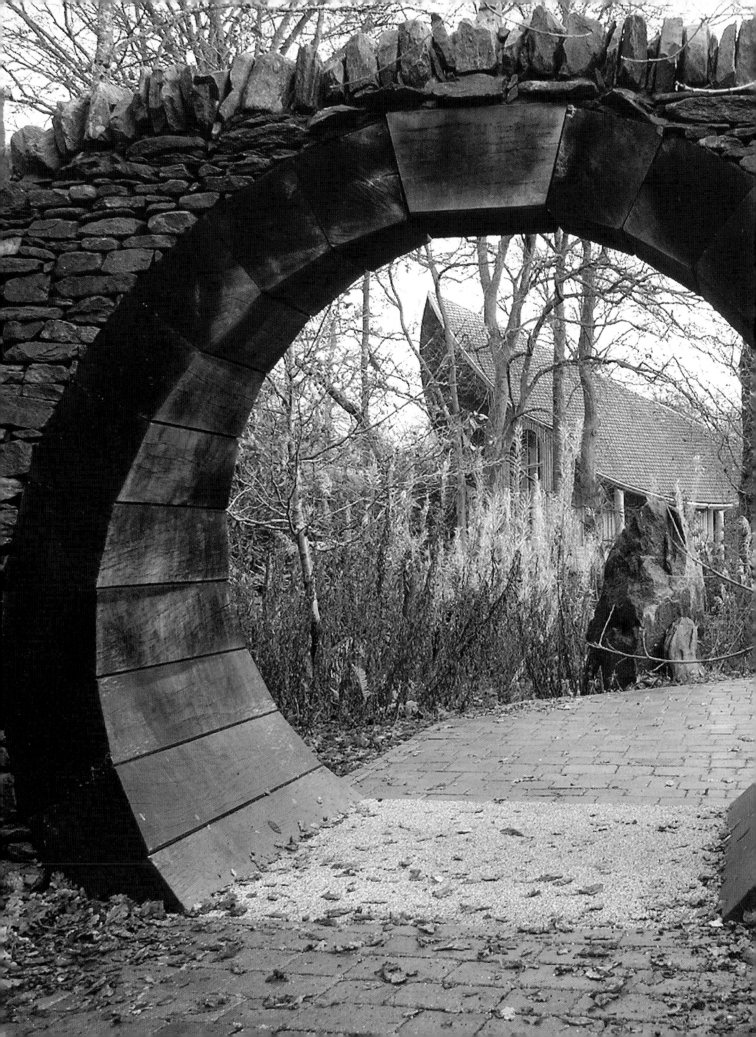

Contents

(Facing page)
**David Douglas Centre,
Pitlochry, Perthshire:**
Scottish Timber Award 2005.
Gaia Architects
(Photo: the author)

(Previous page)
**Bourne House, Weem by
Aberfeldy:**
Winner of UK House of the Year
1993.
Gaia Architects
(Photo: Gaia Architects)

Appraisal tools and techniques

Introduction

Market awareness, legislation, government and private sector policy have provided incentives to improve construction practice and to set in place procedures for continual improvement. This has resulted in development of a range of tools and techniques to promote, assist and measure achievements. The number and type is expanding rapidly.

They range from analytical methods – such as used in modelling performances – to critical path guides, targeting tools, benchmarks, and a wide range of third-party validated labels and certificates which are driving forward practice. At a simple level, checklists, awards, regulatory requirements and policy have a place, albeit they often have limited aspirations.

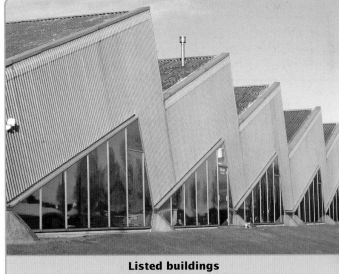

Listed buildings
Until recently building qualities were rarely classified other than according to preservation orders – like this magnificent if redundant A-listed rolling stock factory in Shotts
(Architects: ABK; photo: Michael Wolshover)

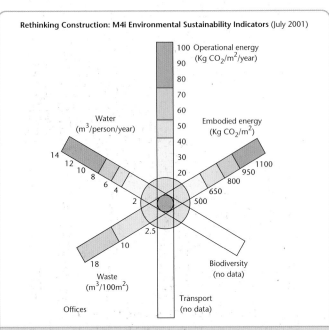

Rethinking Construction: M4i Environmental Sustainability Indicators (July 2001)

Environmental Key Performance Indicators
All appraisal tools and techniques act as both a guide and a measure of performance and therefore have to be developed used responsibly to ensure that what we build is appropriate to the challenges we face

Each approach, in its way, acts as both a measure of achievement and also, importantly, through its selection of parameters and values, as a guide to users. These tools therefore bear a heavy responsibility to address the important issues, and not just the measurable ones, and to inspire adequate action to deal with current threats.

The benefits of appraisal tools and techniques, to a large extent, define the problems with them. For governments, designers and clients with an awareness of international issues and a tendency to register environmental and social concerns, they can be a useful addition to the existing toolkit and mindmap that contribute to a project. To those with scant knowledge they can become a crutch.

Because many of them rely on numbers, in the hands of the inexperienced they can give undue emphasis to what is readily measurable at the expense of broader concerns or discrete interactions. Many take a complex array of issues and weightings to arrive at a single figure, which may or may not always be a fair and contemporary assessment. They therefore need to be used with caution.

It is important that designers and clients are able to understand the breadth and comparative value of different techniques in order to best assess their real contribution to a sustainable future. There is therefore no intention to endorse all of the tools shown here, but to encourage critical engagement with them.

Overview

In order to evaluate the degree to which sustainability objectives are being met it is necessary to find agreement on the issues and the severity of the problems. The UK has set sustainability indicators that act as a guide to the direction of future government policy and there is growing consensus on the issues – but little agreement on priorities and targets. As a result, a vast and expanding variety of tools and techniques to promote and appraise sustainable construction have emerged. There is a hierarchy, but most have a useful role to play.

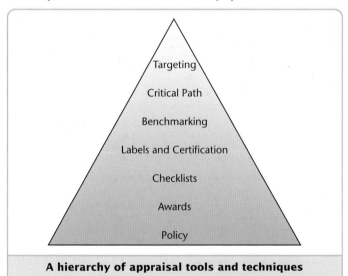

A hierarchy of appraisal tools and techniques

The techniques vary from those that seek to establish sustainable construction as a process conforming to real limitations on resources and impacts, to checklists that do little more than encourage issues to be considered. Award schemes are used to reward best practice, often in a non-systematic way, whilst labelling and certification is more interesting as it demands a degree of traceability and is less fickle. There can be disagreement where a methodology disaggregates factors and then uses weightings that can seem arbitrary. However, professional judgement also has value.

Absolute targets based on known limits are rarely available. Those in common use are generally agreed by consensus with the industry so as to be marginally ahead of regulation. They are unlikely to be adequate to meet current threats. The absolute target for reduction in CO_2 emissions recommended by the Royal Commission on Environmental Pollution (RCEP) is 90%. This sets a precedent in that it is so onerous as to be unimaginable by the bulk of construction practice. Real limitations on use of toxic chemicals, water resources and waste management are unlikely to be more palatable.

The low level of our regulatory benchmark, and its slow improvement, is an aggravation to those at the forefront of design practice who both know how much more is achievable but also have to compete with the non-optimised and poor quality norm. It is notable that other European countries have been more proactive in promoting the continual raising of lowest standards than the UK.

Importantly, there is increasing recognition of the need for process tools to support specialist management of the design and construction process in order to reliably take aspirations through to successful delivery and beyond into genuine long-term sustainability. Anything that stops decision paralysis and the blame culture has to be an improvement.

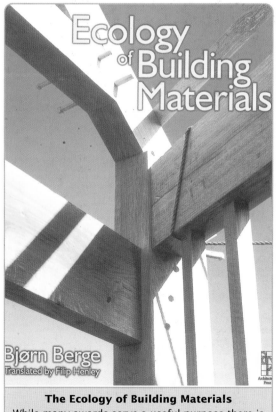

The Ecology of Building Materials
While many awards serve a useful purpose there is sometimes no substitute for individual expertise and judgements, as in the seminal text on building materials by Bjørn Berge, often referred to as the Egon Ronay equivalent guide to ecological materials

Case Study 4.1:

Policy: Ecology Building Society

Silsden, West Yorkshire. Architects: Hodson Architects, 2005

The overall strategy was to produce a building that has very low energy requirements. This is achieved by producing an airtight structure with very low leakage and high levels of insulation. Building regulations state that there should be no more leakage than $10\,m^3$ per hour at a pressure of 50 Pa.

The heating system is designed to run at low temperatures due to the highly insulated nature of the building. It is powered by a high efficiency condensing boiler. Each radiator has a thermostatic control.

The building has a mechanical air-handling unit, which can be used to change the air in the building over as specified period, in winter pre-heating the air on the way in with a heat exchanger extracting the heat from the expelled air. Airconditioning was not installed; instead, there are opening windows and trickle vents to deal with humidity problems.

Mass has been created in the building floor and in the slab that forms the mezzanine, which stores heat and radiates it out when temperatures drop, contributing to an even temperature and further reducing heating requirements.

The HQ won the Bradford and District Design Award for 'Building of the Year' in 2004 and was also a finalist in the Mortgage Finance Gazette 'Innovator of the Year' award. In November 2005 it won Building Magazine's award for 'Sustainable Building of the Year' – for a small project.

Straw bale meeting room

The construction of the circular load-bearing straw bale meeting room demonstrates more radical green building. Building work began in April and was completed in September 2005.

The walls are constructed of locally sourced straw bales, on a lime-crete base with a lime plaster and lime wash finish. The sheep's wool-insulated conical roof is constructed from sustainable timber and will be clad with cedar shingles. The room is not artificially heated as it is highly insulated by the straw bales and requires little lighting due to the large amount of glazing. All scrap wood and metal from the construction process were sorted for reuse.

The room is a green reference library and meeting room for staff, and is available for hire to local community groups and schools. All glass, paper, cans, plastic bottles and batteries are recycled, purchasing policy is Fairtrade, and tea and coffee grinds are composted.

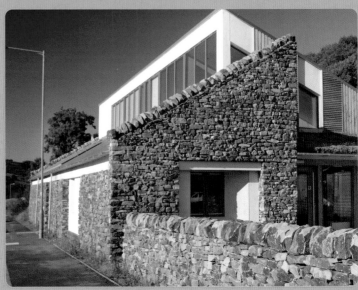

Photo: Ecology Building Society. www.ecology.co.uk

A hierarchy

Policy (the stated priorities, aims and objectives)

Organisations including central and local government, professional bodies and the private sector are increasingly developing policies for sustainable built development. The subject is covered more fully in Chapter 2. Whilst these are welcome as a starting point, they are ineffective unless they have full stakeholder involvement and are accompanied by targets, actions and timescales.

Regulation (the lowest common denominator)

This is an attempt to embrace the issues perceived as relevant and controllable at a pace the industry will tolerate, increasingly used in some countries to support the radical changes required. Despite a number of recent reviews, requirements in the UK still do little to promote a significant step towards sustainable construction and lag behind initiatives by our EU partners. Major changes in regulation are being generated from Europe with, for example, the WEEE directive likely to have a significant impact on the demolition and refurbishment sector, and the new *EU Regulation on Building Labelling* potentially having an impact through clients.

A study by Gaia Research and the University of Dundee looked at *Sustainable Construction and the Regulatory Framework* in the light of the introduction of a new requirement in the Building (Scotland) Act 2003 that the regulations should support sustainable development. It included a review of regulations in other countries aimed at promoting sustainable construction.

Awards (raise awareness of issues)

Many awards aim to promote best practice in specific aspects of sustainable construction, but not in a systematic way. Recently, many civic and professional bodies and environmental agencies have been distributing awards for sustainability considerations in built development and in business operations. This includes attention to design quality and to the social, cultural and business benefits of design interventions and effective environmental management. They include a range of product, professional or business awards, such as VIBES for business practice, Eco-campus for environmental quality and Dynamic Places for design quality.

The UK government has launched an award to recognise projects and initiatives that contribute to making towns and cities better places in which to live and work as part of its sustainable communities initiative. The award 'aims to pay tribute to those people whose commitment and enthusiasm are making a significant contribution, through innovative schemes or ways of working, towards the building of thriving and successful communities'. It also showcases successes and highlights aspects of good practices that have been recognised throughout the assessment process.

Element	U-Value (W/m²K)
Walls	0.10
Roof	0.08
Floor	0.09
Windows	0.85
External doors	0.8
Airtightness = 0.4 air changes/hour at 50 Pascals	

Table 4.1 Swedish Body Heat Standard Specification

Range of tools

Tools exist for appraisal of materials, resources, products, places, occupant satisfaction, components, buildings, professions, processes, social factors, business performance, investment and more.

Issues covered include: energy use; water use; light quantity; emissions; land use; cost; speed; design quality; noise; waste; Volatile Organic Compounds (VOCs); embodied energy; embodied toxicity; quality of place; quality of life; professional competence; indoor air quality; biodiversity; transport; business impact and more.

Case Study 4.2:

Award: Grove Street Primary School, Green Building

Hounslow, London. Architects: Plinke Leaman and Browning, 1993

Sound reduction was the main task faced by the Max Fordham partnership at the school, which is directly under the flight path of London's Heathrow airport. An imaginative low-technology solution was required to restrict noise penetration and provide ventilation without opening windows. The solution involved the redesign of the roof, a standard construction of tiles, sarking and plasterboard. The insulation quilt in the roof void acted as a sound absorber, and the sarking felt and plasterboard were doubled to improve the performance. The floor was a standard concrete construction incorporating a ventilated cavity, but this cavity was used in a novel way, installing flaps in the floor to permit teachers to regulate fresh air intake without opening windows. The school was 1993 Green Building of the Year.

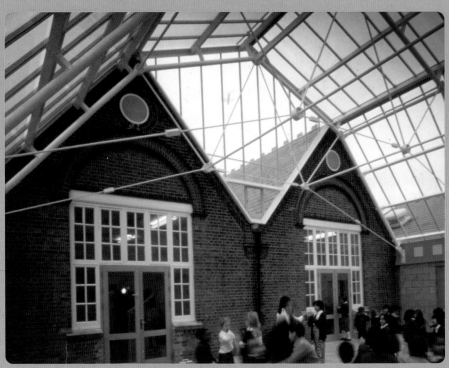

Photo credit: Paddy Boyle (paddy.boyle@tiscali.co.uk); photo permission: Plinke Leaman Browning

Checklists (highlight actions)

These are the simplest way for specifiers to adopt better practice for sustainable construction and there has been a proliferation of them. Examples include Communities Scotland's *Sustainable Design Guide* and many local authorities have followed the *Agenda 21* model and developed checklists including 'green' purchasing strategies to influence building procurement. The *CIRIA Environmental Handbooks* for building and civil engineering are perhaps the most comprehensive of this type of guidance. Checklists are a simple and valuable way to introduce and highlight important and actionable issues, but they are limited because they have no integrating aspect and provide no targets.

Labels and certification (traceable performance standards)

These come in many forms, from a range of product labels for products and services (covering energy efficiency, noise, water consumption, etc.) to labels such as BREEAM, EcoHomes or GreenCalc for whole buildings. The Civil Engineering

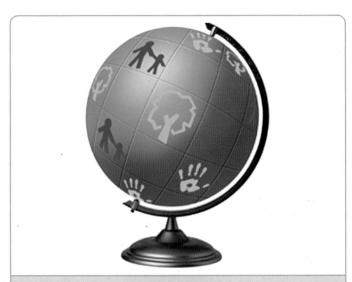

Product labelling
The number of product labels is increasing to cover goods, services and, in this case, ethical investment

Environmental Quality Assessment & Award Scheme (CEEQUAL) is increasingly used for civil engineering projects and the Considerate Constructors Scheme for construction activity. Schemes also exist for materials (Bau-Biology, FSC, Green Guide to Specification).

The recently launched professional evidence-based accreditation scheme for architects in Scotland is the first in the world to acknowledge the practical achievements of designers. These are particularly useful for clients and design teams who recognise that regulatory standards are inadequate and seek to develop significantly better practice.

Benchmarking (enables comparison)

Establishing and measuring performance in relation to agreed indicators allows projects, products and processes to be compared. Examples include the Construction Best Practice Programme Initiative aimed at improving the overall performance of the construction industry using Key Performance Indicators (KPI), and Design Quality Indicators (DQI) and Quality in Design of Schools (QIDS). Benchmarking is, however, consensus based and makes no attempt to establish absolute targets. It cannot be relied upon to promote the necessary or even best possible improvements. PROBE is an example of an initiative that uses other benchmarked performance data in its assessments.

Critical path tools (promote awareness of the process)

These are intended to offer clients, designers and specifiers a means of controlling their design process to improve control, minimise adverse environmental impact and overcome decision paralysis. Examples include the *Environmental Code of Practice for Buildings and Their Services*, the CIBSE log book, the *Green Guide to the Architect's Job Book*, the Sustainable Neighbourhood Audit Technique and the ISO 14 000 Environmental Management Series.

Targeting tools (absolute standards)

These use standards based on the best available science at any time, which changes as information improves. They include life-cycle analysis (LCA) tools such as NABERS, ENVEST, pollution targets and some government indicators. They are increasingly used to set development guidelines in flagship projects aiming to exceed poor regulatory standards. The required development is dynamic modelling to predict behaviour and thereby establish real limits against which to set targets (cf. *Limits to Growth* in the 1970s and 1990s). These would be a vital step forward. Software simulation packages for buildings in their environments are still primitive. Factors 4 and 10 are useful targets, though not based on real limits.

Case Study 4.3:

Checklist: Quality Indicators in the Design of Schools (QIDS)

QIDS was launched in Scotland in November 2002 as a tool for defining and evaluating quality issues in school buildings. It is still at a formative stage and is undergoing a process of testing and feedback by interested parties. Design proposals can be assessed either graphically, using a technique such as spider diagrams, or numerically.

The tool has evolved in response to concerns that design quality has had less attention than legal and financial aspects of the government's Public–Private Partnership (PPP) initiative. It is acknowledged that assessing what are often subjective criteria presents problems and calls for some flexibility.

QIDS attempts to supplement traditional specifications with quality issues and to involve a wide range of stakeholders in defining the aspirations of a new facility in order to engender community ownership. QIDS promotes the appointment of a project advisor with an understanding of the design of schools and the PPP process. The advisor's role is to assist with the compilation of the brief, design vision and business case. They also assist in the preparation of output specifications, assessment of competing proposals and provide advice during the detailed development of design proposals by the successful bidder. The advisor should also prepare feedback for future use.

Design factors are covered under seven headings. However, the intention is that these are looked at holistically, reflecting all relevant social, functional, aesthetic and built performance factors:

1 Uses and spaces
2 Character and form
3 Access
4 Internal environment
5 External environment
6 Social integration, sustainability and ecology
7 Engineered systems and performance.

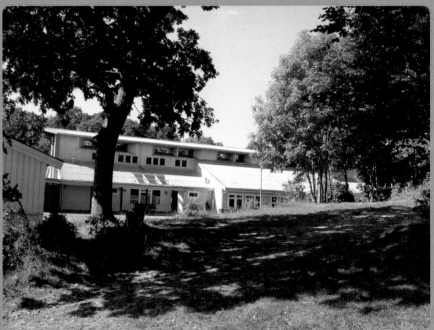

Vanse School, Norway. Architects Gaia Lista; photo Dag Roalkvan

Labels and certification

Certification and labelling is interesting because it provides an objective evaluation of a product's or a process's or a professional's environmental impact. A number of labels and certification systems are described below.

There are schemes available to appraise a wide range of consumer products: from clothes, paints, white goods and food, to construction products, processes and whole buildings.

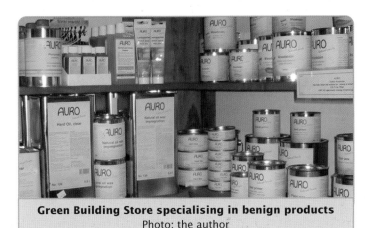

Green Building Store specialising in benign products
Photo: the author

Materials and products

An EU Eco-label scheme was introduced to allow comparability of products on a Pan-European basis, but has made slow progress. Uptake in the construction industry has been particularly slow, with only a few product areas such as paints, varnishes and hard-floor coverings gaining voluntary EU Eco-label status. More well-established national standards, such as the German (circa 1979) and Nordic (circa 1989) eco-labels, cover a much greater range of products. The former currently covers over 3800 products and services and involves 710 companies.

Relatively successful schemes are running for energy efficiency standards in white goods (the European Energy Label) and for sustainable timber procurement (Forest Stewardship Council) and recently UKWAS (The UK Woodland Assurance Standard).

The Green Building Press have developed *GreenPro*, a guide which evaluates products under six categories of impact.

DEFRA has published a *Green Claims Code* and *A Shoppers Guide* for consumers to provide guidance and overcome the tendency for vague and unsubstantiated claims.

Build elements

The Building Research Establishment (BRE) have produced *The Green Guide to Housing Specification*, which adopts benchmark targets of environmental impact for a variety of construction elements such as windows, doors and walls. The guide uses a simple category of A, B or C ratings established by consensus.

It should be treated with some caution, as categories have been disputed in some instances and the predominance of 'A' ratings indicates that there is little discrimination; it includes few examples of really best practice. There are design solutions that are significantly better in every way to any of those considered but they remain unassessed. The emphasis on design solutions, rather than products, is important. The latter generally have proponents to support their appraisal.

The guide does not 'blacklist' despite known adverse impact and even forthcoming legislation, but they do present arguments for avoiding certain materials. In particular, there has been criticism that manufacturing industry has played a defining role in the analysis and has compromised the independence of the assessments. Certainly, it has not evidently pushed UK practice forward.

The vast majority of products and materials used by those specialising in sustainable construction in the UK are manufactured overseas, and either carry recognised labels or are vetted by specialist importers or membership organisations.

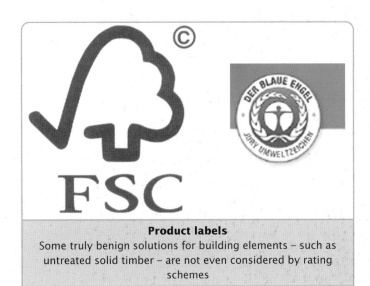

Product labels
Some truly benign solutions for building elements – such as untreated solid timber – are not even considered by rating schemes

Buildings

As with all environmental/sustainability labelling schemes, those for buildings are in a phase of rapid expansion with many countries developing their own national schemes and a number of research organisations attempting to develop overarching schemes. The Building Research Establishment's Environmental Method (BREEAM) in the UK and elsewhere Leadership in Energy and Environmental Design (LEED), The National Australian Building Environmental Rating Scheme (NABERS) and The Green Building Challenge have had limited success in raising standards, although some of these are now increasingly being integrated in client and government procurement strategies.

It is important to realise that any scheme to label a building can only be part of an overall process. They are a very good mechanism for encouraging design teams, particularly those unfamiliar with the issues of sustainable design, to focus on a client aspiration. However, they tend to reward the measurable and they are not sensitive to context so, inevitably, some design teams and clients will feel themselves unjustly penalised.

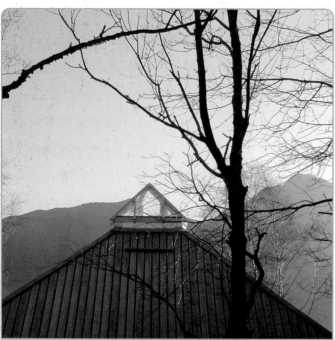

Untreated solid timber roof – Glencoe Visitor Centre. Despite excellent environmental credentials it does not comply with the materials credits of BREEAM which are based on a limited pallette

(Architects: Gaia Architects, photo: Michael Wolshover)

BREEAM – BRE Environmental Assessment Method

The building appraisals series BREEAM was originally developed as a tool to stimulate market demand for 'green' buildings. It provides a label for buildings that can be applied at design and refurbishment stages, or for existing buildings in operation. It has spawned a number of schemes for building types such as offices, supermarkets, housing, hospitals and schools. They offer bespoke appraisals for other building types such as laboratories and libraries.

Assessment covers a range of issues, encompassing the impacts of buildings on the environment at global, regional, local and indoor levels:

- Environmental impacts, leading to protection and perhaps enhancement of the environment by reducing pollution of air, land and water.
- Prudent use of natural resources by: proving durable buildings able to survive changes of fashion and use; selection of materials and products with better environmental performance; encouraging appropriate recycling; encouraging the reuse of buildings; encouraging the reuse of land, water economy, etc.
- Quality of life, with competitive business providing high-quality built environments, buildings and indoor environments to satisfy human and business needs.

BREEAM is building-type specific and outside the existing family of tools it is possible to have a bespoke assessment. Credits are awarded in each area and weightings enable the credits to be combined into a single overall score – of pass, good, very good or excellent.

It is not an absolute standard or completely objective as performance targets and weightings are derived from consensus between the building community, including manufacturers. It also gives low priority to community issues. However, it has shown itself able to respond to criticism and has evolved considerably since its inception in the late 1980s to become a very valuable tool for clients and design team unjustly penalised.

Case Study 4.4:

Label: Osberton Top Bridge refurbishment – CEEQUAL

Chesterfield, Construction: Galliford Try, 2003

This was a joint project between British Waterways and Galliford Try Construction through the BW North East Omnibus contract. The project involved the reconstruction of a redbrick arched accommodation bridge that was in very poor condition. It was not deemed viable to strengthen the bridge and therefore it was demolished and replaced with a similar structure that would complement the local character of the Chesterfield Canal. It was one of the eight projects undertaken during the first trial year of CEEQUAL and was awarded 'Very Good'.

The new structure was built using bricks, selected to match the existing bridges with a similar arch profile, although incorporating additional air draft for user safety. Hydraulic lime mortar was used to construct the arch to allow free drainage and thermal expansion/ contraction of the arch, and then saddled to provide the necessary strength.

Recycled stone steps and copings were obtained and original springing blocks that contained historically important wear marks, resulting from the ropes used by horse-drawn boats, were reused within the new structure.

During construction of the bridge, which lies within a County Wildlife Site, disturbance to surrounding trees and hedgerows was minimised by having a compact site compound.

The hedgerow adjacent to the site was enhanced with locally occurring species after the construction phase. An advance survey had shown that the original structure was used by a protected species, the Daubenton's bat. Following consultation with English Nature and DEFRA, a new roosting habitat was incorporated within the rebuilt structure.

Adjacent to the bridge, eroded canal banks were reinstated and wildlife habitats created using a type of soft bank protection, coir rolls, planted with locally sourced riparian plants (see www.ceequal.co.uk).

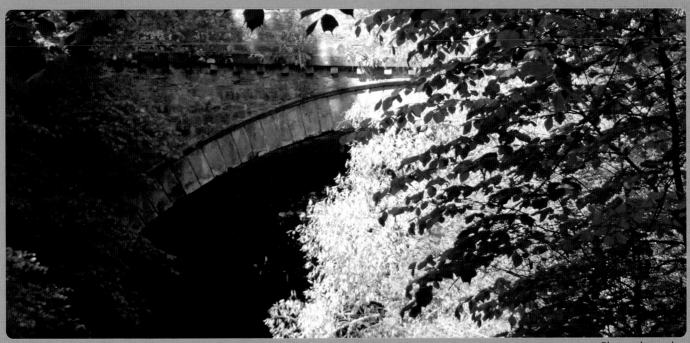

Photo: the author

Process

There are currently two notable certification schemes used to manage the sustainability aspects of the construction process, considerate constructors and CEEQUAL.

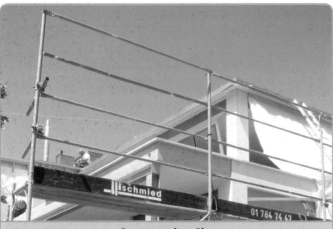

Construction Site
Site activity is increasingly subject to voluntary and mandatory controls such as CEEQUAL and Considerate Constructors
(Photo: the author)

Considerate Constructors' Scheme

Considerate Constructors is a voluntary Code of Practice open to all construction companies; it seeks to:

- minimise the disturbance or negative impact (noise, dirt and inconvenience) sometimes caused by construction sites to the immediate neighbourhood
- eradicate offensive behaviour and language from construction sites
- recognise and reward a contractor's commitment to raise standards of site management, safety and environmental awareness beyond statutory duties.

The Civil Engineering Environmental Quality Assessment Scheme (CEEQUAL)

CEEQUAL aims to encourage the attainment of environmental excellence in civil engineering projects. It specifically sought to overcome some of the weaknesses of schemes such as BREEAM by evolving a system that was respectful of context. CEEQUAL focuses on the processes that enable delivery of best practice and is robust enough to deal with projects of long timescale, making it worthy of consideration for regeneration and other large projects.

Professional practice

Whilst there are numerous checklists, policies and incentives to encourage sustainability within professional bodies there is little by way of third party appraisal. The RIAS Accreditation Scheme for Sustainable Design is an exception.

The RIAS launched an accreditation scheme in sustainable building design in 2005. It allows architects to advance through classes of environmental design, based on demonstration of practical experience. A precedent had been set by the Conservation Architects accreditation scheme operated by the RIAS.

The initiative is timely and in line with the priorities of government, many building clients and all of the major professional institutions. It is hoped that it will be attractive to clients who objectives and for designers providing added motivation for raising the priority of sustainable design on a job-by-job basis. It is peer assessed, making it a professional qualification rather than an academic one, and firmly rooted in practical achievement. It is proving attractive to those applying principles of sustainable construction who wish to demonstrate their skills, and to those who recognise the requirement to develop these skills over time.

Four classes of accreditation (A–D) are designed to allow designers to get onto the first rung of the ladder and to advance over time. Advancement relies on dealing with increased complexity of building design through scale, technical integration, development of interdisciplinary professional skills, and integration of the economic and social factors essential to sustainable construction. Innovation in any class is acknowledged by a star rating.

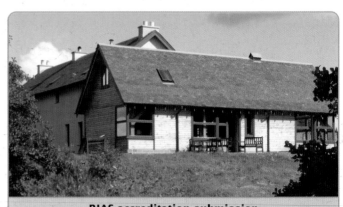

RIAS accreditation submission
Branshogle, Perthshire
(Architects: Simpson & Brown, Photo: Simpson & Brown)

Case Study 4.5:

Award: Colorado Court – Habitat

Santa Monica, California. Architects: Pugh + Scarpa, 2000

Colorado Court is a demonstration building featuring a gas-powered CHP system. It incorporates energy-efficient measures to exceed standard practice, including: passive strategies beginning with locating and orienting the building to optimise the solar and ventilation microclimate; shaping the building to induce buoyancy for natural ventilation; designing windows to maximise daylighting; shading south-facing windows and minimising west-facing glazing; designing windows to maximise natural ventilation; shaping and planning the interior to enhance daylight and natural air flow distribution.

Colorado Court features a gas-powered CHP system that generates the base electrical load and hot water demands for the building, Solar PV panels integrated into the façade and roof of the building supply most of the peak load electricity demand.

Unused solar electricity is delivered to the grid during the daytime and retrieved from the grid at night as needed.

Colorado Court has won many awards and was finalist in the 2003 World Habitat Award alongside Gaia's Fairfield project in Perth.

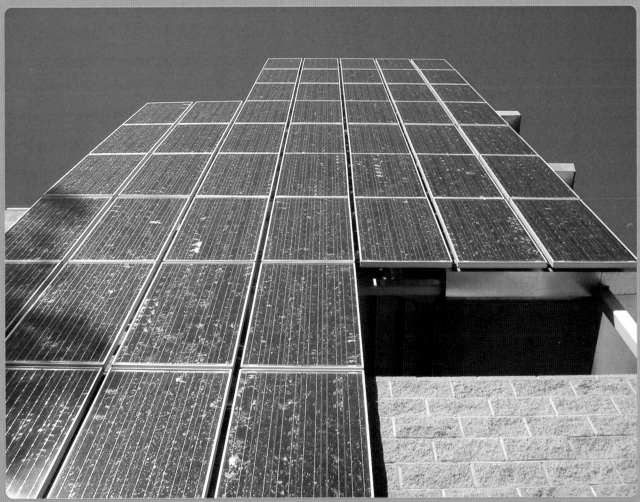

Photo: Pugh and Scarpa

Benchmarking

A benchmark is a reference point to objectively appraise relative achievement and is more indicative of performance than a simple score. Two aspects of benchmarking are described to indicate how benchmarking can be used across a range of issues.

> ### Client satisfaction
> If a construction client rated their overall satisfaction with a project at 6 out of 10, those involved might be reasonably content; unless information gathered from the industry indicated that over 85% of projects provided greater client satisfaction

Key Performance Indicators (KPIs) – rethinking construction

A principal element in the DTI's campaign to improve the performance of the construction sector is the publication of Key Performance Indicators (KPIs). They were introduced to enable firms to benchmark themselves against the rest of the sector in traditional aspects of business performance, cost, time, safety, profitability, etc. and to target improvements. All the major sectors publish annual wall charts of performance. Separate KPIs have been produced for housing, food retail, non-food retail, hospitals, offices and schools. The DTI recently turned its attention to environmental performance and new KPIs cover energy and water use, embodied energy, construction waste and impact on biodiversity. Transport indicators are being developed. Unfortunately, there are as yet no indicators for health or toxicity.

Further information on participating in the KPI process, benchmark curves for the indicators and news of regional workshop events is available from www.kpizone.com.

Design quality

Quality of design is extremely difficult to assess but has been receiving increasing analytical attention with the disturbing tendency for increasing dominance of non-designers at the leading edge of building procurement. The Design Quality Indicator (DQI)

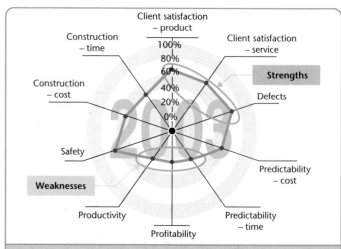

> ### Strengths and Weaknesses
> The KPIs could also serve as a useful tool for client organisations wanting to measure and benchmark performance in existing premises

was launched as a web-based tool in September 2003 following a year-long pilot scheme with 100 participating organisations. It focuses on assessing and measuring the value of a completed building and acts as a comparator and indicator, by allowing comparison of results on the basis of three main headings:

1. Build quality – relates to the engineering performance of a building. This includes structural stability and the integration and robustness of the systems, finishes and fittings.

2. Functionality – concerned with the arrangement, quality and inter-relationship of space and the way in which the building has been designed to be used.

3. Impact – refers to the building's ability to create a sense of place, and to have a positive effect on the local community and environment. The impact of the materials used, together with the character and innovation of the design, is also a consideration.

The technique is being moved forward in some sectors to cover specific build types. In Scotland a tool called QIDS (Quality Indicators in the Design of Schools) is being applied to schools.

Case Study 4.6:

Benchmark: Wessex Water – ENVEST

Bath. Architects: Bennetts Associates, 2000

Wessex Water are a waste and water company based in the south-west of England. When they set about building a new office building for their 500 staff, they were keen that it reflected their commitment to sustainability and energy conservation. The resulting 10 000 m² building comprises office space, a café and meeting/ training rooms. It is naturally ventilated with energy-efficient lighting, solar hot water heating and rainwater harvesting for non-potable uses. It achieved an excellent rating through BREEAM.

Bennetts Associates also worked with ENVEST to generate LCA data that would enable them to compare options for materials and specifications based on their potential environmental impacts over the life of the building.

Designers input their building designs (height, number of storeys, window area, etc.) and choices of elements (wall, roof covering, etc.). ENVEST then draws on environmental impact data to identify those elements with the most adverse impact and the effects of selecting different materials. It also predicts the impact of heating and cooling strategies and building operation. It considers climate change, ozone depletion, minerals and water extraction, pollution to water, air and land, waste disposal and toxic impacts on humans.

ENVEST assessment results in a single score of environmental impact measured in eco-points: 100 eco-points are equal to the impact of one UK citizen for one year. 1 eco-point is equivalent to any one of the following:

- 320 kWh of electricity
- 1000 baths or 83 m³ of water
- travelling 65 miles by truck
- landfilling 1.3 tonnes of waste
- manufacturing 250 bricks
- moving 540 tonne-kms by sea
- 1.4 tonnes of mineral extraction.

ENVEST results are presented as a single composite rating, which allows clients and designers to compare different designs and specifications directly and to determine those elements of the building that had the most adverse impact on the environmental performance.

This means that they can focus on interventions that generate the greatest benefits. Comparison of the floor and ceiling finishes highlighted the significantly higher impact of the former and a range of alternative options were considered, leading them to select one with a high recycled content. Results are provided in impacts/m² of building gross floor area. A typical building having no consideration for environmental impact would be expected to score approximately 40 points/m². It is possible to compare results from buildings.

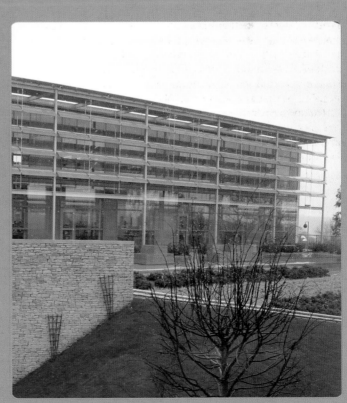

Photo: Bill Bordass, William Bordass Associates

Critical path tools

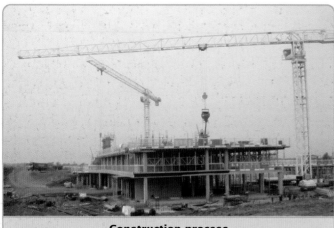

Construction process
The Green Guide to the Architect's Job Book has been used by Gaia Research to guide the development of the Queen Margaret University Campus in East Lothian (Photo: Carillion)

Insufficient attention is normally given to the problems associated with the design, construction and handover process. Yet it is well known that it is from scheme design onwards that sustainability objectives are particularly vulnerable. Tender strategies, cost cutting, and building management and operation have the potential to undermine a project's aspirations and it is important that sustainability is maintained high on the agenda throughout if the benchmark objectives are to be achieved. An increasing number of guidance documents have begun to address this aspect of sustainability and are designed to provide realtime guidance as the project progresses. The requirements are wide-ranging, but amongst the tasks are:

* preparation of tender documentation to respect sustainability objectives
* establishing controls within the routine of the site and building operations
* maintaining records compatible with sustainability objectives
* training in sustainability and unusual elements of the design
* assessing changes to minimise adverse impacts on sustainability
* ensuring that good records are maintained to assist in the process of handover
* training and involvement of users and operation/maintenance staff.

Amongst the available critical path tools are the *Green Guide to the Architect's Job Book*, the *Environmental Code of Practice* and the CIBSE *Building Log Book Toolkit*.

The *Green Guide* and the *Code of Practice* outline the critical steps required to ensure the right approach to the design of the built environment. These are primarily aimed at architects and engineers respectively. They attempt to ensure the process of sustainable design is correctly followed through by all involved. They do not attempt to evaluate sustainable construction per se, but provide a 'route' rather than 'rules'. Building log books are the latest addition to critical path guidance. Part L of the *English and Welsh Building Regulations* includes requirements for log books in new and refurbished buildings, and when major items such as boilers are upgraded/replaced. These are intended to bring together the design and facilities management communities to set down in simple terms how a building is meant to work, and provide somewhere to log performance and maintenance. They are seen as an essential tool to promote more energy-efficient operation through improved understanding, management and operation, resulting in more sustainable buildings with lower running costs. Building occupants also stand to benefit as the provision of information will contribute to enhanced occupant comfort, satisfaction and productivity. The log book should be an easily accessible focal point of current information for all those working in the building.

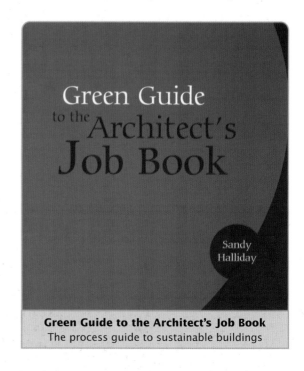

Green Guide to the Architect's Job Book
The process guide to sustainable buildings

Case Study 4.7:

Critical path: Regeneration Study – SNAP

Paisley. Gaia Planning, 2000

In the course of moving community architectural projects in peripheral housing estates towards the aims and objectives of *Agenda 21* – both before and since its formal adoption in 1992 – the Gaia Group have been developing methodological tools to support their work.

One empirical technique, devised during the Paisley regeneration process and subsequently developed in other projects, may have a significant role to play in the construction of sustainable communities.

The sustainable development tool aims to assist communities to participate in the process of sustainable community development, and to enable designers and other professionals to develop a more holistic approach to the development of sustainable communities.

Sustainable construction is taken to include social and economic criteria as equivalents alongside physical interventions. Without this context the built environment cannot be delivered with a guarantee of sustainability.

Summary

Relevant issues originate from both the global context (top down) and the local situation (bottom up).

Local issues are identified through community workshops, and placed on the matrix under Work, Folk and Place headings.

Global issues are defined under three key headings, each subdivided into general headings:

- *Community (Folk) issues* – social equity, amenity, health and safety, and nutrition and fitness
- *Economic (Work) issues* – employment, local economy, affordability, and waste and recycling

- *Environmental (Place) issues* – global pollution, local pollution, biodiversity/ecology and resources.

Proposals for action – identified as the means of resolving both the global and the community requirements – are placed centremost.

These constitute the interventions which would be a step towards sustainable community development.

The framework provides a mechanism for then identifying appropriate resources and importantly for monitoring improvement.

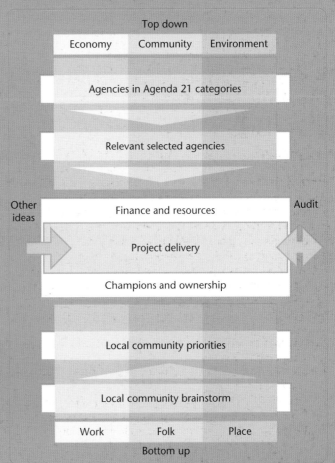

Targeting tools

The strength and value of targeting tools is that they set quantifiable standards based on some known measure, which may be existing building regulations of, more radically and more relevantly, an ecological footprint.

Flagship projects

One of the most significant recent advances in the field of appraisal tools is the development of localised performance standards that go beyond mandatory requirements. A number of regional authorities and clients throughout Europe are establishing new minimum requirements that are intended to be appended to building regulations on specific – often large – projects, and by precedent and inference then set a new 'flagship' standard. The Netherlands has a family of national packages in which various sustainable building measures are proposed and these form the basis of negotiated agreements between client and contractor. Other flagship projects in Finland, Sweden and Germany have been established and monitored.

The indicators are intended to be cross-cutting and there is no specific indicator in relation to sustainable construction, although a number can be potentially related to it. A key dilemma in determining appropriate indicators is the difficulty in sourcing real data on impacts and limitations. On a global basis, there are now hundreds of sets of indicators for sustainable development and with the number continually growing, attempts to harmonise them are increasing. There are plans to harmonise the indicators across the UK.

The UK website includes links to all relevant publications and reference to key international initiatives and organisations, and the most up-to-date information on the headline indicators. You can access the data behind the indicator, the regional version and technical details. The objective, relevance and background to each indicator are also outlined, along with key references and an assessment of progress for each indicator in relation to the objectives.

Viikki – Plan
The development of an eco-suburb on the ouskirts of Helsinki

Sustainability indicators

The UK and devolved administrations have each defined sets of indicators with specific targets to measure progress towards sustainable development. They are comparable to the accepted economic indicators that are used to monitor how the economy is performing.

They are intended to inform policy decisions and to contribute to understanding the consequences of action by individuals and business. They cover social, economic and environmental issues.

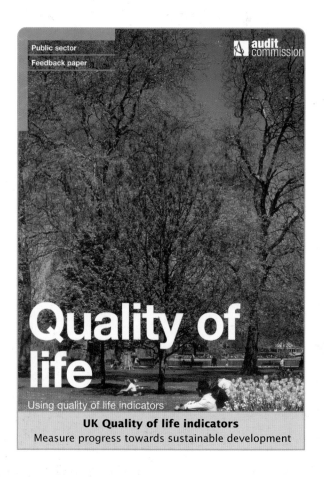

UK Quality of life indicators
Measure progress towards sustainable development

Case Study 4.8:

Targeting tools: Government office – GreenCalc

Haarlem, The Netherlands, 2001

NIBE Consulting in the Netherlands to assess and compare the 'environmental sustainability' of buildings. It is divided into four modules: materials, energy, water usage and transport.

- The *materials module* calculates the environmental impact (including the total embodied CO_2) of materials during the lifetime of the building (including maintenance). Products, elements and whole buildings are evaluated as comprehensively as possible using quantitative data obtained from LCA studies or qualitative information taken from international literature. It is subdivided into raw materials, pollution, waste, nuisance, ecological effect, energy, reusability, reparability and lifespan.
- The *energy module* calculates the consumption during the lifetime of the building and consists of building use, heating, ventilation and hot water demand, lighting, use of renewables, etc. These parameters are the base for the so called EPC value, the regulatory norm, which is being reduced in successive reviews (see Sustainable Development and the Regulatory Framework at www.gaiagroup.org).
- The *water module* calculates the water consumption during the lifetime of the building, including drinking water or the substitution by 'grey water'.
- The *transport module* calculates the mobility-related hidden environmental costs associated with commuting during the building's life. The location of the building is considered in relation to infrastructure, connections and distance to public transportation.

The environmental impact is translated into costs per m^2 for the total life cycle of the building (construction, use and demolition).

The government office in Haarlem received a total index of 245, making it a factor of 2.45 more sustainable than a reference building from 1990.

Buildings such as the DTO Mecanoo building have been the subject of visioning design studies for construction by 2040 and have been assessed at a factor 14.5 more sustainable than the reference.

Recent buildings are achieving more than 400.

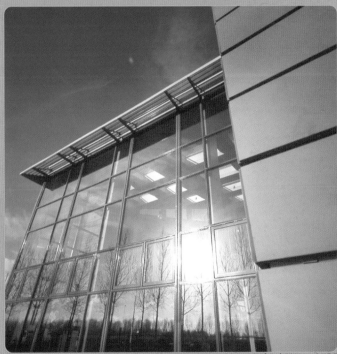

Photo permission: Michiel Haas, NIBE

Case Study 4.9:

Targeting tools: Eco-suburb – PIMWAG

Viikki, Helsinki. Late 1990s

Since 1931 there has been a small teaching and research facility at Viikki, 8 km from the centre of Helsinki and 20 minutes from the airport. In the late 1990s, a decision was made to construct a new city district in the area in such a way as to retain the existing rural landscape. It was also felt that, in keeping with the trend for increased environmental responsibility, the development should be undertaken with these considerations at the core. The intention was that the area should develop a population of 18 000 by 2025, with an additional 6000 employees at the science park and a similar number of students.

Along with considerations that might be expected to be undertaken in a project of this scale, minimum performance standards were defined to allow proposals to be assessed against specific ecological criteria. The requirements were intended to serve as a guide for design and implementation, and to be appended to building regulations on all city-owned sites such that all designs meet the minimum requirements. The criteria cover pollution, natural resources, health, diversity and food production. The system (called PIMWAG, an acronym of the authors' names) recognised that capital cost implications, estimated at 5%, are not intended to be onerous. The criteria were intended to save on running costs over the project's life.

Minimum standards were set that improved significantly on the current building standard – defined by a conventional apartment in the district of Helsinki. Additional points accumulated for improvements on the base level, with 10 of 30 possible additional points considered excellent and 20 requiring excellent innovation.

- *Pollution* – building less, more efficiently (energy use and traffic), durable and recyclable structures.
- *Natural resources* – better or less building, renewable resources and recyclable materials.
- *Health* – favourable microclimate and healthy conditions inside, local control, banning materials known or thought to be toxic, external comfort, healthy and comfortable internal space.
- *Natural diversity* – leave as large a part as possible unbuilt, high density, access for animals, diverse planting.
- *Food production* – resident allotments and use of topsoil.

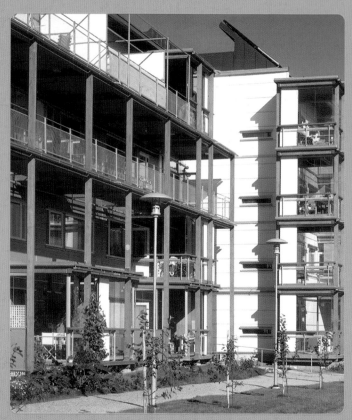

Photo: Chris Butters

Factor X

The expression 'factor X' is used to describe the efficiency with which we use environmental resources. GreenCalc takes a figure of factor 20 – based on a calculation by the American ecologist Barry Commoner – as the requirement for our resource use by the year 2040, taking the base year as 1990. In other words, the environmental impact per unit of product or service must be 20 times lower. Factor 20 therefore corresponds to an environmental index of 20 x 100 = 2000.

The current environmental index of most projects is between 100 and 200. Leading projects achieve 250 and a few exceptions are higher. On the basis of linear growth from 1990 to 2040, we should by now be at an environmental index of around 500.

Practical experience has shown that the environmental gains from technical measures, such as using environmentally friendly materials and renewable energy, are limited. At constant accommodation costs, these measures do not bring the environmental index above about 200. After that the costs rise rapidly. If we are prepared to pay the additional costs, an environmental index of around 500 is what can be achieved by utilising all technical options. A different approach is therefore needed in order to achieve factor 20 (environmental index of 2000).

In order to achieve factor 20, the scope of the exercise has to be extended from the design phase – where the technical measures come into play – to the initiative phase of a project, and in particular to the concept that underlies the design. We can reduce the need for new construction – and consequently the environmental impact – by gearing the concept to intensive and protracted use of a building, such as the introduction of hot desking and the multi-functional use of space. Reusing existing buildings is a step in this direction.

The replacement of the conventional forms of accommodation through these new concepts requires constructive dialogue between all the parties involved at the beginning of the project in order to ensure that the concept is commercially feasible and at the same time has a high environmental index.

Ecological space (e-space) and ecological footprints

The concept of e-space was developed in 1992. It estimates the space claimed by an average citizen in any given country based on the global resources they consume in a year. From this, limits to per capita resource use have been developed based on an equitable and sustainable distribution of global resources between countries. The model can be used to calculate the global share of construction resources and energy use on a per capita basis for comparison with the actual distribution and setting targets for reduction.

The 'ecological footprint' – developed in 1994 – is the area of productive land needed to meet the consumption of a single person and to absorb the waste produced. In 1996, the average North American needed 10–12 acres of productive land to support his or her lifestyle, whereas an average citizen from a developing country only needed about 2 acres. The world average is 5.2 acres. It would take four planets the size of the earth to enable the whole population to enjoy an American lifestyle. It is possible to estimate the ecological footprint of an entire population or economy to calculate the amount for an individual building or person.

Bibliography

Indicators, regulation and policy

DETR (1998) *Sustainability Counts* (www.sustainable-development.gov.uk/indicators).

Audit Commission (2002) *Quality of Life* (www.audit-commission.gov.uk/pis/quality-of-lifeindicators.html).

ODPM (2002) *Annual UK Performance Measured in Relation to Quality of Life Indicators* (www.dti.gov.uk/energy/inform).

Morse, S. (2004) *Indices and Indicators in Development – An Unhealthy Obsession with Numbers.* Earthscan.

Movement for Innovation – www.m4i.org.uk

Checklists

CIRIA (2000) *Environmental Handbook*: Vol. 1, *Design and Specification*; Vol. 2, *Construction*.

Stevenson, F. and Williams, N. (2000) *Sustainable Housing Design Guide for Scotland.* Stationery Office. Labels and certification.

Labels and certification

Anderson J. and Shiers D. (2004) *The Green Guide to Specification* Blackwell Publishing

Department for Communities and Local Government (2006) *Code for Sustainable Homes* www.planningportal.gov.uk/uploads/code_for_sust_homes.pdf

BREEAM – www.bre.co.uk

EcoHomes – www.breeam.co.uk/ecohomes

FSC – www.fsc.org

GreenPro – www.newbuilder.co.uk

LEED – www.usgbc.org/LEED/

NABERS – www.nabers.com.au

RIAS Sustainable Design Accreditation Scheme – http://rias.mmidev.co.uk/content/default.asp?page=s3_9

UKWAS – www.ukwas.org.uk

Benchmarks

CIRIA (2003) W005, *Biodiversity Indicators for Construction Projects.* CIRIA Design Quality Indicators (www.DQI.org.uk e-mail: dqi@cic.org.uk).

DTI (2005) *A Complete Housing KPI Toolkit.* CBPP.

DTI (2005) *Construction Industry Key Performance Indicators.* CBPP.

Quality in the Deisgn of Schools (QIDS) – www.rias.org.uk.

Critical path tools

Halliday, S. P. (1994) *Environmental Code of Practice for Buildings and their Services.* BSRIA.

Gaia Architects (2002) *Sustainable Neighbourhood Audit Process* – www.gaiagroup.org.

BRE, GPG 348 (2003) *Building Log Books.* BRE.

Halliday, S. P. (2007) *Green Guide to the Architect's Job Book.* RIBA Publications.

CIBSE Log Book – info@cibse.org or www.cibse.org

Targeting tools

Meadows, D. et al. (1972). *The Limits to Growth.* Signet.

von Weizacher, E. and Lovins, A. L. (1997) *Factor 4 – Doubling Wealth and Halving Resources.* Earthscan.

Ecological Footprints – www.myfootprint.org; www.redefiningprogress.org; www.ecouncil.ac.cr

ENVEST info and Benchmarking Club – envest@bre.co.uk or 01923 664380

Factor 4 – www.rmi.org; www.wuperinst.org/factor4

Factor 10 – www.factor10-institute.org

NABERS – www.deh.gov.au

NIBE – www.nibe.nl

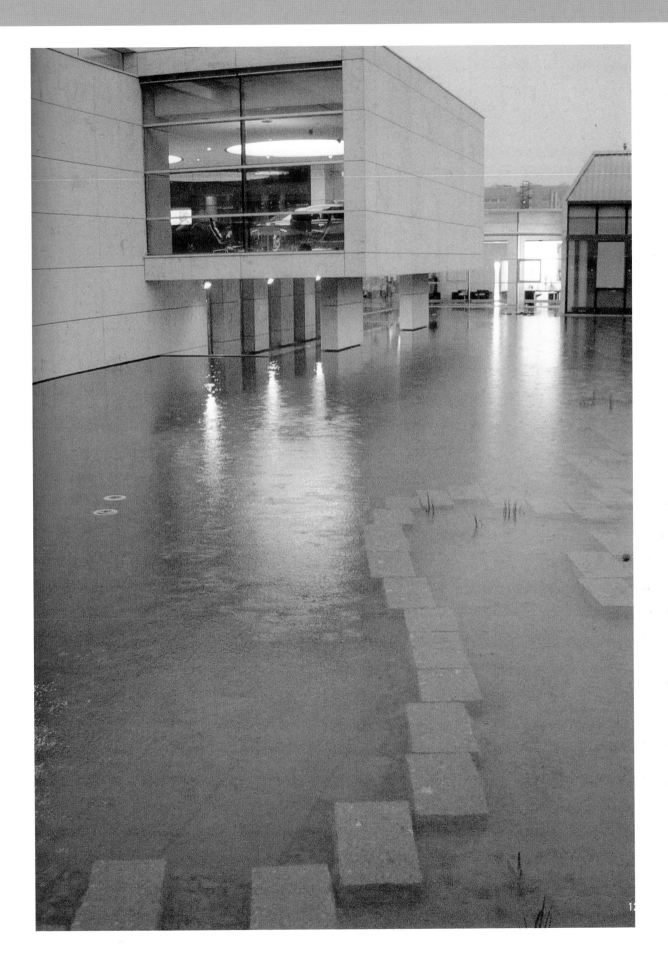

Chapter 5
Materials selection

In which we seek to give the reader a sound and broad grasp of the issues and priorities affecting materials selection in the design of sustainable places, buildings, services and objects and a realistic perspective on the range of issues, including their invisible qualities, which should affect decision-making.

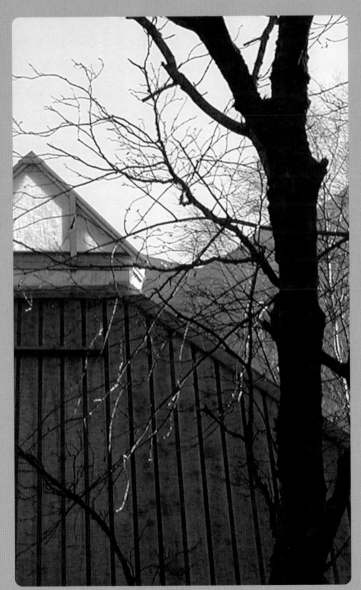

'Hygroscopic building materials are 9 times more effective than mechanical ventilation in controlling indoor relative humidity'

VTT Espoo Finland

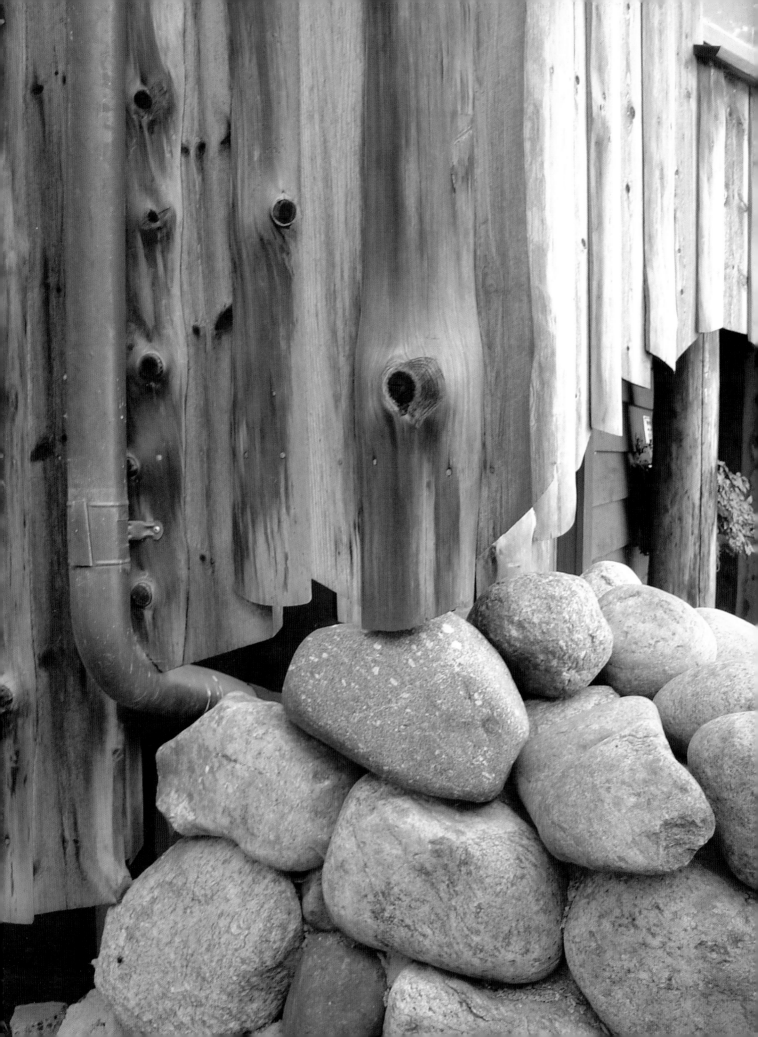

Contents

(Facing page)
Andersen House
The moisture from the building is vented behind this sacrificial timber layer (Architects: Dag Roalkvam and Rolf Jacobsen; photo: Dag Roalkvam

(Previous page)
Solid timber roof at Glencoe visitor centre
(Photo: Michael Wolshover; photo permission: Gaia Architects)

Materials selection

Introduction

Ecological building design is characterised by the use of natural materials with a minimum of processing and transportation; and an emphasis on healthy, non-toxic specification to minimise pollution. Ideally materials should also contribute to passive forms of environmental control.

Many attempts have been made to create a coordinated and comprehensive analysis tool for materials in the construction industry that can enable those specifiers, who are minded to do so, to make objective decisions about material selection. Many of these take a life cycle approach. A number of the techniques are helpful, and there is ongoing improvement as information evolves, but none are comprehensive. Nor are they ever likely to be so.

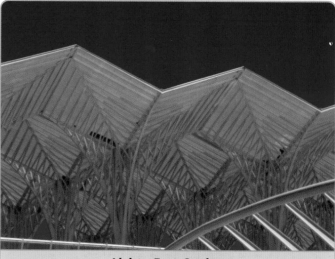

Lisbon Expo Station
Materials selection does not exclude any architectural style
(Architect: Santiago Calatrava; Photo: the author)

In part this is because of the complexity of the issues but also because the 'sustainability' of most materials owes much to the sourcing and handling, the way in which they are used, and the care that goes into their detailing and maintenance. This cannot as yet be completely covered by any analytical process that is reliant on being uniformly applicable.

A contributory factor is doubtless to do with the relationship between products and design, and the opportunities for added value. There is still widespread ignorance about how to use materials in their natural state and many manufacturers prefer to avoid scrutiny.

The most valuable approach in most circumstances is to be cogniscent of the issues and have access to up-to-date guidance. It will generally be necessary to compare options and relative impacts in a particular circumstance. These issues therefore remain within the realm of compromise and judgement, a realm familiar to designers. However it extends the territory such that distance, manufacture, human rights, biodiversity and pollution might all be part of a balanced judgment. Importantly this should not be restrictive on design, if thought about intelligently, but should open up new creative opportunities. For example thinking about the future of a rare or energy intensive material is as important as looking at its past

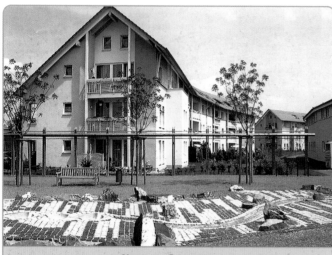

Kamen, Germany
Housing development, part of Emscher Park regeneration designed using 100% eco-labelled materials
(Architect: Joachim Eble Architects; Photo: Howard Liddell)

The life cycle approach

The main questions to ask of a material specification choice are:

1 *What is the Resource Base?* – Where is it from and how much is left?
2 *What is the Embodied Pollution?* – What has been done to it and by whom? – There is often an ethical component.
3 *What is its Impact in Use?* – What effects does it have on people and the wider environment?
4 *What is its Final Destination?* – What will happen to it at the end of its life?

In general it will not be practical, or possible, to arrive at definitive answers to all or any of these considerations. Nor is it feasible for most specifiers to assess each and every component against each and every consideration. In the face of such limitations, more important is a genuine commitment to achieving the best result. A basic knowledge of the issues and opportunities can readily lead to sensible assessments and substitutions. Conversely, a basic disregard for good sense, pollution and ethics undermines the serious advances that are possible. Ultimately, the assessment is made by the environment.

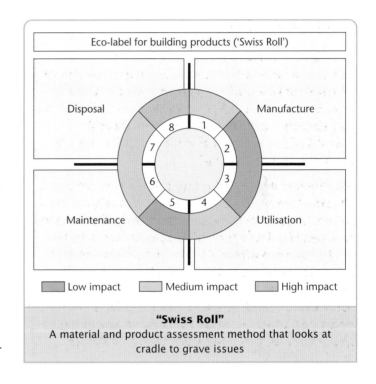

Eco-label for building products ('Swiss Roll')

Disposal · Manufacture · Maintenance · Utilisation

8 1 2 3 4 5 6 7

Low impact · Medium impact · High impact

"Swiss Roll"
A material and product assessment method that looks at cradle to grave issues

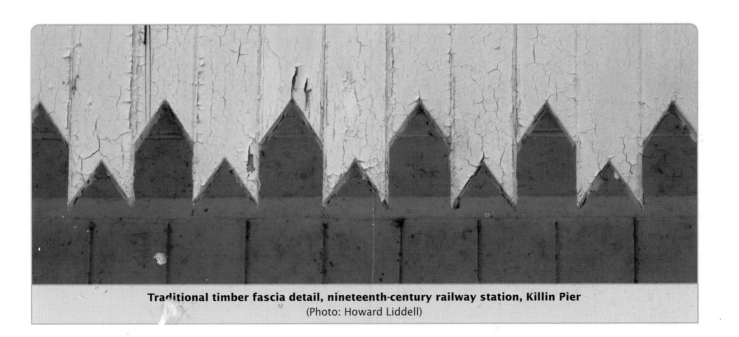

Traditional timber fascia detail, nineteenth-century railway station, Killin Pier
(Photo: Howard Liddell)

Resource base

Certain resources are becoming extremely rare and the use of remaining stocks should be treated cautiously, especially where they are known to support threatened habitats or where there are known to be uses that should take precedence.

Most rare materials used in construction can be substituted by other, less rare or renewable materials. However, there are few absolutes. These guidelines have to be taken within the context of what is appropriate and possible.

- Renewable materials should take precedence over non-renewable ones.
- Reused or recycled materials or components should take precedence over equivalent 'virgin' elements.
- Sourcing of materials from areas that are particularly fragile – in respect of their aesthetic, community or ecology should be avoided.
- Materials with significant reserves remaining should be used in preference to those with smaller reserves.
- Materials should be used as efficiently as possible and allow for their eventual reuse or recovery – especially where using a material with minimal reserves.

Many metals commonly used in the construction industry have extremely limited estimated reserves. World Resource Institute estimates suggest that we may have only a further 10–12 years supply of lead and zinc. This compares poorly with an estimated 210-year supply of bauxite – the main source of aluminium, which would be a good substitute in most circumstances. Also, recycling of aluminium is extremely well developed.

Most plastics derive from the world's oil reserves. The use of recycled plastic components makes environmental sense, except

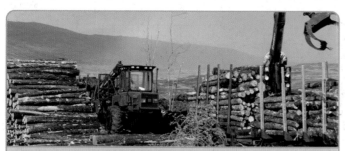

Materials selection, timber
Timber from a local source, used in an untreated form and detailed for long life, is a good choice. However, if brought huge distances, treated with polluting materials such as CCA and poorly detailed, it is not (Photo: Howard Liddell)

where recycling contributes to additional and avoidable pollution. However, many recycled materials remain more expensive than 'virgin' equivalents and meeting appropriate building standards may require pre-planning, which should be allowed for.

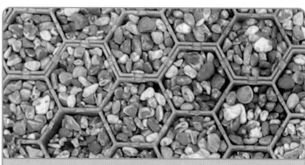

Embodied Toxicity
Plastic is being recycled into a range of useful components, such as this 'squidgy tarmac', but we have to be careful about embodied toxicity (Photo: the author)

Embodied pollution – what has been done to it and by whom?

Huge damage is done to the local and global environment and to the health of workers and others through the extraction, production and distribution that make up the construction industry supply chain. Some manufacturers are involved in ethically questionable practices, whilst others have explicit and forward thinking policies on environmental and social issues and may be willing to provide good information on their impacts, and strategies. It is up to the specifier to determine the relevance and priorities. It is notable that purchaser power is increasingly responsible for changes in government policy and that increasing numbers of companies are developing guidelines to address their responsibilities.

All materials contain embodied energy, which is a form of embodied pollution, but many conventional building materials also contain additional elements, as a consequence of chemical processing, which are known to be toxic to humans and or wildlife.

This includes concrete, PVC, MDF, most glues, paints and finishes. This "embodied pollution" can impact throughout the product life; on employees in the manufacturing process, to building occupants through off-gassing or leaching in use and eventual pollution through recycling or disposal.

Case Study 5.1:

Timber College, Lyss

Architects: Itten and Brechbuhl, 1998

This forest training centre in Switzerland was visited in 2005 by a group of Scottish and Scandinavian building designers interested in new developments in wood construction.

The building, occupied in 1998, is owned by a foundation from 11 cantons. It was originally intended to be a concrete construction but, with the timber industry in decline, the director insisted on a timber construction.

The primary construction comprises 300 silver fir columns with steel consoles. The floor construction comprises suspended MDF acoustic ceilings below rough pine roundpole and cheap tiles made of recycled materials. All the furniture is red heartwood beech. In total, about 2000 m³ of timber was used, equivalent to 1.7 hours Swiss forest growth. It is heated from a wet wood biomass boiler using in total 650 m³/annum.

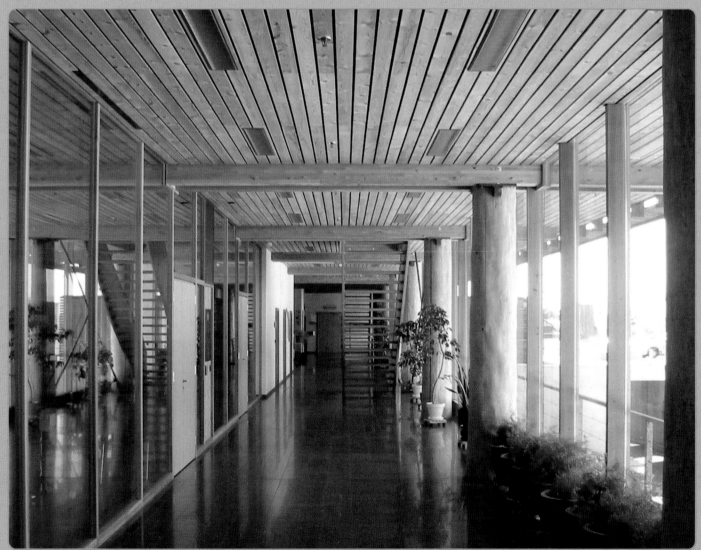

Photo: the author

Case Study 5.2:

Prisma mixed development, Nuremberg

Architects: Joachim Eble Architects, 1997

Despite being in the centre of a German city and having to comply with stringent building control and fire regulations, this nine-storey mixed development manages to achieve a very high standard of specification in terms of environmentally sound materials – notably the finishes. Where possible, floors are of mass timber to form an equivalent to concrete beam and block flooring. Concrete is used only where absolutely necessary. Timber finishes are used throughout, and the paint and other surface treatments are all low or zero emission.

This is probably the world's largest complex that can be defined as an ecological design project. The ground floor is a shopping precinct, the next three floors are offices and the top floors are residential.

The inner courtyard offers a secure environment for a kindergarten, which serves the on-site housing. All the commercial properties get their preconditioned ventilation from the large solar atrium.

Passive solar and natural ventilation strategies utilise water flows and planting in atrium spaces. The water strategy is based on catching, conserving and recycling on site.

This scheme sought to use as many recycled or reclaimed materials as possible, sourced within budget and time constraints. The aluminium roof has the potential to be reused as a high value material in perpetuity but there may be energy penalties.

The housing scheme comprises a three-storey block of flats, a row of houses and cottage flats. The block of flats face south and the L-shaped plan forms a semi-private enclosed garden and children's play area.

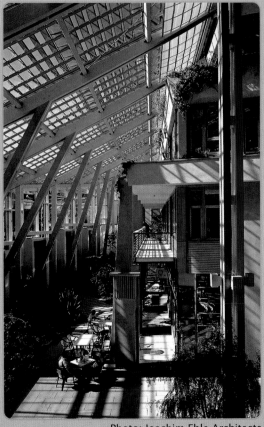

Photo: Joachim Eble Architects

Extraction

We need to be aware of the effects from pollution that extraction/mining/harvesting will have on the immediate natural habitat, the flora and fauna, landscape character, pollution of ground and surface water and reduced water table, and any particular cultural or environmental features of note. Also be aware of what effect site workings may have on the health and wellbeing of workers on site. There may also be implications for the local population in terms of noise, dust, local transport problems, disruption or nuisance generally.

Certain extraction processes are inherently efficient in resource use, whereas others are extremely inefficient and lead to significant waste. The primary energy used in some extraction processes is extremely high, whereas others use almost none at all. This figure is part of the overall 'embodied energy' of a particular material.

Attention to waste has led to development of new manufacturing opportunities, based on waste and offcuts, and also to improvements in technology. There is often considerable scope for designing out waste. Reconstituted slate and fibreboards are examples of new products from waste. The use of a waste product in manufacturing is clearly environmentally advantageous but should be considered in totality. Recent improvements in stone-cutting technology, for example, are both less polluting and hugely more efficient in turning 'raw' rock into useful product, whilst the opportunities for specifying less polluting and recycled products have increased enormously.

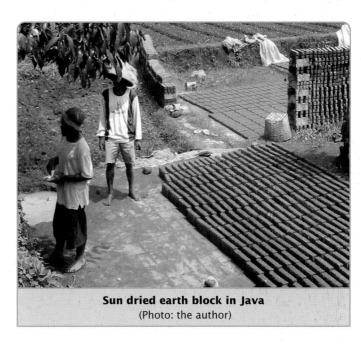

Sun dried earth block in Java
(Photo: the author)

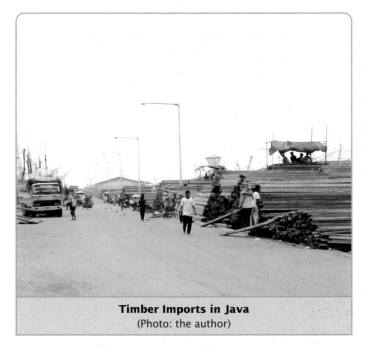

Timber Imports in Java
(Photo: the author)

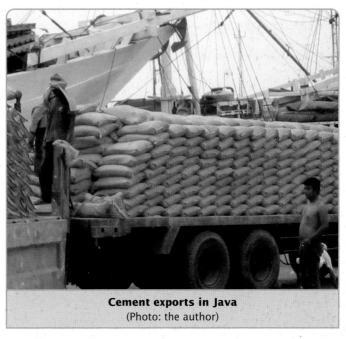

Cement exports in Java
(Photo: the author)

Processing and production

Pollution also results from the process or processes of producing a material or product. These can adversely affect the immediate and the wider environment. Pollution may be airborne – via chimneys, for example, or waterborne – via watercourses, due to seepage from buried waste for example. Highly processed components are generally to be avoided where a lesser processed product can fulfil the same function.

Many industries have poor credentials when viewed in terms of worker health and safety. Some existing practices deserving better precautions remain acceptable and this is particularly so in developing countries when the most disadvantaged might be exploited. It is often best to look at those forms of production that are inherently least hazardous.

There may be great economic benefits from local manufacture and less mystery in terms of the impacts. Labour intensive operations are favoured by some specifiers but situations should be considered on their merits. Recent proposals to shift the burden of taxation onto resource consumption, and away from taxing people, are to be welcomed but it may be some time before these are implemented.

The energy used in manufacture alone renders some materials unacceptable to certain specifiers. However producers are not ignorant of the opportunities for savings and minds have been focussed by the increasing cost and by taxation of fossil fuel energy. Highly energy intensive aluminium production is located to exploit hydropower and several British brick manufacturers use a proportion of bio-gas in firing their bricks. The issues are rarely straightforward. Finally, whilst many of the worst practices have been outlawed in developed countries, this is not the case in some developing countries where labour costs are also cheaper, and can be a contributory reason for avoiding imported materials.

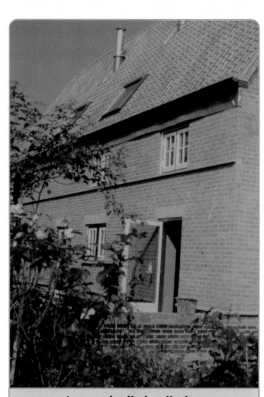

Low embodied pollution
At the Autonomous House in Southwell the selected bricks were fired from landfill gas (Architects: Robert and Brenda Vale; photo: the author)

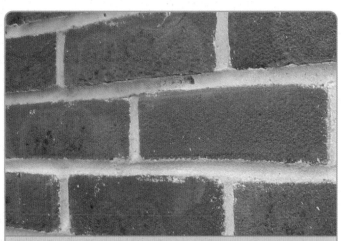

High embodied pollution
The embodied energy of these fired bricks compares poorly with the autonomous house, where bricks fired from landfill gas were used and with ARC Architects house at Dalguise, Perthshire which used earth blocks
(Photo: the author)

Assessing impacts of even one material is extremely complex. It has been calculated that it takes approximately 75 times more energy to import softwood than using local air dried sources. In terms of embodied energy by volume, local timber is one of the very best options, while imported timber is one of the worst materials. The situation is compounded when countries then import energy intensive and polluting materials locally.

Case Study 5.3:

Linacre College, Oxford

Architects: ECD Architects, 1995

The main ambition for this project was to use materials that required little processing. Low embodied energy was an integral part of a general low-energy strategy. The specification also includes recycled materials (roof tiles, copper piping and hardcore), natural finishes, organic paints, timber from traceable sustainable sources and no ozone-depleting insulants. The building was also one of the first to investigate the aspect of forestry planting and CO_2 trading.

The building was framed in a context of low CO_2 emissions and had a number of passive design features, including the use of passive controls. Heat recovery and grey water usage were included. This project achieved Green Building of the Year status and was an early example of a high-scoring BREEAM building. The materials side was less ambitious than many later projects, but green for its time in the UK and very thorough in its approach to selection.

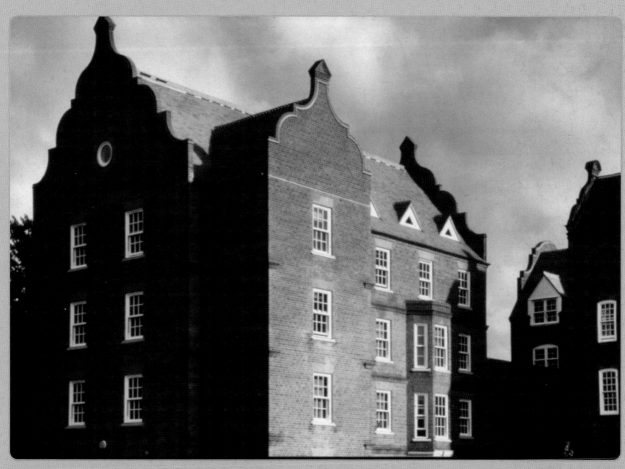

Photo: the author

Waste

Certain manufacturing processes, such as paint production, are hugely inefficient in resource use and produce considerable amounts of waste, which is both toxic and has little or no further use. In contrast, processes such as the production of earth blocks has almost no associated waste, and any that there is can be readily returned to the site without damage to natural habitats. Sometimes by-products can be used as input to other processes and reduce the overall waste associated with a process.

Recycling

A number of production processes incorporate the use of either recyclate (e.g. glass) or the waste from other processes (e.g. the use of gypsum from coal-fired power stations in plasterboard). Whilst there may be a number of concerns regarding reprocessing some of these materials, an overall reduction in resource use results.

Transportation

In many cases, there are considerable transport requirements between the site of extraction and the site of processing/ production. For some composites there will be a corresponding accumulation in 'transport miles' and the consequent embodied energy and pollution.

Distribution

Transportation of products from processing plants, to further processing plants in the case of composite elements, to holding yards, to wholesalers or regional distribution centres, to Builders' Merchants and finally to site can contribute in excess of 50% of the overall embodied energy of a particular element. It is generally high for imported materials. Smaller, regionally based plant and distribution, and more local sourcing, will generally improve the overall environmental burden of any particular material.

Packaging

A considerable amount of packaging material is used in the distribution of building materials, very little of which is biodegradable or can be safely burned. This represents a significant waste of resources. Whilst some materials need to be carefully protected in transit and others may be moisture sensitive etc., there is room for improvement in the overall materials flow. It is worthwhile requesting information from suppliers on packaging materials and overall environmental policies.

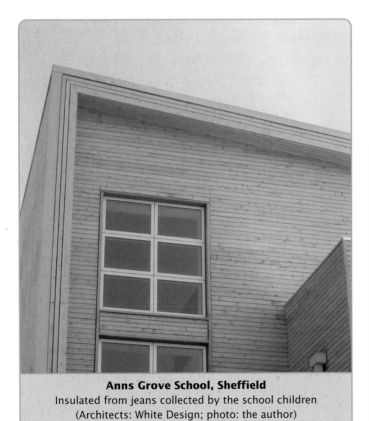

Anns Grove School, Sheffield
Insulated from jeans collected by the school children
(Architects: White Design; photo: the author)

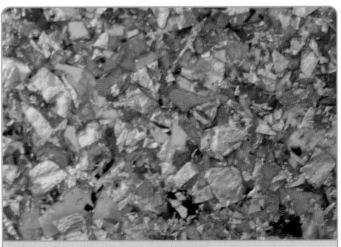

Recycling
Packaging can be recycled for a limited number of uses, like this school pinboard (photo: the author)

Impact in use

The aim is to minimise and, if possible, remove the harmful effects of materials on occupants and the environment through the life of a building. Beyond this, it is desirable to design the indoor climate to actively benefit the health of occupants.

Detailing

Timber framed windows, for example, are intrinsically more insulating than metal framed windows, but these advantages can be rendered meaningless if the frame to wall junction is detailed incorrectly. Timber will cope with a range of adverse climatic conditions provided it is properly detailed.

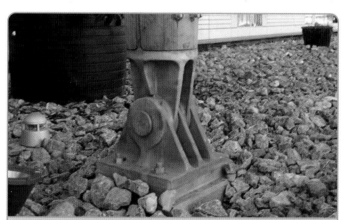

Timber detail Mont Cernis Akademie, Herne, Emscher Park
(Architects: Jourda Architects, Paris and HHS Planer + Architekten BDA, Kassel, Germany; photo: the author)

Proper detailing of appropriate timber obviates the need for treatments. Much of the justification for treatment of timber is based on a history of poor detailing that led to moisture sitting and giving rise to mould and rot. The use of inappropriate weather proofing materials – generally plastic paints – worked in opposition to the natural movement of wood in response to climate. Timber is resistant to climate as long as it does not stay wet. Alternatively, it is robust when used completely under water – as in Venice – and cannot get dry.

Toxicity

A wide range of commonly used products contain substances which adversely affect the health of occupants of a building. It is often the case that the extent and severity of the risks are contended, and the precautionary principle insufficiently invoked. Some substances that are banned in other countries remain freely available in the United Kingdom. Others known to be harmful are policed by health and safety initiatives such as the COSHH regulations.

Work undertaken by Fanger in Denmark brought about a sea change in the way that we look at the indoor environment. The biggest single source of pollutants was shown to be ventilation systems – this is covered in detail in a later chapter. At the time smoking was common indoors and was responsible for significant pollution, however that aside the second biggest source was from materials used in the indoor environment.

A concern often voiced is that product information relating to health hazards is usually derived from tests conducted on otherwise healthy people under laboratory conditions using only one substance. The affects on those potentially most vulnerable to such toxins, such as the elderly, children and the unborn are rarely considered. Also in reality, much of the risk to health comes from the unknown 'cocktail effect' of the many chemicals present in buildings and so information on health risks associated with isolated substances is insufficient.

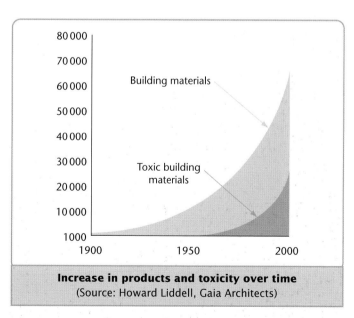

Increase in products and toxicity over time
(Source: Howard Liddell, Gaia Architects)

Building products that are considered harmful include:

- many forms of paint and varnish,
- formaldehyde in resin bonded boards, like plywood, chipboard and some foam products,
- vinyl products such as flooring tiles,
- most timber treatments.

Case Study 5.4:

Glencoe Visitor Centre, Glencoe, Argyll

Architects: Gaia Architects, 2001

This was built for the National Trust for Scotland as a replacement visitor centre with several associated works. The £3 m centre is primarily timber. All the timber was procured to a strict set of principles to ensure that its use represented genuine ecological best practice. The timber was:

- Sourced from Scotland only, with the relatively small embodied energy this would entail, and the associated economic benefits to both the timber industry and woodland viability. Completely untreated (this meant that durability was achieved by the careful choice of species and careful detailing based partly on Scandinavian best practice).
- Sourced from certifiably well-managed forests.
- Designed to be easily maintained, repaired and ultimately replaced and/or reused. This meant the development of careful layering detailing and a 'nail-free' construction system. With no chemical treatment of the timber nor synthetic coatings, it could also be safely

composted or burnt at the end of its intended life. It was designed to be as simple and user friendly as possible. The buildings are part of the interpretation strategy for the project and its environment. The style of a clachan of low-lying bothies and the slate and lime render finish that predominates on the entrance side of the building transforms into timber walls and roofs on the reverse (wooded) side. It is superinsulated and cellulose insulation is used with sheep's wool for detailing around windows where movement could occur.

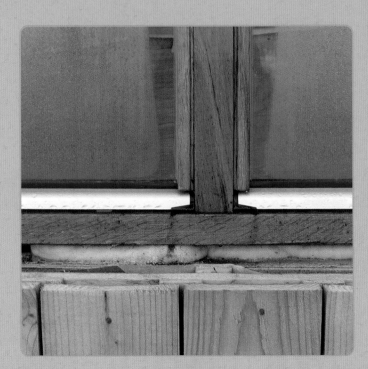

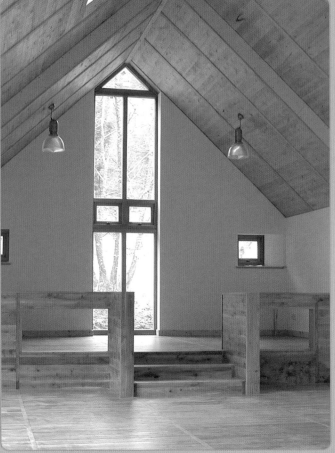

Photos: Gaia Architects

Passive environmental control

An important aspect of achieving comfort in buildings is attention to thermal and moisture mass.

Thermal mass

Sustainable design places an emphasis on maximising comfort and energy efficiency simultaneously and, in combination with appropriate ventilation requirements, preventing those conditions that are associated with ill-health. This can be aided by the appropriate, climate dependent, use of thermal mass. The thermal storage capacity of materials and the concept of thermal mass, are widely understood. Human beings sense temperature as a combination of air temperature, modified by the air velocity, and radiation from, or to, surrounding surfaces.

Heavyweight materials can be used in a building (earth is ideal) to regulate and balance the thermal fluctuations in a building and to avoid rapid swings in temperature. Creating warm surface temperatures allows for lower air temperatures, creating fresher environments and reduced ventilation heat loss. Avoiding cold surfaces, especially vertical surfaces, also avoids draughts. Warm surfaces also reduce the risk of surface condensation and mould.

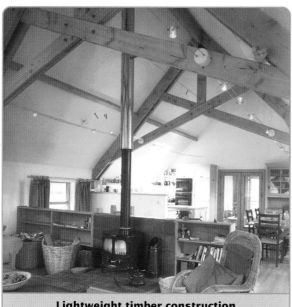

Lightweight timber construction
Ledliath, Culkein-Drumbeg, Sutherland
(Architects: Gaia Architects; photo: Howard Liddell)

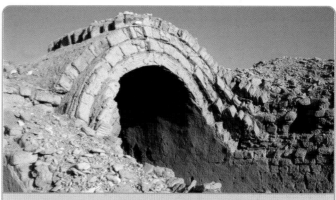

High thermal mass
The oscillation in outside temperature from day to night is buffered by the thermal mass of the earth construction to provide a comfortable internal temperature throughout 24 hours
(Photo: Howard Liddell)

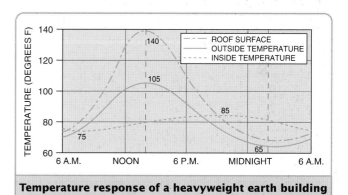

Temperature response of a heavyweight earth building

In contrast, heavyweight buildings take longer to heat up and cool down, but this 'thermal lag' can be designed to complement the occupancy patterns and can be usefully combined with passive solar design. In general heavy thermal mass is most appropriate for buildings that are occupied for long periods, and in particular where overheating is a problem.

Lightweight constructions tend to heat up quickly and cool down quickly, and are therefore ideal for quick response situations where heating is not needed all the time.

Hybrid structures exist where thermal mass is incorporated into an otherwise lightweight structure, such as a solid ground floor or central core. These buildings, if correctly designed, can possess the best characteristics of lightweight and heavyweight construction.

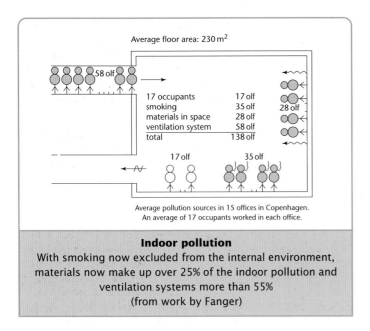

Average floor area: 230 m²

58 olf

17 occupants	17 olf
smoking	35 olf
materials in space	28 olf
ventilation system	58 olf
total	138 olf

28 olf

17 olf   35 olf

Average pollution sources in 15 offices in Copenhagen.
An average of 17 occupants worked in each office.

Indoor pollution
With smoking now excluded from the internal environment,
materials now make up over 25% of the indoor pollution and
ventilation systems more than 55%
(from work by Fanger)

Moisture mass

The indoor environment is dealt with in more detail in Chapter 10 but it is worthwhile to highlight the important link between materials and the indoor environment through the parallel concept of moisture mass.

Moisture mass works in a similar way but relies not on density, but on hygroscopicity. Hygroscopicity is the capacity of materials to absorb and re-emit ambient moisture vapour. This capacity enables certain materials to regulate the relative humidity in the indoor climate, by absorbing moisture when the humidity rises and emitting it when the air becomes dry, smoothing out peaks and troughs, in much the same way as thermal mass regulates temperature. As extremes of relative humidity are linked to a number of health problems, moisture mass performs a valuable function in health terms.

Moisture regulation reduces the potentially harmful developments of organisms and atmospheric conditions which occur at the extremes of relative humidity. Materials such as timber, plaster, earth and textiles have hygroscopic properties, but it is important that these are not impaired by inappropriate, impervious coatings, such as conventional varnishes, paints, stabilisers and others.

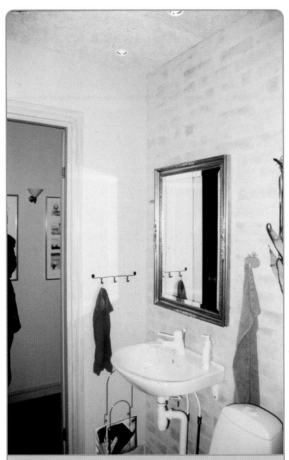

Hygroscopic mass
The effect of hygroscopicity was well demonstrated by the clay finish in this Swedish bathroom, which passively prevented the steaming up of the bathroom mirror. The same effect was achieved in a Japanese bathroom through a significantly more resource-intensive use of embedded electrical heaters. Gaia now use clay finishes in bathrooms as a standard detail in private and social housing projects
(Photo: the author)

Moisture transfusive construction

Another strategy for maintaining a balanced relative humidity – in addition to adequate ventilation – is the use of moisture transfusive, often mistakenly called 'breathing' external fabrics. They are more accurately 'sweating constructions' and the concept is most simply understood by comparison with the human body.

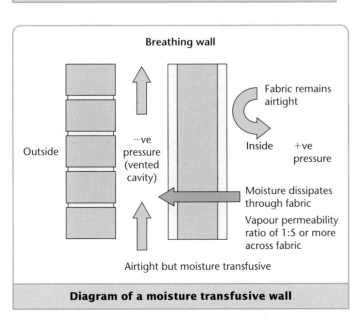

Moisture transfusive construction
An otherwise traditional school designed using moisture transfusive construction, a technique now increasingly common Brenzett, Romney Marsh, Kent, 2001 (Architects: Mouchel Property Services; photo: the author)

Without porous skins we would die. We are most comfortable in clothing that allows moisture to pass through it and the sportswear industry has developed fabrics to deal with this. Similarly from an ecological perspective the ability of a building to allow and encourage moisture to move from inside to outside using natural forces of vapour pressure gradient enables a significant reduction in mechanical systems.

These natural forces allow moisture to naturally and passively diffuse from the inside to the outside of a building in response to a vapour pressure gradient. This relies on the surfaces being left uncoated, or coated in vapour permeable finishes.

Local issues

The choice of building materials can be affected by a range of factors. The vernacular traditions of an area may affect what will be acceptable to local planning authorities or there may be a desire to enhance the 'sense of place' and local distinctiveness by the use of local and traditional materials whilst helping a new building to sit well with its neighbours. Certain regions maintain particular skills or crafts, often intimately connected with a particular local material, and this can form an important part of the heritage and ongoing culture of an area. A desire to support local skills can assist in determining the choice of materials.

An ecological approach would tend to encourage sourcing of local materials whilst recognising limits to scope, availability and the constraints on creativity and expression. It does not encourage pastiche!

Breathing wall

Outside

−ve pressure (vented cavity)

Inside   +ve pressure

Fabric remains airtight

Moisture dissipates through fabric

Vapour permeability ratio of 1:5 or more across fabric

Airtight but moisture transfusive

Diagram of a moisture transfusive wall

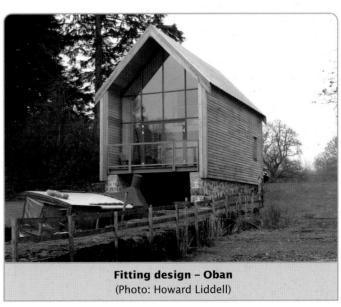

Fitting design – Oban
(Photo: Howard Liddell)

Case Study 5.5:

Edinvar Housing Association, Edinburgh

Architects: Gaia Architects, 2005

Refurbishment of a tenement block into low allergy, affordable flats.

All toxic materials and potential asthma and allergy triggers were removed and replaced with natural materials. Gaia first carried out a feasibility study for Edinvar Housing Association looking into the possibility of achieving a 'state-of-the-art' green refurbishment exploring the twin areas of refurbishment and ecological design, in particular with regard to listed buildings where planning constraints are onerous.

The refurbishment considers community aspects, with a communal sitting area and clothes washing facilities, amenity (particularly relevant for a building that provides no access to external

space), energy conservation, water conservation, healthy indoor climate, healthy materials and an approach to the construction process that deals with the logistics of building sustainably on a tight site.

Only benign materials have been used in the refurbishment that places its emphasis on the creation of a healthy indoor climate.

Materials with hygroscopic properties and breathing walls were specified in order to aid moisture management and combat moulds and mites. Specification and details were refined as required following the results of Gaia's research project into low allergen/trigger environments at Fairfield's Toll House Gardens.

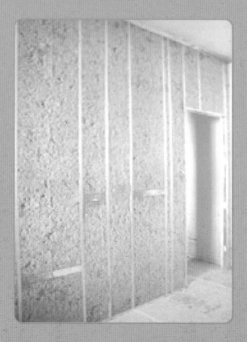

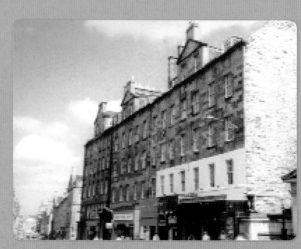

Photos: Gaia Architects

Final destination

The construction industry is the second largest consumer of raw materials, after the food industry. There is a considerable amount that could be done to reduce the consumption rate. In addition the majority of materials are highly processed with additives that are unstable and may present problems at the end of their useful life.

There is significant untapped potential to reduce the overall impact of materials by:

- innovation of new or traditional materials that are non-polluting at the end of their useful life;
- improved detailing such that materials do not require to be treated in such a way as to be difficult to deal with at the end of their useful life;
- increasing the inherent durability of buildings and components;
- reducing waste through improved design and construction processes;
- extending the useful life of materials by the re-use and recycling of materials and components.

To achieve this, a systematic approach to material specification and design is needed. The order of preference is: innovate, reduce, repair, re-use, recycle and lastly, energy recovery.

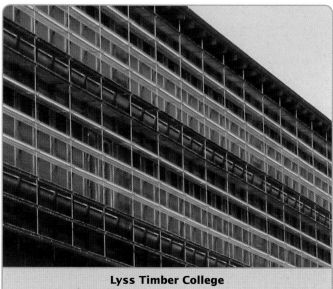

Lyss Timber College
Multi-storey timber construction (Photo: the author)

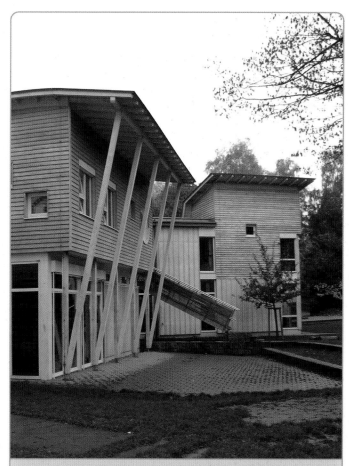

Pfennikäcker, near Tübingen, Germany
A modern ecological timber school with water-based paints that allow the wood to breathe (Architects: Joachim Eble Architects; photo: Ian Cameron)

Durability

It is important to look at the inherent durability, and the quality of a material, and to detail it so as to enhance the durability as far as possible. There is good information available on detailing to enhance durability, but materials and components have got to be worth reusing, and this places an emphasis on the specification of good quality materials in the first instance.

Maintenance

'Maintenance free' buildings are increasingly sought by clients anxious to minimise the running costs associated with built developments. This is not surprising given the backlog of poorly detailed and inappropriately managed buildings that resulted in a legacy of high maintenance.

A relevant example is poorly selected, detailed and inappropriately treated timber, which unfortunately gave a bad reputation in the 70s and 80s to an essentially benign material that is easily maintained if properly selected, detailed and treated, if at all, with moisture open finishes. This became a significant maintenance issue because remediation invariably involved a difficult process of paint removal using even more toxic substances and then re-application so that the cycle could begin and fail again.

Some designers have returned to designing with timber basing their detailing on traditional techniques from countries where timber use is the norm such as Norway.

Sadly timber itself has now become design rhetoric for those wanting to be seen to be delivering sustainable buildings and most of this is being undertaken without adequate selection, detailing and treatment experience. This is increasingly resulting in a return to the poor appearance and high maintenance that we have seen before and is highly likely to feed another inappropriate over-reaction against it.

It is vitally important that the industry recognises that planned maintenance is likely to be an essential pre-requisite of sustainability for most products and services. 'Maintenance free' often describes components that are simply 'non-maintainable' and need to be disposed of in total when one part fails. Common examples of this are uPVC joinery and cladding panels, as opposed to timber joinery elements and cladding boards. It is infinitely preferable to use the appropriate materials, components and treatments in such a way that they are easily maintainable and which, with a little attention, will tend to be much more durable (and cost effective) than their maintenance free counterparts.

Lifespans

A building can be viewed as a series of layers with different lifespans. The overall structure might be expected to last 100 years or more, the external skin 50 years, the internal partitioning 20 years, and elements of the services 10 years. Fit-out, decoration and equipment cycles are often less than 5 years.

Ideally a building could be conceived and detailed in a series of technically discreet 'layers' to reflect these lifespans. This would optimise the potential for maintainability and re-use, and avoid the risk of elements of the building being removed prematurely. The elements with shortest lifespan could be adjusted or replaced without unduly affecting more durable layers. This principle can also be usefully applied to areas of a building – internal or external – that suffer differential levels of wear and tear such that they can be maintained or replaced independently.

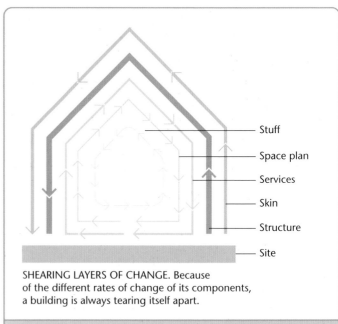

SHEARING LAYERS OF CHANGE. Because of the different rates of change of its components, a building is always tearing itself apart.

Building 'layers'; from *How Buildings Learn* (Brand 1994)
A building has to be designed to deal with the different rates of change of its component parts.

When no re-use or recycling is envisaged for a component, it is better to opt for organic, that is, biodegradable materials so that these can be re-absorbed into the earth by the natural cycle of decay, at the end of their useful life. It is very important to note that many coatings and preservatives transform otherwise 'natural' materials into toxic waste (e.g. most conventional preservative treated timber) that is no longer harmlessly biodegradable and must be disposed of by regulated means.

Choices – the 5 Rs

The options available to designers can be summarised as the 5 Rs: Refuse, Reduce, Re-use, Recycle, Repair.

Refusing represents the ultimate sanction – setting guidelines on what is and is not acceptable based on best possible information. It may involve declining unethical work or establishing and overseeing a policy. Examples include the Tübingen Policy referred to in Chapter 2 or the exclusion of uPVC for the Sydney Olympic Stadium.

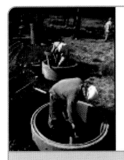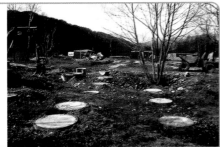

Spot foundations
At Glencoe the building was placed on spot or pad foundations rather than a massive concrete slab
(Architects: Gaia Architects; photos: Gaia Architects)

Architects, engineers and others in the construction industry will tend to consider solutions to problems in construction-related terms, but a building is not always the best solution to a perceived need. It is worth establishing the true nature of the requirement before embarking on a building related solution. Alternatives might include moving premises, reorganising internal arrangements, re-organising the client organisation (be it a company or a family) or re-addressing priorities – even something so mundane as a thorough tidy-up and clean. It may well be the most cost effective solution and the lowest impact of all. If building work is required, the lowest impact may be refurbishment, although this is not necessarily the cheapest option nor involve the least upheaval. Another aspect to bear in mind is to build as small as practicable to minimise adverse impact.

Reducing the amount of any resource: materials, space or elements, need not detract from a good design solution. Reducing the amount of mechanical services is increasingly a design aspiration.

Reuse of buildings and materials is a serious resource issue. It requires attention to flexibility, the opportunities for future extension or reduction and awareness of the different layers of a building and how they wear. Design for re-use involves consideration of the material and jointing technique so as to enable re-use and replacement of components, either in part or in whole. Components have to be worth reusing to enable a market for re-used goods to develop, and easy enough to re-use to make it profitable to do so. These considerations tend to favour modular construction. A good example is the use of lime mortar which enables bricks to be re-used, whereas cement mortar is often too hard and makes such re-use extremely difficult and not cost effective.

It is significantly easier to reclaim components when attention has been given to this at the design stage.

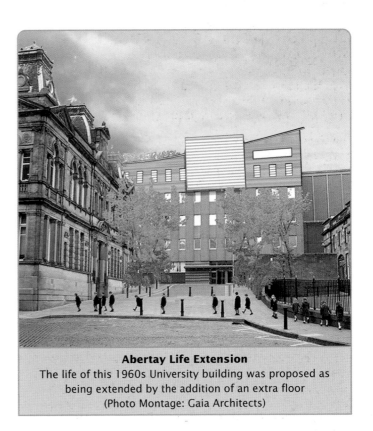

Abertay Life Extension
The life of this 1960s University building was proposed as being extended by the addition of an extra floor
(Photo Montage: Gaia Architects)

Recycle – Where the re-use of a component is not possible, it may be possible to recycle it in whole or parts. Glass, copper and zinc are examples of materials that are partly recycled, and paper is increasingly used as in insulation material, but there is huge scope to increase this. Building using recycled materials is a matter of much current attention. The government Wrap programme is setting voluntary guidelines on quantity by value.

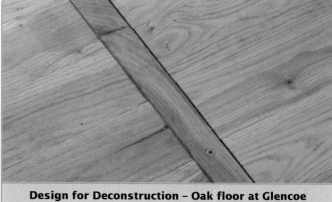

Design for Deconstruction – Oak floor at Glencoe
(Detail: Dag Roalkvam, Gaia Lista Photo: Michael Wolshover)

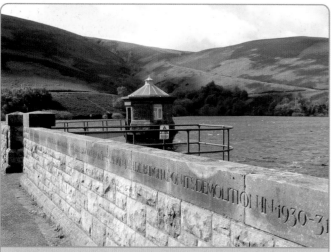

Care for valuable resources used to be commonplace
The message reads *"The arch of this bridge and the walls of the water course which it spans were brought from the Calton Jail Edinburgh upon its demolition in 1930-31"*
(Photo: The author)

Anything can be recycled, but the ease, value and toxicity issues are important. The potential for recycling is significantly reduced if components are inappropriately coated, or laminated or connected in some way that makes cost effective acquisition of any one material impossible. A ubiquitous example is the sandwich panel that is enamel or powder coated on both sides, with resin bonding of the metal sheeting to the insulation. This renders it practically impossible to recover those parts that could be recycled. Recycling can add embodied pollution and expense.

There are serious questions to be asked about the extent to which the construction industry should be prepared to take waste from other sectors – in particular polluting waste – and thereby allow the waste streams to continue unabated.

Repair – We have grown used to a culture in which we expect minimum maintenance of our habitat – buildings and gardens. In truth this is unrealistic and not just in the field of ecological design. However, a consequence of our expectation is reduced life of many components – which is wasteful – and the substitution of polluting materials such as PVC and timber treatments and coatings in place of regular care.

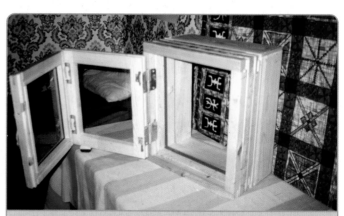

Timber-triple glazed window
When many multi-glazed windows (including those with gas fillings) were shown to leak after short periods of time, the architects at Gaia Lista designed their own cleanable and maintainable window – a sustainable alternative to uPVC
(Design: Gaia Lista; Photo: Howard Liddell)

Case Study 5.6:

Fairfield, Perth

Architects: Gaia Architects, 2003

The extent of eco-design specification of materials (and other principles) increased with each phase of development at Fairfield. This started in the late 1980s with attention to non-toxic timber treatment – both zero and borax treatment methods – to replace copper–chrome–arsenic (CCA). Later phases (mid-1990s) added moisture-transfusive wall construction with use of high levels of cellulose fibre insulation, timber flooring rather than chipboard, organic paints and finishes, and an encouragement for tenants not to use carpet or vinyl finishes. The single most important aspect of the project is that the 'green' specification elements were delivered within the Scottish Homes cost yardsticks.

It is often thought that ecological design is not a high priority for communities whose prime concern is to rid themselves of slum conditions. However, in this project the continuity of design and management teams over two decades has built up a trust and dialogue where the cooperative has been open and positive to such principles. The most significant aspect lies in the major social improvements, which are essential as part of the total picture of sustainability.

The extension of the aims at Fairfield to produce an allergy-free specification are discussed in relation to social costs and the environment in Chapter 3.

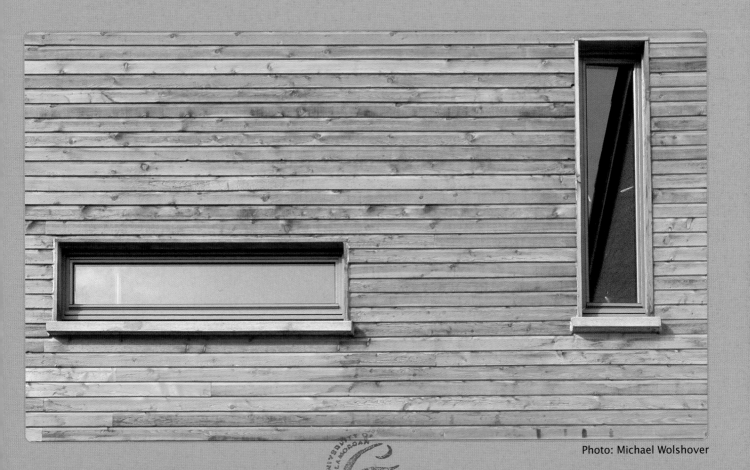

Photo: Michael Wolshover

Materials – handy hints and tips

Process

- Use the *Green Guide to the Architect's Job Book*.
- Materials selection needs to be approached in an interdisciplinary manner, in order to integrate the design of structure, services and landscape.
- Planning permission sometimes requires an early decision on materials selection.
- The form of a building will predetermine the materials choice.
- Use of recycled materials should be undertaken with consideration of any adverse health implications and should not encourage the built environment to become a depository for unsustainable practice by other industries.
- Design for flexibility, repair and deconstruction. It will need forward planning.
- The culture of clients requesting eco-products and services is less advanced in the United Kingdom than in mid-Europe and Scandinavia. Construction professionals need to take a lead.

Local Economics

- In most cases the use of local materials (timber, bricks, recycled materials) contributes to reduced embodied energy but will also benefit the local economy.
- It is worthwhile considering what sustainable materials are locally available – including recycled materials – and what skills, prior to starting to design.
- In some areas the benefits may lie in utilising locally available skills/trades and/or materials.

Health

- What does it say on the tin?
- Avoid materials that give off fumes. An increase in materials with toxic emissions – many of them above the levels recommended by the World Health Organisation – has followed the increase in man-made materials incorporated into buildings.

- The ability of materials to deal with indoor moisture is important – especially in the airtight constructions necessary to meet energy targets.
- Many manufacturers have sought to 're-market' unsound products rather than change them or mitigate negative properties. Seek third party approvals rather than advertising claims for a product's suitability to sustainable design.

Management

- Is it maintainable? We need to move to a culture of ongoing maintenance and maintenance free often means unmaintainable.
- Does the selection match user and management needs and requirements?
- Does the handover plan include for adequate training?
- Designers experienced in ecological design have found that 'green' materials need not cost more albeit specification inevitably requires more professional time to deal with innovative aspects, climb the learning curve and keep abreast of new information.

Affordability

- Does the materials choice minimise excessive financial liabilities through long life and low maintenance?
- Have you investigated the supply chain adequately to ensure that you are paying the right price without inappropriate add-ons due to specialist requirements?

Building Services

- Appropriate choice of (e.g. low emission) materials can reduce the ventilation and relative humidity regime in a building. This is an accepted trade off under the Norwegian building regulations.

Safety

- Can the installation be installed, cleaned and maintained easily and safely? This is increasingly a requirement of legislation.
- Have materials harmful to users and the environment been minimised?

Bibliography

Indispensable

Holdworth, W. and Sealey A. (1992) *Healthy Buildings.* Longman. Sadly out of print, but might be available from a library.

Brand, S. (1994) *How Buildings Learn.* Viking

Berge, B. (1999) *Ecology of Building Materials.* Architectural Press.

Gaia Group (2005) *Design and Construction of Sustainable Schools*, Vols 1 and 2. Scottish Executive. Free from Gaia.

Simonson, C. J., Salonvaara, M. and Ojanen, T. (2001) *Improving indoor climate and Comfort with wooden structures.* VTT Building Technology, Espoo.

GreenPro, the directory of what is available by way of products and services, is available at www.newbuilder.co.uk on subscription.

Guidance Notes on materials and products from Construction Resources at www.ecoconstruct.com.

Various Information sheets on materials and systems at www.cat.org.uk.

Informative

Fanger P.O. et al. (1990) *A simple method to determine the olf load in a building, Fifth International Conference on Indoor Quality and Climate (Indoor Air '90)*, Vol. 1, pp. 537–42.

Whitelegg, J. (1993) Transport for a Sustainable Future: The case for Europe. Belhaven.

Maxwell, I. and Ross, N. (1997) *Traditional Building Materials.* Historic Scotland.

David, A., Boonstra, C. and Mak, J. (1998) *Handbook of Sustainable Building: An Environmental Preference Method for Selection of Materials for Use in Construction and Refurbishment.* James & James.

Woolley, T. (1999) *Green Building Handbook*, Vols 1 and 2. E & F. N. Spon

BRE (2000) *Ecohomes.* The Environmental Rating for Homes.

CIRIA (2000) *Environmental Handbook*, Vol. 1. *Design and Specification.*

Pearson, D. (2000) *The Natural House Book*, Gaia Books.

For information on specific materials

Bramwell, M. (1976) *The International Book of Wood.* Mitchell Beazley.

Liddell, H., Kay, T. and Stevenson F. (1993) *Recycled Materials for Housing.* Scottish Homes.

Houben, H. and Guillaud, H. (1994) *Earth Construction.* Intermediate Technology.

Steen, A. S. W. and Bainbridge, D. (1994) *The Straw Bale House.* Chelsea Green.

Greenpeace (1996) *Building the Future: a Guide to Building without PVC.* Greenpeace.

Stungo, N. (1998) *The New Wood Architecture.* Laurence King.

Gaia Research (1999) *Roundpole* www.gaiagroup.org/roundpole.html and CD.

English Heritage – information on conservation limestone, and other materials at www.english-heritage.org.uk/.

Historic Scotland Technical Advisory Notes – various including lime and earth at www.historic-scotland.gov.uk.

Chapter 6
Low-impact construction

In which we look at evolving approaches to ecological design, many of which are based on the use of locally sourced, traditional, natural and benign materials, often used in innovative ways, and the construction techniques that follow from them.

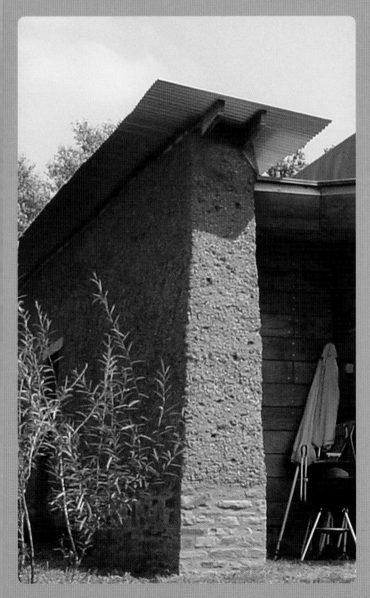

"What will eat your building?"

Paul Hawken

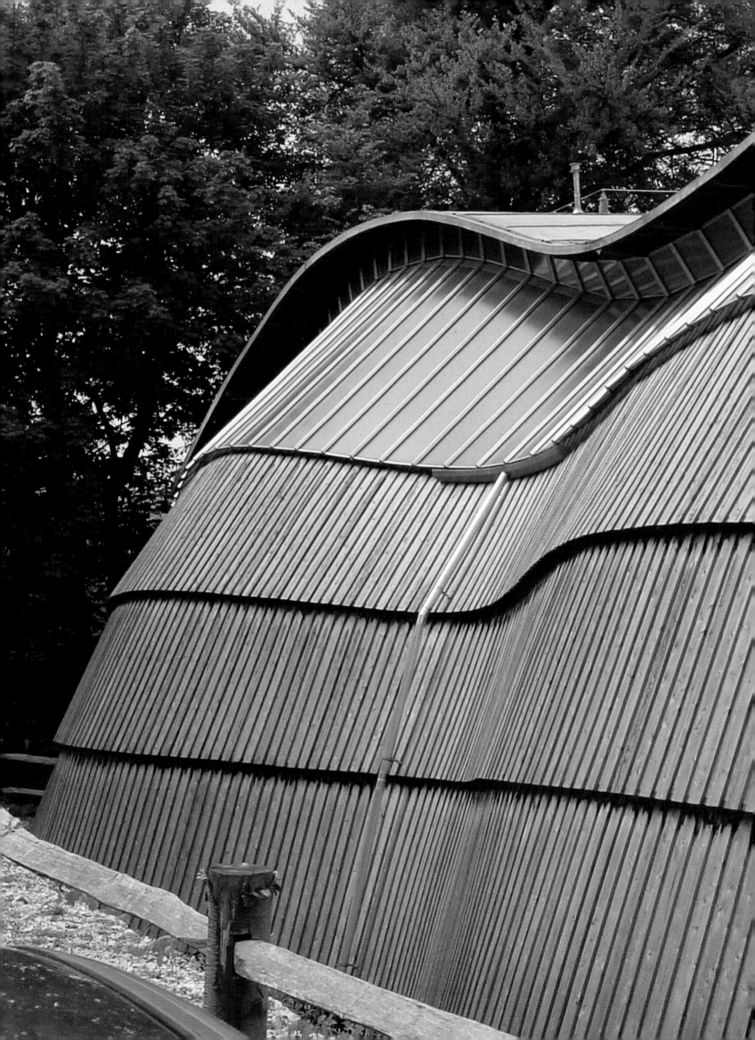

Contents

(Facing page)
**The Downland Gridshell,
Singleton, Chichester**
(Photo: ©Buro Happold/Adam
Wilson)

(Previous page)
Cobton House, Worcester
(Photo: Bill Bordass)

Low-impact construction

Introduction

Mainstream construction practice is putting in place policies and process management techniques to enable it to improve its sustainability performance. This is resulting in incremental improvements in many sectors of the industry. The previous chapter looked at issues concerned with the vast majority of contemporary building materials and how to minimise their adverse impacts.

Low-impact construction as described in this chapter looks at a tiny minority of wholly natural materials and how their use in construction is evolving. It is a marginal area in practice, but of great research and development interest to many. The resulting buildings can challenge contemporary approaches to materials, maintenance, labour and contract management.

Many of the techniques are both rooted in tradition and simultaneously at the forefront of research interest. Further knowledge could potentially provide a significant contribution to the delivery of sustainable buildings.

With few exceptions, contemporary examples of low-impact construction are small-scale and rural. This presents the risk that the materials and techniques are dismissed as irrelevant to larger-scale projects and/or urban design. However, historically many of them were used at a larger scale and in urban areas. If anything, technical advances should mean that we are better positioned to use them than before, but the knowledge gap has expanded in recent years, not least because of the ease with which mechanical and chemical manipulation of materials can take place. As a consequence the research emphasis has been on new materials rather than better use of existing ones.

There is also a significant issue of architectural perception. Sadly, too few contemporary examples of 'low-impact construction' are architecturally appealing. Only rarely is it possible to point to twentieth-century work with straw bales, earth or roundpole timber and see any real architectural merit. Indeed, the association of these materials in construction with poor design has encouraged distancing from conventional practice. This is changing as the use of the materials evolves, as they are taken

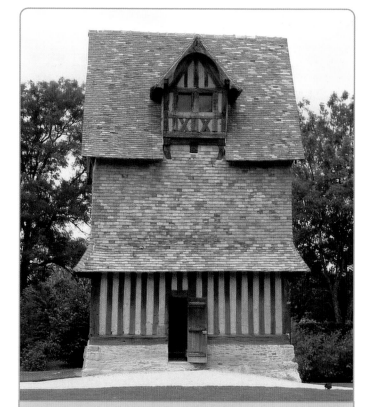

Traditional Building
Until recently there was only a limited pallet of materials available and these were all of natural origin. If the materials were used, and buildings designed and maintained, appropriately then this could ensure both a long life and eventually safe disposal or recycling
(Photo: Cat Button)

more seriously by conventional practice, and the architectural opportunities are better exploited and respected.

The recognition of human factors in sustainable design means that the self-build and skills development aspects of much low-impact design is gaining a resonance. The materials are often cheap, but the shift of emphasis to time means that the techniques are attractive to self-builders. This fits with the most advanced thinking in sustainable economics, which aims to shift the emphasis of taxation from people to resources and create a more level playing field for this approach to building.

Brettstapel construction has made the transition from a peripheral enquiry on the part of ecological structural designers, to a cost-effective, elegant, benign material, manufactured in huge quantities and with great potential as a substitute for contemporary materials. But is it still low impact?

Context

Most, but not all, current best practice in sustainable construction tends to rate improvement by small changes, giving an incremental reduction of environmental damage and perhaps some improvement in human aspects.

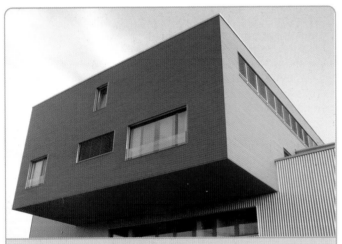

Brettstapel Construction
Office of Pirmin Jung Engineers, who specialise in brettstapel construction, including the design of their own office in Rain, Switzerland (Photo: the author)

An argument in favour of low-impact construction is that challenging the construction industry status quo, through the use of unconventional technical and contractual frameworks, can deliver improvements and efficiencies measured in orders of magnitude. The use of natural materials and innovative construction types also often enables dramatic cost savings. It is the low costs of materials such as clay and straw bales that explains their popularity with selfbuilders and those with relatively little money. By applying an element of self-build these materials can be used to deliver buildings at a fraction of the cost of conventional buildings, with improved environmental performance and markedly lower running costs, despite the additional maintenance required.

Because of their intrinsic ecological properties, the opportunities for local skill development and sourcing they offer a very direct route to realise significant economic, social and ecological benefits.

Set against this potential, simply meeting or exceeding building control, or other standards, appears a meagre aspiration. However, for many of those involved in low-impact construction, it is also part of an approach toward sustainability that demands deep-rooted change in social and business structures, and delivers more local empowerment.

In most conventional construction there are formal and informal systems of checks, which are designed to identify potential problems and prevent building failure. There may be significantly less information, knowledge and experience around to support low-impact construction. Any building must be subjected to the building control process, but with low-impact construction it is likely that few of those involved will be familiar with any innovative techniques and few organisations will offer guideline details. The designer and/or constructor will therefore be required to fill the knowledge gap for others involved through research and/or demonstration of experience.

Materials used in low-impact construction, such as earth and clay, are widely and readily available; others, including many crops, are renewable. Many crops could be grown ecologically on a large scale to produce much more, by volume, of the bulk materials used in building construction.

Other largely natural materials – stone, slate, baked clay, bricks and tiles – also have an important role, though these materials are well understood generally and well documented.

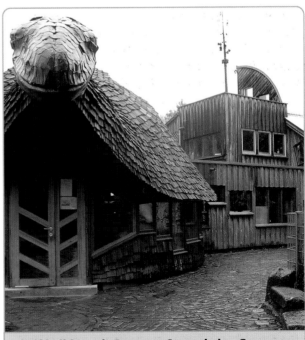

Self-build Youth Centre at Stammheim, Germany
Designed and built by local youth with Hübner Architects
(Photo: Howard Liddell)

Back to the future

Low-impact development now comes in many guises. David Lea's cottage presents a typical example of a building generated from its surroundings. Findhorn, near Inverness, is a large community that has developed into a multi-million pound enterprise with a collection of varying impact houses, from reused whisky vat houses to the 'Field of Dreams' – a new 'eco'-development.

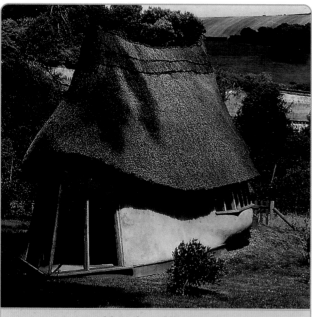

David Lea's Studio Cottage
Local, very small diameter saplings were lashed into a grid shell, rendered and thatched to form a simple, stable and very cheap building (Photo: Peter Blundell Jones)

But, as sustainability exerts an increasing influence over design and construction, approaches that once appeared radical are permeating mainstream practice. Glencoe Visitor Centre is a multi-million pound visitor centre designed to fulfil the National Trust for Scotland's desire for a building that would evidence its claim to be the country's principal conservation organisation and have the lowest footprint it was possible to have. It involved many innovative approaches to design and procurement. It could lay claim to be at the forefront of the development of low-impact construction, using benign materials in innovative and architecturally stunning ways and challenging traditional procurement methods by detailed attention to sourcing or materials, products and fuel.

General issues on materials

Sourcing

An important aspect of low-impact construction is that the sourcing of materials is not always straightforward. Specifiers conventionally choose materials from brochures produced by manufacturers and agents, which give a lot of information, including performance criteria, best practice details, relevant guarantees and so on. Contractors source these same materials from known, nationwide industry networks. Many materials mentioned in this chapter cannot be sourced in this way and this raises important issues. It makes more sense to undertake an audit of locally available materials, and perhaps skills, rather than to decide on a material and then look for it.

The most appropriate local source of a material may be the site itself (earth), a nearby farmer (straw), forestry operator, estate manager or sawmill (timber) or any number of other options.

Some materials, particularly those related to agriculture, may only be available, or only available at a reasonable price, at certain times of the year and it may be necessary to arrange appropriate storage until the right time in the construction programme. There may be no obvious price strategy for some otherwise waste material.

Notably, straw bale construction originated from the use of waste straw as a temporary construction element with surprisingly long life.

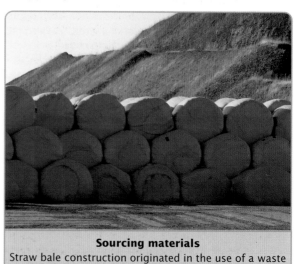

Sourcing materials
Straw bale construction originated in the use of a waste material but it is no longer conveniently packaged as building blocks (Photo: Michael Wolshover)

Performance

Many low-impact materials are not standardised. It is therefore important to identify performance characteristics at the outset as this may have implications for the design, contract cost, planning, building control approvals and so on.

Whoever supplies the material may or may not be in a position to certify or guarantee its performance, or even size, in the way that might be expected of a conventional manufacturer or supplier. This puts the onus onto the buyer to ascertain the nature of the material, and on the designer to allow for possible weaknesses or problems so that they can be readily remedied if need be.

When properly designed and if left uncoated, or coated in vapour-permeable finishes, all the natural materials described in this chapter will behave hygroscopically, as described in Chapter 5, and contribute to a moderated healthy indoor climate. Constructions such as Brettstapel using open-ended wood in the indoor environment offer a huge surface area for moisture absorption. All of the materials can also be used as part of a 'moisture transfusive' wall design.

Maintenance

For many construction materials in conventional use, maintenance is seen as something to reduce to a minimum or remove if possible, and there is an increasing preference for components to be 'maintenance free'. This has hidden disadvantages. Very few materials are naturally exempt from the ravages of weather and time. In attempting to escape the natural order of decay and weathering, these materials often require finishings or the introduction of invasive chemical treatments which cause considerable environmental damage in manufacture, through leaching in use, and when ultimately returned to the ground.

Despite this, a few conventional materials or components escape the requirements of maintenance, which can then be more difficult to administer because it has not been planned for. Often, when damage occurs minor repairs are impossible and whole components need to be scrapped; uPVC windows are an example of this. This has given rise to a concern that 'maintenance free means unmaintainable'.

The UK experience with timber has been that plastic paints intended to protect the wood fail to do so. The timber naturally expands and contracts and tries to breathe, leading to paint invariably flaking off. This looks untidy and the maintenance involves intensive work to remove and then re-apply additional finishes. In Norway, where use of timber is widespread, the tendency is to either leave it unfinished or to paint it for decorative purposes in easy-to-apply, water-based paint – repeated on a reasonably regular basis. Hence, whilst in the UK

the use of timber boarding is rare, it is a common site even on the rain-pounded west coast at Stavanger and Bergen.

In low-impact construction it is accepted that maintenance is necessary on a regular basis and that, if conscientiously undertaken, a small amount of maintenance will prolong the life of most components indefinitely at minimum environmental or financial cost. The design aims to facilitate ease of maintenance rather than its avoidance.

The most important job is to make regular checks for moisture, cracks, or particular erosion or failures such as delamination which might betray a more serious durability threat. Simple visual checking is often all that is required, but it should be thorough and regular.

Plants or detritus should be kept clear of wall surfaces to avoid build-up of material that could prevent adequate ventilation. Surfaces, such as window sills, should be kept clean to avoid mould build-up, and gutters cleared of leaves, eaves and verges checked for insects, etc. In this way almost all serious problems can be spotted early and dealt with cheaply and simply. Every five years or so, repainting of external surfaces may be necessary and, occasionally, repair of components and replacement of elements are also needed.

Labour and skills

An important aspect of much low-impact construction is the significantly different cost ratio between materials and labour, compared to conventional modern construction. In most low-impact construction, labour intensity offsets much lower material costs.

For this reason, low-impact construction is often of interest to the self-build sector, and proponents often use unconventional methods to produce buildings, such as workshop groups for certain work stages, and in some cases linking the additional labour required to financial incentives for site-based training. Not all low-impact construction is necessarily more labour intensive, but it is worth bearing this in mind when planning a building to assess the appropriate design or construction type/programme response.

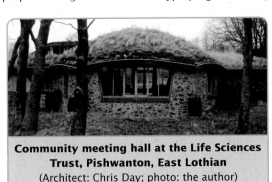

Community meeting hall at the Life Sciences Trust, Pishwanton, East Lothian
(Architect: Chris Day; photo: the author)

Earth

Unfired earth contrasts markedly in appearance and embodied energy with our contemporary tendency to reduce fire-bricks to cinder.

More than a third of the world's people live in unfired earthen homes of one sort or another. Relatively little energy is used to acquire the raw material and there is rarely any pollution associated with its extraction, manufacture or disposal. In its unfired form it also has considerable potential for the passive environmental control of buildings. Many different techniques have been created and some common types are described here.

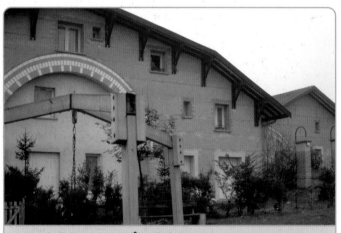

Earth housing at Île d'Abeau, near Lyons, France
Construction of a experimental earth housing centre in the 1980s. The project was undertaken by a range of architects including Hugo Houben and has had a major influence on the revival of interest in earth construction
(Photo: Howard Liddell)

- The thermal mass of the earth brick walls contributed significantly to the thermal comfort of the house by storing passive solar gains and moderating peak temperatures within a slow response heating system. Ventilation patterns adopted by the residents had a major effect on the amount of energy used to heat the house.
- The earth bricks were locally sourced and easy to use, though they suffered minor shrinkage cracking, probably caused by moisture absorbed in transport.
- The clay plasters achieved an attractive finish, but minor defects demonstrated that their different working qualities require specialist training to achieve a good finish.
- Very little waste was produced by the earth materials, both in manufacture and on site, where the small amount of waste produced bio-degraded into the site soil.
- The earth materials had very low embodied energy and carbon, approximately 14% of ordinary brickwork.
- The earth materials controlled the risk of condensation in the building without the need for membranes. No condensation occurred within the fabric. Their ability to absorb excess air moisture made the bathroom extract fan effectively redundant.
- The owner/occupiers were very happy with the house and content with the limitations on decoration of the walls necessary to maintain vapour porosity.
- The earth masonry worked well in combination with the structural timber frame. Good detailing and quality control are important at junctions with other materials.
- Earth masonry has the potential to improve building quality, reduce the environmental impact of construction and create healthier homes within current affordable housing market conditions. While these materials are relatively easy to use by non-specialists, the market is not well developed. Technical research, product development and contractor skills are areas that require further investment, etc.

Modern Earth Construction

A new house built in Perthshire in 2003 aimed to use earth bricks and clay plasters to improve indoor air quality, reduce construction waste and carbon emissions, and achieve a good quality of building at an affordable cost. A monitoring programme showed that:

- The earth materials passively controlled moisture in the building, generally to below levels known to be a major cause of asthma and mould-related disease.

Case Study 6.1:

Autonomous Environmental Information Centre, Machynlleth

Architect: Pat Borer, 2001

The building forms the major part of some 450 m² of new development at CAT. It provides an Information Centre along with staff accommodation and new toilet facilities. The building was designed following a 'Planning for Real' exercise to arrive at a consensus view and is one of the most significant new ecological buildings in the UK. The materials were all carefully selected for their local availability, sustainability, and health and environmental impact.

The external walls are highly insulated timber frame with woodwool boards as partial bracing, with a lime render finish. Rammed earth is used internally to act as thermal capacity. The earth for the rammed earth columns came from a quarry near Oswestry and was screened down to 6mm for the project, making a usefully homogeneous material; 8% powdered clay was added to bring the clay content to 15%. Lime was added in the top and bottom few inches to stabilise and strengthen the mix. Self-coloured clay plasters are used internally over reinforced plasterboard in preference to gypsum. The roofing and other panels are from local and sustainable timber sources (larch and oak).

All finishes are low emission and natural materials. The building features other innovations, such as:

- the use of unstabilised, non-reinforced, rammed earth elements as load-bearing supports internally (as well as thermal mass)
- the on-site manufacture of 1700 compressed earth blocks for use in the toilet block, which feature low-flush WCs, a dry composting toilet, waterless urinals, and an Aquatron waste separator (in a situation where no sewage infrastructure is available) for on-site sewage treatment and rainwater recycling
- sheep's wool insulation within the 325-mm-thick timber-framed external walls
- the complete exclusion of cement from the entire development (largely substituted with lime-crete, which contains roughly half to two-thirds of the embodied energy, but also completely alternative solutions)
- the 120 m² array of solar water panels, linked to a heat main which is also supplied by a biomass-fuelled boiler.

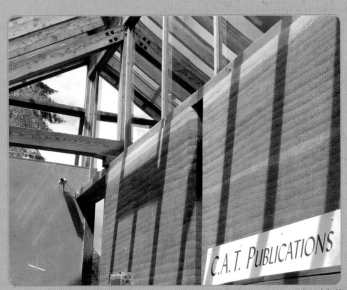

Photo: Howard Liddell

Earth techniques

Adobe

Adobe is the name for sun-baked or dried bricks, more or less hand made, and containing a relatively thick, dry and malleable mud mix to which straw is often added. These are stacked, as per conventional construction, to form load-bearing external and internal walls, ceiling vaults, They are usually finished with an earth- or lime-based plaster or render on both sides. Adobe is usually associated with Central America, Africa and Asia, but is applicable anywhere.

Where mechanical compression is used, this drives out more moisture than sun baking and enables the blocks to take on considerable compressive loads. Compressed earth blocks are generally larger.

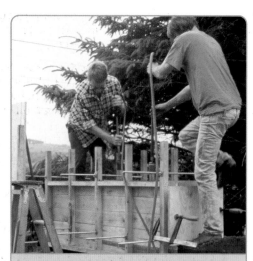

Tamping Rammed Earth Wall At Gaia Lista's Office
(Photo: Gaia Lista)

Rammed earth

Rammed earth requires a strong formwork, often of metal-reinforced plates, and tamping down a fairly dry earth and sand mix to form heavyweight monolithic load-bearing walls. The tamping may be by hand, but the technique has been significantly developed over the past 25 years, and is now often carried out in a largely mechanical site process by specialist construction companies.

Cob

Cob is the English term (mudwall the Scottish) for stacked earth – the most common earth construction method in the UK. It uses fairly wet mixes (compared with rammed earth), usually with straw for reinforcement, placed or stacked on a wall and trampled or hand-tamped into a monolithic wall construction. It is capable of taking considerable loads in compression, but not to such a degree or to such a calculable extent as the more mechanised procedures.

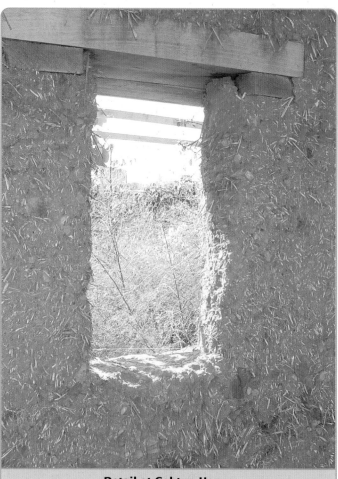

Detail at Cobtun House
(Photo: Bill Bordass)

Wattle and daub

Wattle and daub is the English term (stake and rice in Scotland) for a fairly wet mix applied to a (usually) timber frame as infill. A principal frame is usually fitted with a secondary, smaller-scale

Wattle and daub construction, Oxfordshire
(Photo: Oxley Conservation)

lattice, or series of armatures, to which to secure the earth mix. Straw or other fillers or reinforcements are needed to control inevitable shrinkage in a wet, clayey mix. This was traditionally

used where timber was an abundant resource. The other methods tended to develop in regions without significant timber resources.

Light earth construction

Light earth is the generic name given to a method of construction whereby straw, wood-chip, hemp or some other suitable 'fill' material is coated with clay slip and set within shuttering as simple infill for walls.

Light earth is never used in a load-bearing capacity, but is set within a structural frame to which shuttering, services, joinery, etc., are fixed. Light earth is usually made in situ, but can equally be constructed from blocks/infill panels. The surfaces are normally rendered on both sides with lime-based or earth renders.

Light earth construction as practised today was only recognised in the middle of the twentieth century as a discrete technique and was first documented in Germany in 1933.

The technique did not develop widely until the 1980s, when it was promoted and developed by enthusiasts, particularly in Germany, but later across the world. Recent research by Gaia Architects produced the first major work on the subject in English.

The thermal properties of light earth are intimately linked to its density – the lighter the mix, the greater is its insulation capacity, while a higher clay content improves its ability to store heat (thermal capacity). The lighter mixes, which are reasonably insulative, can be used in the UK for external walls.

Light earth construction operates as a moisture transfusive construction, as long as the finishes used are vapour permeable, and so it is inherently protected against the risk of interstitial condensation due to the vapour permeability and hygroscopicity of the materials used. In addition, the ability of these materials to absorb moisture allows light earth walls to moderate internal humidity levels. This has considerable indoor environmental benefits. Light earth is difficult to ignite, but is officially combustible, where the fill material is combustible.

Even without plaster coatings, its resistance to fire is good, but the presence of plaster coatings allows it to be used for all situations under the Building Regulations, except those requiring non-combustible materials only.

Case Study 6.2:

'The Cabin', Melrose, Scotland

Architects: Gaia Architects, 2002

This light earth outbuilding using straw-clay and woodchip-clay for the external walls is the first in the UK to be awarded Building Control approval for this form of construction. It is just less than 50 m² in plan and cost about £40 000. There was a substantial element of self-build, which mitigated the cost of high-quality finishing materials used, such as an oak floor and imported clay finishing plaster.

The building is suspended off the ground on timber beams spanning between steel columns with a suspended floor. Both the floor and ceiling use 250 mm of sheep's wool insulation in a 'breathing' construction. The internal finish to the ceiling is rough-sawn softwood, while the floor is of oak boards over a 50 mm lime/sand screed between battens. Within this screed heating pipes are run to create an underfloor heating system, which is continued into the 25 mm depth of wall plaster to create low-level heated walls. This is designed to optimise the thermal comfort characteristics of the building and capitalise on the mix of insulation and thermal capacity offered by the light earth wall mix.

The project was undertaken as a research project and the research report is available from Gaia.

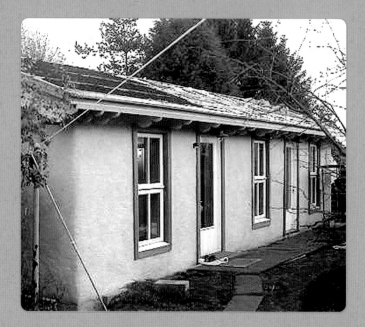

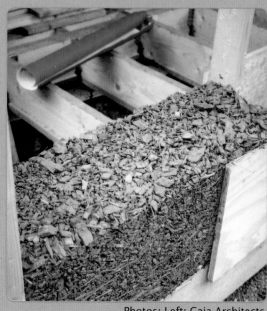

Photos: Left: Gaia Architects,

Right: Steven Downie

Straw bale

Straw bale construction has a number of advantages. It is a quick and very simple construction method, ideally suited to self-build. Bale costs are low compared to other wall materials and bring direct income to farmers. Straw is often a waste product, it is entirely renewable, and the resultant walls are non-polluting, biodegradable, eventually, and very well insulating. It is vitally important to keep bales dry at all times, and to use breathable or moisture transfusive coatings, especially on the external surfaces. Clay and lime are preferred. Wide overhangs are advisable, along with total protection from rising damp.

Honesty Window
It is a long-standing tradition to expose a part of the structure in straw construction – a technique that has become known as an honesty window
(Photo: the author)

Straw bale walls may be infill, with a structural frame of any suitable type or material, or load-bearing. The historical US bale buildings are load-bearing and this method is preferred by many, as it dispenses with a framework. However, it is more complex to construct and is less flexible should subsequent problems arise.

The walls are laid in a staggered manner like conventional masonry, but without mortar (in general).

They need to be stitched or bound to each other and to adjacent frames and joinery such as windows and doors. It is useful to plan the building around bale size modules to minimise the need to break bales or create special sizes. But be warned, bales are not standardised – they come in different sizes! Bales can be used on edge but are usually (and for load-bearing walls, preferably) laid flat. At approximately 450mm wide, plus plaster depths, they do take up a lot of space on plan, but equally provide pleasantly deep reveals akin to many older vernacular buildings, and excellent insulation.

Hemp

Hemp has a reputed 25,000 uses, including foodstuffs, fuel, biodegradable plastics, textiles, cosmetics and building materials. Like bamboo, described below, it has an enormous potential to contribute to the construction industry. It is as yet almost wholly unused. Possible hemp composites include insulation, screed levellers and underlays. As a crop, hemp is extremely hardy, productive and easy to grow in a range of climates, and resistant to disease and pests. There is no requirement for fertilisers. In addition, it tends to inhibit weed growth. The tap roots aerate the soil and the leaves produce a rich mulch, such that it is a good rotational crop, benefiting subsequent crop yields. Therefore, its ecological benefits mean that hemp represents a good low-impact building material.

Hemp/lime construction

The use of hemp fibres with lime is an established form of construction, particularly in France. Hemp fibres are also used on the Continent as insulation, though they require fire retardant treatment. Hemp/lime construction is very much like light earth construction in practice, though the use of lime rather than clay reduces the hygroscopicity of the mix. It is generally denser than a light earth mix.

Some research has indicated that the compressive strength of certain mixes may be enough to dispense with, or at least reduce, the timber framing required. In general it is used as infill only. The treatments and importation of hemp increase the embodied energy, but the potential to develop UK-based options exist. Prototype houses have been built in Suffolk. The relatively unimpressive 'U' values do not reflect the actual thermal performance of the buildings. This has been borne out by the BRE monitoring of properties built in Suffolk by Modece Architects.

Case Study 6.3:

Straw bale office, Dunning, Perthshire

Architects: Gaia Architects, 2000

The client, an architect and member of the UK Sustainable Construction Forum, decided to build a garden office and approached Gaia Architects for a truly sustainable construction.

The project provided Gaia with the opportunity to innovate based on recent research into roundpole construction, carried out for the Northern Periphery Programme. A local materials audit led to investigation of the potential of straw bale. The resulting building has a roundpole frame, walls of straw rendered on both sides with lime plaster. The sheep's wool-insulated roof was covered with turf to replace the displaced garden space removed. All the materials, including recycled windows, were sourced from within 20 miles.

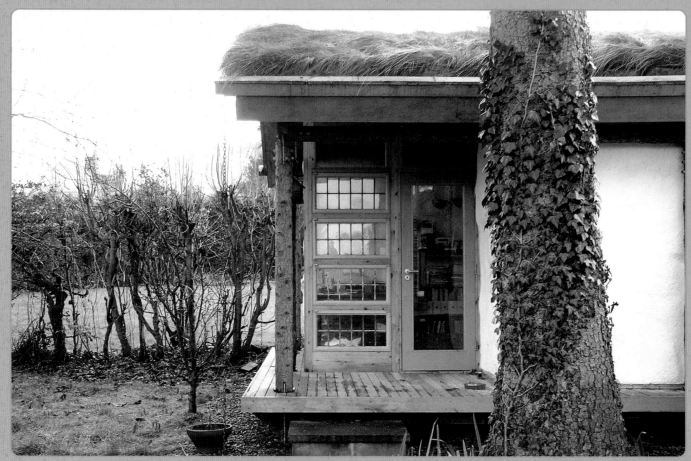

Photos: Gaia Architects

Case Study 6.4:

Hemp houses, Suffolk Housing Society, Bury St Edmunds

Architects: Modece Architect, 2001

A French company, Isochanvre (www.isochanvre.com), have developed two prototype hemp/lime houses in Suffolk, in partnership with Suffolk Housing Society and Modece Architects.

These have been monitored by the BRE against two otherwise identical conventional houses.

The imported hemp fibres used are 'mineralised' in a commercially secret process to render them rot-proof, non-flammable and inedible to rodents – the difficulty in achieving this in an environmentally benign way is bound to raise questions about the net benefit of hemp as a construction material.

The BRE Report concludes that the hemp/lime homes are more expensive than conventional houses, with comparable waste minimisation, thermal and durability performance, while acoustic performance was poorer but condensation generation was less.

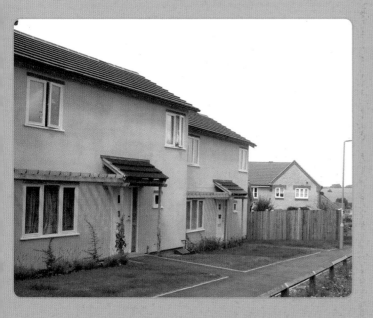

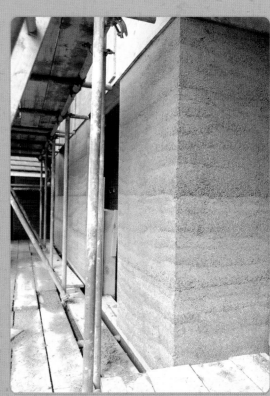

Photos: Modece Architects

Case Study 6.5:

Rowardennan Visitor Centre, Loch Lomond, Scotland

Architects: Simpson and Brown/Richard Shorter, 2001

The Rowardennan Visitor Facility sits in a tranquil woodland setting on a small rise between the Loch and the foot of Ben Lomond. The building straddles the path from the pier that leads to the Ben and forms part of the West Highland Way. Visitors can walk straight through or stop for shelter, toilets, changing facilities, bin-store and an exhibition area providing local information. A park warden is also based there.

Designed to be in sympathy with its setting, the building is constructed using locally sourced materials. It has gently curving walls and a swept roof form. The traditionally made peg-jointed oak frame, assembled from trees felled within a few hundred yards of the site, supports a timber roof structure covered with reused Aberfoyle slates.

Initial attempts to reopen the Aberfoyle quarry proved fruitless, but slates became available during the investigations. There are no damp-proof membranes in the building, so it is a completely breathing structure, the floor being lime concrete on a free-draining stone base. The low stone walls are built off the formation level in lime mortar.

Above the stone base the external walls are formed in traditional cob: clay, sand and straw mixed together and forked onto the wall head, trampled in place and trimmed. They are finished externally with lime harling and lime wash, and internally with clay plaster. Natural oil-based paints are used on the joinery work.

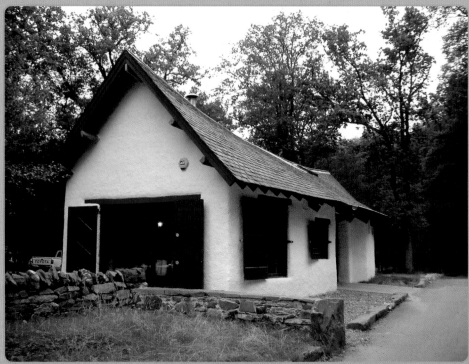

Photo: the author

Timber

For many, simply using timber automatically transfers a sense of environmental credibility. Unfortunately, this is far from the case and, depending on the circumstances, some timber specification can be worse than almost any other material. Consider, for example, hardwood, culled from old growth forest where logging companies displace local, perhaps indigenous, people and where the forest is either not replanted or is replanted with a single age monoculture. This timber is then shipped across the world, where it is then heavily machined, treated with toxic chemicals to increase its durability and then used in a building with poor detailing which, despite its preservative treatment and inherent durability, leads to early decay. After, perhaps, 10 years, it is discovered to have 'failed' and is disposed of, either legally as toxic waste or illegally, where it pollutes the soil and groundwater.

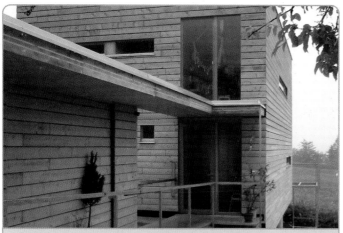

House at Batchuns, Austria
One of an increasing number of houses built to a passive standard from Brettstapel constrruction
(Architect: Unterrainer, Photo: the author)

For timber to form part of a sustainable approach to specification and design of building, sustainable management of the forest resource is vital. There are several definitions, but importantly the timber should not be old growth – there is little enough left. It is now common practice for 'Scandinavian' or 'Baltic' timber, which is largely Siberian old growth forest, to be imported into the UK via the Baltic states. The forest structure should be of mixed age, or building toward that state. A largely native and sound ecological replanting system should be in place. Some cultural or social recognition of the local landscape should be evident, along with policies to protect and enhance existing wildlife in the area. Ideally, the timber is from as close a source as

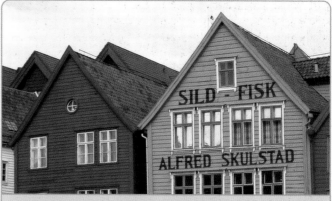

Timber detailing
Wooden houses are common in exposed coastal regions in Norway where timber is selected, detailed and maintained properly. The UK experience of poor timber, bad details and plastic paints have undermined its longevity
(Photo: Cat Button)

possible and certainly not imported. It is not treated unless absolutely unavoidable (which is extremely rare), machined as little as possible and is used efficiently, detailed well to achieve durability and is able to be easily repaired, and eventually safely composted. Some types of timber use take advantage of some of these principles to realise lower impact timber buildings.

A number of systems have been set up to enable specifiers to be confident of their timber source, but these systems are difficult to police, albeit worthwhile. The FSC is one such scheme. In the UK, simply stating that the timber should be UK sourced is reasonably sound.

Local sourcing

The main value of sourcing timber locally is to reduce the pollution associated with its transportation. Attention should be given to finding the most locally available source of appropriate timber with the more local specification desirable. Support for UK forest and timber economies encourages the sustainable management of UK forests.

It may be useful, and can have cost advantages, to assess the characteristics of local timber supply prior to starting a design, as with other aspects of materials. This means that opportunities may be taken to design to what is available. In Scotland, for example, it is difficult to source long lengths of timber, so designs based around the use of short timber lengths make it easier to achieve local supply at a reasonable cost.

Timber techniques

The most popular technique for co-self-builders was developed by Walter Segal. It originated, rather like the development of straw bale construction, from the construction of a temporary shelter that then stood the test of time. It is a rigorously simple technique that is logical and extremely resource efficient. It is only truly low impact when the materials are appropriately sourced and treated, and attention is given to the health aspects of the design.

'Green' timber

The designed use of 'green' timber involves constructing part of the building (largely associated with oak structural framing) with timber that is only recently felled and machined. The timber then seasons 'in situ'. This invariably involves movement and must be accommodated by subsequent elements. This use of 'green' timber cuts out the need for kiln drying and saves energy. Visually it is likely to result in 'organic' shapes. Clearly, building with 'green' timber (inadequately dried) without taking account of future movement leads to structural failure and/or interstitial water that can lead to mould and subsequent health problems.

Gridshells

Gridshells are made from small-section material that is formed into curved shell-like shapes. This gives them huge strength and they can span large distances without intermediate support. They are relatively low impact because of the small amount of material needed to span such lengths so effectively.

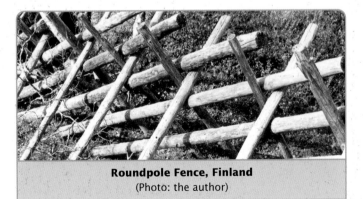

Roundpole Fence, Finland
(Photo: the author)

Roundpole

In recent years there has been significant investigation of the use of timber in the round because it is strong. With roundpole the

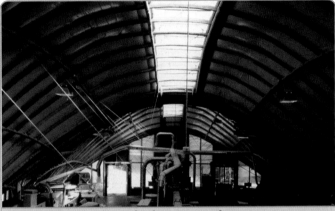

Roundpole construction
Much of the early work on roundpole construction was undertaken at Hooke Parke by ABK and Buro Happold
(Photo: Howard Liddell)

fibres are uncut; hence, the round sections are as strong as rectangular 'beam'-shaped section timbers cut from much larger logs with discontinuous fibres. As in theory no machining is needed, it is accessible to remote communities as a building material and avoids either the need to purchase machinery or to transport the timber to central treatment areas.

Much of the early work on roundpole construction was undertaken by Buro Happold at Hooke Park. The achievements in manipulation and the resulting forms were truly stunning, but some fundamental problems of ecology were not resolved, namely in the glues, fixings and roof membranes.

One project, undertaken by a partnership between the Gaia Group in Scotland and practices in Norway and Finland, looked specifically at the use of roundpole in the northern periphery areas of the European Union. The aim was to investigate opportunities to add value to logged timber in the northern periphery whilst maintaining an ecological silviculture. This might, for instance, include the use of relatively young trees for structural timber. Liberating valuable timber at an earlier stage could theoretically increase the value of forestry.

Inevitably, the biggest problems are in making connections between non-planed surfaces and this often involves some machining to create a strong joint. The alternative is to use glues, which in general are less benign the stronger the connection. There are a number of examples that resulted from the research and development of this technique at Hooke Park in Dorset by the Parnham Trust, with engineers Buro Happold.

Case Study 6.6:

The Downland Gridshell, Chichester

Architects: Edward Cullinan Architects, 2002

Weald and Downland is an open-air museum showcasing historic English buildings from the thirteenth to the nineteenth centuries that have been carefully restored and placed on the site.

In 2002, the Downland Gridshell was completed to help with this conservation work. The award-winning building is the first timber gridshell to be built in Britain and houses the museum's collection of artifacts from rural life in the climatically controlled basement and a building conservation workshop space, where timber-framed buildings can be laid out for conservation, under the gridshell roof.

The gridshell is a lightweight construction method that allows a large area to be covered with low impact on the site and minimal materials use. The gridshell has the strength of a double curvature shell but without having a solid structure. It is made of oak laths finger-jointed into standard 6 m (20 ft) lengths and then joined together to make 36 m (120 ft) laths, using high levels of carpentry skills.

The structure is double layered for strength whilst retaining flexibility and then triangulated by an additional layer. The diagonal grid was initially made flat and then slowly bent into shape to form the curved shell.

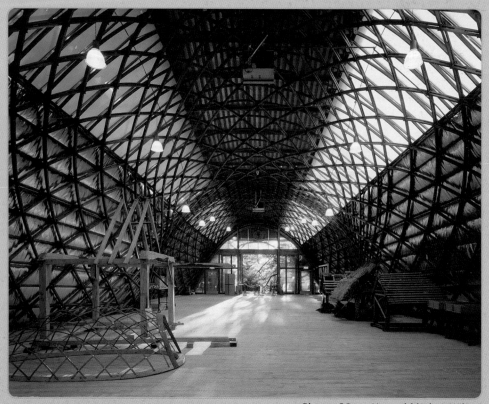

Photo: ©Buro Happold/Adam Wilson

Brettstapel

Brettstapel is the commercial version of an idea developed by Natterer in Germany, involving the use of planks, or thicker sections of wood, laid on edge and connected together into wide panels of solid timber. It is a resource hungry method, which is best suited to using low-value timber – of which we in the UK have a great deal. The resultant brettstapel panels are strong and useful. They will span 12 m at little more than 150 mm deep. The major advantage in ecological terms is adding value to low-value timber, which would otherwise be used only for paper, matches, pallets, etc.

It is now in widespread use in Germany and factories have developed in a number of Scandinavian counties. An issue of relevance is that spread of flame is not a significant issue on the Continent. The use of brettstapel in the UK would require a properly fire-engineered approach, otherwise it would be necessary to treat the panels against fire, or cover with plasterboard or plaster, either of which would undermine both the simplicity and the environmentally benign nature of the visible timber finish.

The latest developments in factory construction of Brettstapel buildings offer an interesting link between relatively high technologies for the construction industry such as computer numerically controlled (CNC) programming and healthy, resource-efficient approaches to building design.

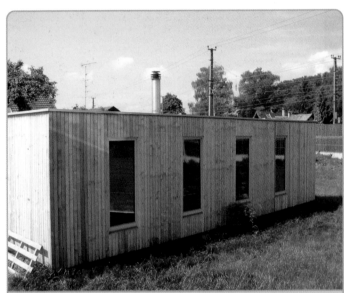

Mader School, Austria
A simple plan for a very cheap temporary, selfbuild and movable structure. Walls and roof are made of white pine massive wood construction with orthogonal dowels. The result is very cheap but with nicely detailed finishes
(Architect: Walter Unterrainer; photo: the author)

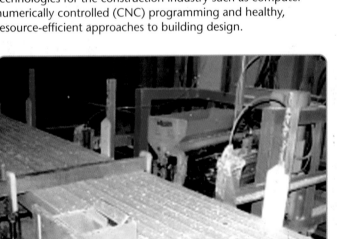

Sohm Diagonaldubelholz Factory, Austria
Factory construction of solid timber panel, 8–30 cm thick, up to 16 m long and 620 cm wide. Glueless bonding using dowels rammed under pressure into holes drilled orthogonally in two directions to resist movement. Wall elements have one side of finished quality, making a high quality, ecologically sound and healthy building material
(Photo: the author)

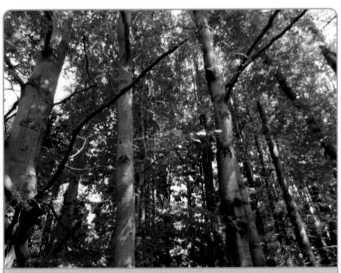

Timber resources
Use of some timber threatens biodiversity and human habitats whilst other timber resources, such as Sitka spruce that could supply a brettstapel industry, are undervalued and underused
(Photo: the author)

Case Study 6.7:

Pfennigäcker Nursery School, near Tübingen, Germany

Architects: Joachim Eble Architects, 1998

The building is organised around several separate two-storey 'houses', which act as homes for classes of children throughout their time in the nursery school. The structurally separate buildings are joined by a central area, which acts as the 'public space' for joint activities, such as lunchtimes and recreation.

Each building is completely constructed from 'brettstapel' panels of dowelled timber planks on edge, forming large, solid timber elements. These are used for floors, walls and roof elements, covered externally with insulation and cladding as necessary, and exposed internally. When it was originally conceived, 'brettstapel' was very much seen as an innovative 'low-impact' material. It has since become a commonplace ecological approach to building throughout Europe, except the UK.

The timber used is relatively poor-quality softwood, but used in this way is structurally very strong (floor spans of 12 m are possible) and self-bracing. Gaining value from low-quality timber helps the economic case for well-managed forestry.

The solid wood, with a density of around 750 kg/m, is both thermally massive and reasonably insulative, though additional insulation is placed externally. In this way the internal surfaces are relatively warm, thereby reducing the radiative heat loss from occupants and allowing for lower air temperatures, reducing stuffiness.

Natural pigmented plant-based paints and stains are used internally, which enable the panels to absorb and desorb moisture from the internal climate, regulating the indoor relative humidity and creating a healthy, balanced climate for children and staff.
Colour specialist: Lasuveda.

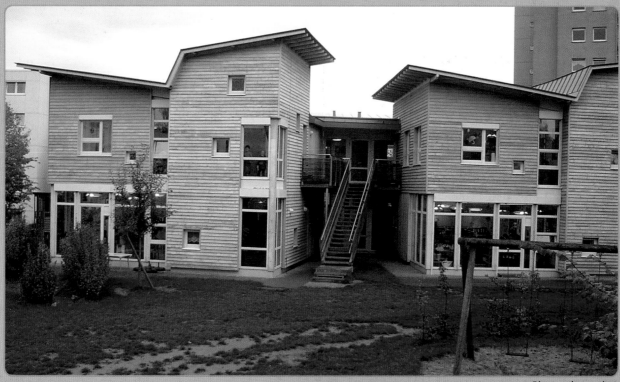

Photo: the author

Bamboo

Bamboo grows extremely quickly in many environments. In places where timber is scarce, it is a strong, lightweight option that avoids the deforestation associated with logging in marginal areas. Like roundpole, the difficulties in using bamboo are to do with connections between circular section poles. Architect Simon Velez has developed a modern tradition of bamboo architecture, with many new buildings demonstrating the technique, including the ZERI pavilion at the Hanover exposition.

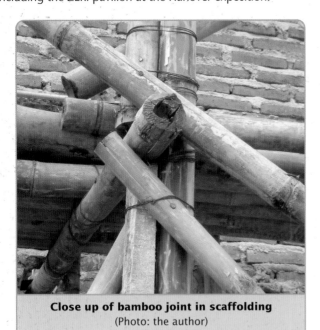

Close up of bamboo joint in scaffolding
(Photo: the author)

Cardboard

Cardboard is almost entirely made from recycled material and so represents a benign material that is essentially non-polluting and biodegradable. A recent school extension was built using mostly cardboard, by volume, with recycled plastic film for water protection and some non-toxic (and recoverable) additives for protection. The panels and tubes used provide structure and protection from the elements.

Construction using reused, recycled materials or waste

Construction and other waste generation is a major issue in the UK and we lag far behind many countries in recycling and reuse.

The creative reuse of materials is still a largely untapped resource despite the efforts of a few motivated individuals and organisations. Lowest impact options are non-polluting materials that can be simply reused. Recycling and reuse of polluting materials that would be destined for landfill is creditable, but ultimately the final destination must be a consideration and hence the manufacturing processes which create polluting materials must be challenged. It is important that the use, and potential for reuse, of benign materials is built into everyday detailing so that today's building materials do not become tomorrow's waste.

Reused products, such as doors and fire surrounds, are often of high value; so, it is worth reusing them. Note labour costs may also be high. However, floorboards, bricks, tiles and slates are often only available in batches. Products are available that have been recycled, into similar materials (metals, glass cullet, etc.) or something quite distinct (certain plastics can be converted into building boards).

Architects such as Michael Reynolds in the United States have incorporated the use of waste into their designs as an integral part of their overall low-impact strategy (see Case Studies 6–9 on 'earthships'). Reynolds's design relies heavily on tyres and cans, which are widely available across the globe, so the idea is universally applicable, but adaptable to suit local conditions. The potential use of construction as a depository for other industries' waste is a concern, and also that many of these materials do not positively affect occupant health.

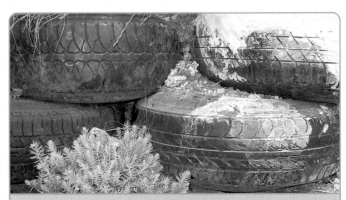

The Fife Earthship
Building with waste materials should not challenge us aesthetically or endanger our health. Building with the toxic waste of other industries is unwise
(Photo: the author)

Case Study 6.8:

Cardboard School – Westborough Primary School, Westcliffe-on-Sea, Essex

Architects: Cottrell and Vermeulen Architecture, 2001

The Primary School at Westcliff-on-Sea, completed in 2001, uses cardboard panels and tubes within the walls, roof and structure. The design aims to challenge people's perception of the materiality of cardboard. By going against the material's inherent characteristics, the building immediately becomes a point of interest and an education tool in itself.

The two main problems faced by card are that it burns very easily and loses structural integrity when wet; to minimise the effects of fire and water on the building, the cardboard used is combined with other materials.

The building is made up of two basic cardboard components, structural tubes and panels. The tubes were manufactured by Essex Tubes and are made by winding strips of recycled paper tightly around a metal-centred column. Once the tube is the desired width and length, the centre column is removed and reused. The paper used is made water resistant by a waxy layer, which

is applied prior to being wound; it is also possible to varnish the completed tubes for double protection.

The panels used in the walls and roofs are manufactured by Quiton & Kaines, who specialise in cardboard building components. Panels are made to suit the application; in this case, a composite panel of 15 mm solid card sheets and 3 x 50-mm-thick card honeycomb was used. The honeycomb provides insulation by trapping warm air. The individual panels are finished with a wooden frame for protection and ease of assembly.

A thin plastic layer and water-resistant chemical were applied to the internal walls of the building to prevent moisture from inside the school affecting the card. Externally, the panels were clad using a wood pulp nd cement mixture, which also provides protection from footballs, stones and general damage.

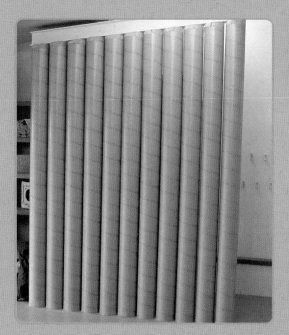

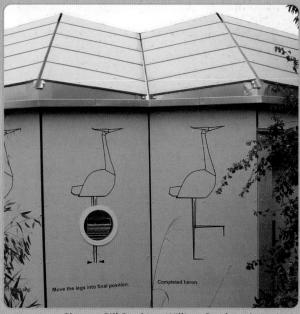

Photos: Bill Bordass, William Bordass Associates

Case Study 6.9:

Earthship, Fife, Scotland

Architect: Michael Reynolds, 2004

An earthship is a passive solar building with thermal mass. This project in Fife is the first demonstration of the earthship concept in the UK.

It is made from natural and recycled materials, including earth-rammed tyres and aluminium cans. It is powered by renewable energy, catches its own water supply from rainwater, and treats and contains its own sewage in planter beds. It is a concept, not a set design, and can be adapted for any climate worldwide.

The building has been developed as a Demonstration Centre and has full planning permission and five-year building warrant approval. The body of the building was completed in a series of workshops during 2002, and the self-sufficient services and internal finishes were completed during 2003.

The retaining walls of the earthship are constructed with tyres, which are then filled with earth. The UK consumes 140 000 tyres every day and there is no satisfactory disposal method in place. Some are incinerated causing air pollution. The rest are landfilled or informally dumped. However tyres are highly suspect from a toxicity perspective and this casts real doubt over the project value. Cans are used to fill the subsequent depths in the surface and the internal face is covered in a clay-based plaster. The 'wing' walls are clad in stone. The floor is of solid lime-crete – concrete with lime instead of cement. Full height glazing admits light and heat that is stored in the thermally massive flanking walls and floor. There is no additional heat source.

It advertises itself as the first autonomous building in the UK, disregarding the experience of the "Street Farmers" and the Autonomous House at Southwell – both of which were lived in, whilst this is essentially a small office.

It is promoted as offering people the opportunity to build their own homes, however the health risks of the construction materials and final indoor climate need to be appraised. The effectiveness of this strategy is being monitored over a three-year period to assess its performance and its relevance to construction in Scotland.

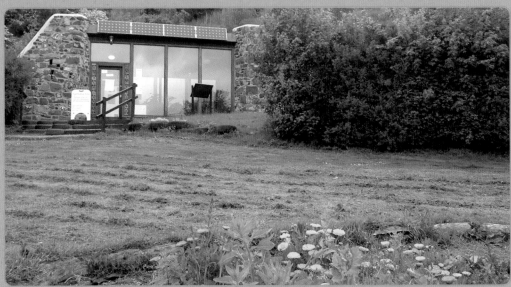

Photo: the author

Planning and low-impact development

In considering low-impact buildings, it is useful to understand the context within which these buildings may be conceived and developed. Simon Fairlie's book *Low Impact Development* looks at the planning process in the UK, with a view to promoting the development of low-impact structures and ways of life. An organisation known as 'The Land is Ours' has developed 15 criteria which form a basis for understanding the conceptual and practical context for low-impact buildings. Fairlie notes that few buildings will conform to all criteria, but that significantly low-impact buildings are likely to conform to many and that the criteria act as a useful checklist for assessing the impact of any proposal. The 15 criteria are:

1 The project has a management plan which demonstrates:
   – how the site will contribute significantly towards the occupiers' livelihoods
   – how the objectives cited in items 2–14 below will be achieved and maintained.
2 The project provides affordable access to land and/or housing to people in need.
3 The project provides public access to the countryside, including temporary access such as open days and educational visits.
4 The project can demonstrate how it will be integrated into the local economy and community.
5 The project can demonstrate that no activities pursued on the site shall cause undue nuisance to neighbours or the public.
6 The project has prepared a strategy for the minimisation of motor vehicle use.
7 The development and any buildings associated with it are appropriately sited in relation to local landscape, natural resources and settlement patterns.
8 New buildings and dwellings are not visually intrusive nor of a scale disproportionate to the site and the scale of the operation, and are constructed from materials with low embodied energy and environmental impact, and preferably from locally sourced materials, unless environmental considerations or the use of reclaimed materials determine otherwise. Reuse and conversion of existing buildings on the site is carried out as far as practicable in conformity with these criteria.
9 The project is reversible, in so far as new buildings can be easily dismantled and the land easily restored to its former condition.

10 The project plans to minimise the creation of waste and to reuse and recycle as much as possible on site.
11 The project has a strategy for energy conservation and the reduction, over time, of dependence on non-renewable energy sources to a practical minimum.
12 The project aims over time for the autonomous provision of water, energy and sewage disposal, and where it is not already connected to the utilities shall make no demands upon the existing infrastructure.
13 Agricultural, forestry and similar land-based activities are carried out according to sustainable principles. Preference will be given to projects that conform to registered organic standards, sustainable forestry standards or recognised permaculture principles.
14 The project has strategies and programmes for the ecological management of the site, including:
   – the sustainable management and improvement of soil structure
   – the conservation and, where appropriate, the enhancement of semi-natural habitat, taking into account biodiversity, indigenous species and wildlife corridors
   – the efficient use and reuse of water, as well as increasing the water-holding capacity of the site
   – the planting of trees and hedges, particularly in areas where the tree coverage is less than 20%.
15 The project can show that affordability and sustainability are secured – for example, by the involvement of a housing association, cooperative, trust or other social body whose continuing interest in the property will ensure control over subsequent changes of ownership and occupation.

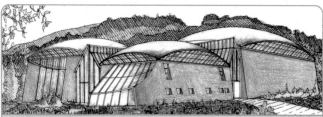

The original design for Drumchapel Leisure Centre, Glasgow
Gaia Architects' design in 1994 was based on the principles of earth, air, fire and water. It was to be modern earth construction
(Image: Gaia Architects)

Case Study 6.10:

Animal architecture

Elements of animal architecture have been used to develop concept designs for a range of building types. The project aimed to bring animal building to the attention of the construction industry in order to encourage innovation.

An area of particular interest is to explore new ideas and research needs within the context of sustainability and to address biodiversity, environmental pollution and protection, which are key aspects of Government Sustainable Construction objectives.

Animals are responsible for some impressive, experienced and environmentally sensitive architecture. Like humans, they construct in order to transform their environment, improve their quality of life, and provide safety and security for their young. Their achievements in structural form and strength, microclimate creation, material exploitation, membrane design, ventilation and pest management are immense. However, we still know very little about these achievements, the underlying physical principles and how we might apply them. In contrast to animal builders, humankind uses significant mechanical and chemical resources to create and transform our habitat. It is argued that use of these resources has been a principal element in our species' success, but how optimised is our performance? And how significant and predictable are the problems which we are introducing for future generations?

These issues were explored by Gaia Research in a project to design a building based on animal architecture principles.

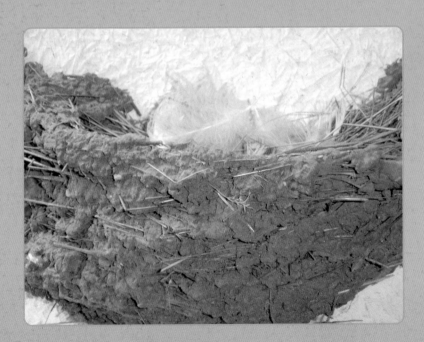

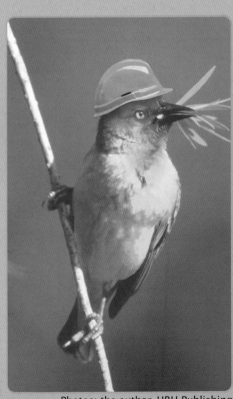

Photos: the author, HRH Publishing

Bibliography

General Texts

Stulz, R. (1983) *Appropriate Building Materials – A Catalogue of Potential Solutions.* SKAT Swiss Centre for Appropriate Technology and Intermediate Technology Publications, St Gallen, Switzerland.

Shoard, M. (1987) *This Land is Our Land.* Paladin.

Mollison, B. (1990) *Permaculture: A Practical Guide for Sustainable Living.* Island Press, Washington, DC.

Fairlie, S. (1997) *Low Impact Development: Planning and People in a Sustainable Countryside.* Jon Carpenter Publishing, Charlbury.

Maxwell, I. and Ross, N. (1997) *Traditional Building Materials Conference.* Historic Scotland.

Mitchell, M. (1998) *The Lemonade Stand – Exploring the unfamiliar by building large-scale models.* The Centre for Alternative Technology Publications, Machynlleth, Wales.

Elizabeth, L. and Adams, C. (2000) *Alternative Construction, Contemporary Natural Building Methods.* John Wiley, New York.

www.segalselfbuild.co.uk – UK trust helping people to build their own homes using the Segal method, with an emphasis on low-impact healthy materials.

Earth construction

Houben, H. and Guillaud, H. (1994) *Earth Construction: A Comprehensive Guide.* Intermediate Technology Publications, London.

Dachverband Lehm (1999) *Lehmbau Regeln (Earth Building Rules).* Vieweg & Sohn, Wiesbaden.

Minke, G. (2000) *Earth Construction Handbook Building Material Earth in Modern Construction.* WIT Press, Southampton.

Little, R. and Morton, T. (2001) *Building with Earth in Scotland Innovative Design and Sustainability.* Scottish Executive Central Research, Edinburgh.

Light earth construction

Laporte, R. (1993) *Mooseprints: A Holistic Home Building Guide.* Robert Laporte, New Mexico.

Volhard, F. (1995) *Leichtlehmbau Alter Baustoff – neue Technik (Light Earth Building, Old Building Material – New Technique),* 5th edition. C. F. Mueller, Heidelberg (in German).

Westermarck, M. (1996) *The Manufacture and Use of Nature-Based Building Materials as a Secondary Livelihood for Farmers,*

1st English Résumé. The Unit for Nature-Based Construction, Helsinki University of Technology, University Publication, Helsinki.

Gaia Architects (2003) *Light Earth Construction* (www.lightearth.co.uk). Gaia.

Straw bale construction

Steen, A. and Steen, B. (1994) *The Straw Bale House.* Chelsea Green, Vermont.

www.strawhomes.com – USA.

www.thelaststraw.org – USA.

www.strawbalefutures.org.uk – UK site run by Amazon Nails.

Timber construction

Bramwell, M. (1976) *The International Book of Wood.* Mitchell Beazley.

Broome, J. and Richardson, B. (1991) *The Self-Build Book.* Green Books.

Stungo, N. (1998) *The New Wood Architecture.* Laurence King.

Gaia Research (1999) *Roundpole* www.gaiagroup.org/roundpole.html and CD.

Waste and recycled materials

Liddell, H. et al. (1993) *Recycled Materials for Housing.* Scottish Homes.

National Recycling Forum – www.nrf.org.uk/buy-recycled

Salvo News and Salvo Guide – www.salvo.org.uk

Lime

Centres of excellence on lime, running hands-on courses – www.thelimecentre.co.uk

Animal Architecture

von Frisch K. (1975) *Animal Architecture.* Hutchinson & Co.

Hansell M. (1999) *The Animal Construction Company.* The Hunterian Museum and Gallery.

Rudofsky, B. (1995) *Architecture Without Architects.* The Museum of Modern Art, New York.

Halliday S.P. (2000) *Anarchi – Animal Architecture.* Gaia Research

Chapter 7
Heating

In which we assist building designers to extend their existing skills so as to be better equipped to deliver high-quality buildings which have a low heating demand, that can be efficiently met, and retain a positive effect on health and well-being.

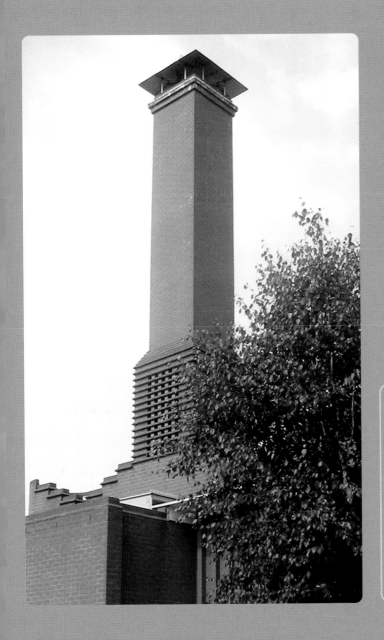

'If you put a frog in a pan of hot water it will immediately jump out rejecting its inappropriate environment. If you put the frog in a pan of cold water and gently heat it, it will slowly cook to death.'

Gaia Atlas of Planet Management, Pan Books (1985)

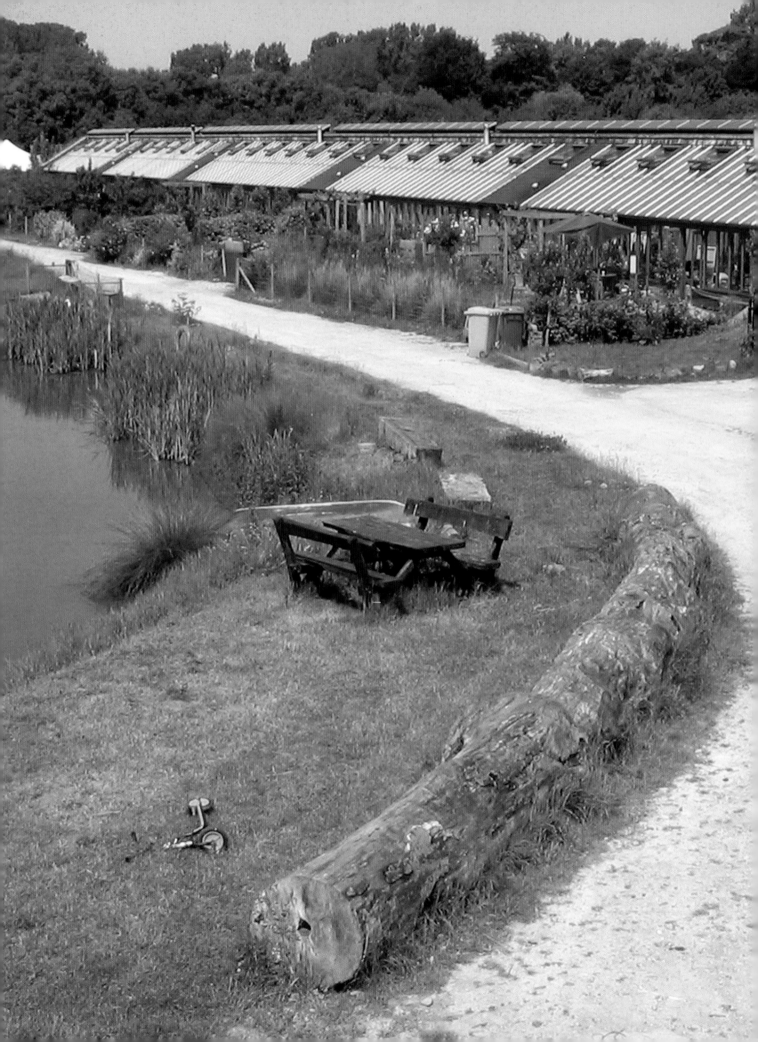

Contents

(Facing page)
Earth-sheltered housing at Hockerton
(Photo: Hockerton Housing Project)

(Previous page)
DeMontfort University
(Photo: the author)

Heating

Introduction

All designers attain at least a basic knowledge of underlying principles of thermal comfort, heat transfer and energy flows. However, this is not always readily translated into design practice. As issues of energy security and the unknown, but potentially devastating, impacts of climate change have been acknowledged, legislators have begun to make conservation of fuel and power a priority. In order to best deliver this, we need to pursue an integrated approach to heating design. It is no longer acceptable to design buildings that squander fossil fuels.

Our buildings use far more energy for heating than is required, due to less than optimal attention to basic aspects of build quality and management. Significantly improved environmental performance can be achieved by attention to the building envelope, with added benefits of enhanced durability and comfort. Being attentive to the building context is vitally important to make the best use of available resources and minimise heating demand, as is fuel sourcing, equipment specification and controls.

The answer to affordable sustainable heating is not roof-mounted wind turbines and ground-source heat pumps for the few. This is equivalent to trying to fill a bath with the plug out. At least in the first instance, the answer lies in quality passive design and attention to detail in all housing. Much can be achieved during the early stages of new design development, but opportunities abound in existing buildings. Indeed, these are vitally important if we are to limit energy consumption to sustainable levels.

An energy audit as a precursor to physical improvements and the implementation of good management and maintenance practices can enhance comfort and energy efficiency whilst reducing running costs. Even small investments in energy-saving equipment or education can result in short-term paybacks.

If we are to create sustainable environments then we have to marry the demand for reduced pollution with affordability and social responsibility. Heating can be a significant expense for individuals and families on low income. Where it is outside a family's means to maintain adequate thermal comfort and hot water for basic needs, then the resulting damp and cold conditions are an ideal breeding ground for moulds and mites that cause health problems, particularly breathing-related disability such as asthma. The problem has been exacerbated by a generation of houses that were designed with inadequate ventilation. As low-income families occupy a disproportionate amount of the worst quality housing in the UK, the issue of fuel poverty is not trivial.

It is more important than ever for the professions to work together. Aspirations and information need to be shared to achieve a good result, which will work well in the long term. There is emerging good-quality guidance and an abundance of case study publications.

Though energy consumption continues to increase, it is not predominantly as a result of heating. Some positive change is evident. This chapter therefore aims to highlight the priorities and direct designers to the fundamental issues, contemporary tools and guidance to assist and encourage implementation of very best practice. The case studies here attempt to highlight innovative approaches and best practice.

Thermal image of County Hall, London
Thermal photography highlights the parts of buildings where heat is escaping through poorly insulated elements such as windows, inadequate seals or thermal bridging
(Image: www.irtsurveys.co.uk)

Pollution – the global context

In most UK buildings, space heating and hot water account for the largest annual consumption of delivered energy and hence CO_2 emissions. The energy is most commonly generated from burning non-renewable carbon-based fuels – either directly or after conversion to electricity. The potential impact of the waste products of combustion – CO_2, SO_x and NO_x – has been known for decades. Carbon dioxide is a principal contributor to global warming and oxides of sulphur and nitrogen contribute to acid rain. The issue is far from new.

The predictions for global warming made in the early 1970s are not dissimilar to figures now accepted and used as the basis of policy setting. With rapid industrialisation and exploitation of fossil fuels in developing countries, it seems unlikely that a problem that could have been dealt with by the last generation can realistically be dealt with by the next. Ironically, at a time when many experts agree that climate change is inevitable, international governments have at last committed to address the problem. As part of this commitment, the UK aims to return CO_2 emissions to 20% below 1990 levels by 2010.

In order to achieve this target, it is vital that we improve the fundamental design of buildings, the efficiency with which energy is used in them and shift to cleaner fuel sources. Tackling existing buildings is a crucial part of the solution. Space heating and domestic hot water are primary targets for improved efficiency. Electricity is a particular cause for concern because of the inefficiencies in conversion. Other contributory technical

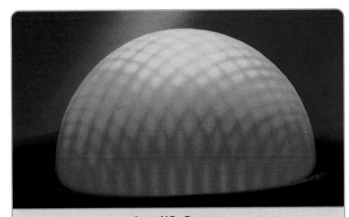

Low NO$_x$ Burner
Technology has advanced considerably to improve the efficiency of fuel burning and minimise pollution: clean burn technology winner of green product award 1995
(Photo: the author)

aspects such as ventilation and cooling are dealt with elsewhere, whilst critical issues such as location and the relationship to transport and amenity are dealt with under urban ecology.

If it is inevitable that the climate will change dramatically, a particular concern in the UK is that our dependence on the Gulf Stream means that we cannot predict the outcome. This does not justify inaction. As with many global issues, local impacts can be a determining factor in decision-making. Environmental improvements whether from the Clean Air Act, with its dramatic impact on health and well-being, radical reduction in heating requirements for buildings, or congestion-charging are historically resisted, but ultimately, extremely popular public measures precisely because they improve the quality of our lives locally. The next few decades will be interesting as we see the extent to which developing countries respond to such issues.

Minimising demand

A major contribution to reducing the adverse environmental impact of buildings is to be attentive to energy efficiency at the outset. Passive systems should always be considered for achieving energy efficiency prior to active systems and alongside life-cycle costing of other heating options. The tendency remains to seek answers in add-ons, with questionable payback and potential high maintenance, where more attention is required to physics, form and fabric, orientation, physical planning, massing, microclimate use/creation and to the possibilities for mixed use, which allow for overall better utilisation of space and energy.

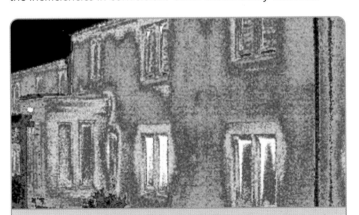

Thermal image of a house
Showing leakage through and around doors and windows and badly sealed edges
(Image: www.irtsurveys.co.uk)

Passive design

- *Form and fabric* – how can the building envelope minimise heating requirements?
- *Context* – how can infrastructure, orientation, layout and microclimate best be exploited?
- *Fuel* – what is the least polluting source of affordable energy?
- *System design* – what equipment offers the best opportunity for efficiency and good control?
- *Controls* – how can controls minimise heat requirements whilst maintaining comfort?
- *Management in use* – what tools are available to improve building management?

Integrated design is vital. Selection of materials, heating and ventilation should be considered together, as there may be implications for:

- indoor air quality
- management
- fabric
- long-term performance
- thermal response.

A healthy indoor environment should never be compromised. For example:

1 The ability of materials to deal with indoor moisture is important – especially in airtight constructions.
2 The choice of low-emission materials can affect the ventilation requirements in a building. It is an accepted trade-off under Norwegian building regulations.

> **Anecdotally, a Swedish friend claims that his zero-heated house was on the cold side until he had a housewarming party!**

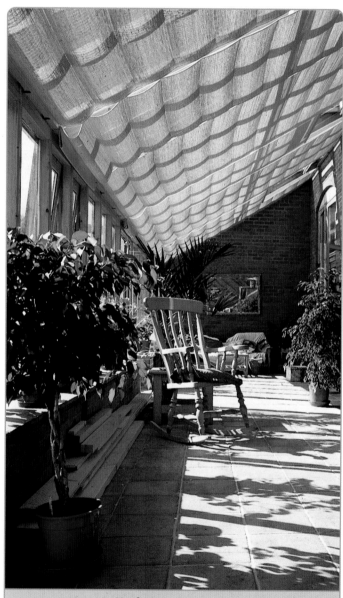

Hockerton Sunspace
Good examples of passive solar atria and sun spaces can contribute to thermal efficiency if appropriately designed, orientated and then managed. If not then they can overheat and lose more energy than they gain
(Photo permission: Hockerton Housing Project)

Form and fabric – how to minimise heat requirements

Good fabric design minimises the need for services, and hence running cost and adverse environmental impact. There is a need to consider thermal insulation, thermal mass, choice and location of openings, and quality of construction details.

Emslie Morgan's Wallasey School was the first notable UK building to seek a passive heating standard (albeit with an overemphasis on lighting inefficiency) and no-heating solutions have since been achieved in a significant number of commercial buildings, e.g. supermarkets and exhibition centres. These need to be judged on their genuine merits. In many of these it is the high levels of internal heat gains, including lighting, that meet all the heating requirements, and overheating is the biggest problem.

Energy use for domestic heating is being addressed by changes to the building regulations in the UK and by a series of voluntary codes of best practice, such as EcoHomes and the Code for Sustainable Homes. However, it is worth noting that we still lag significantly behind many of our neighbours.

Passive standard

The current move towards the passive standard (no heating), increasingly common in northern and central European housing design, is interesting. Such standards are increasingly specified in best European practice. German practice now incorporates a range of options (e.g. Energieplus and Minergie standard) and there are loan incentives for people to adopt the low standards. A significant number of houses are now being constructed to the Minergie standard, which takes into account occupancy patterns and body heat. Problems have been encountered where occupants' lifestyles are other than predicted or buildings simply don't perform as intended.

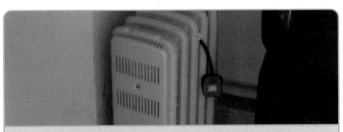

Under the stairs in a zero energy house
If passive / low energy houses are not well designed then occupants will take matters into their own hands
(Photo: the author)

Technical strategies that contribute to delivery of passive standard housing include:

- use of super-insulation
- airtight construction (pressure tested) with adequately controlled ventilation
- passive design incorporating solar layouts and perhaps stack ventilation
- consideration of internal heat generation.

Good-quality guidance is emerging, and designers, clients and builders are increasingly conscious of the need for contractual agreements and post-construction tests to tie down aspirations, because claims do not always stand up to scrutiny. Evidence from northern Europe indicates that occupants can, and do, undermine the design intention with heaters if they are too cold.

The challenge is to achieve a passive standard and deliver healthy indoor air quality. Ventilation is vitally important, and it requires attention to the materials specification and products to be vetted for their toxicity during their installation and use. The material properties relating to humidity control are of significance, as the humidity of indoor air is absolutely crucial to health in a tightly constructed building.

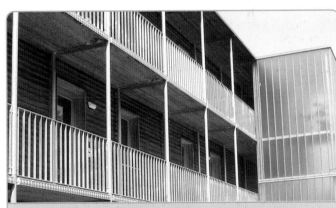

Oelzbundt housing, Austria
This project was one of the first apartment blocks designed to Minergie standards, requiring half the energy for heating of those designed to building standards. Despite problems with heating (they were estimated on the basis of internal gains by families but were occupied largely by single people with different occupancy hours and habits), they did stimulate other such projects and were fundamental in developing acceptability for the approach to be mainstreamed. Similar problems have been encountered in the first generation low energy houses – and if the heating is inadequate then residents will resort to high impact solutions (Photo: the author)

Thermal insulation

Thermal insulation is amongst the most cost-effective means of improving performance.

More insulation reduces the size of heating system required and delivers capital cost savings – to balance against additional insulation cost and running cost – during the building's lifetime. The location of insulation affects the thermal response:

- Internal. Structure is cold, leading to greater likelihood of interstitial condensation or frost damage. It can be avoided with extra ventilation and/or heating to raise surface temperatures, but with an energy cost.
- Interstitial. Risk of condensation or excess heat loss due to thermal bridging at openings or junctions with internal walls and floors.
- Composite structure. Fixing details are critical to avoid thermal bridging, particularly where masonry penetrates insulated components.
- External. Structure remains warm, with low risk of surface condensation. The full benefit of the thermal capacity is obtained.

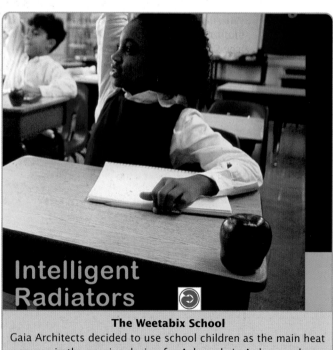

The Weetabix School
Gaia Architects decided to use school children as the main heat source in the passive design for Acharacle in Ardnamurchan
(permission: Mulberry Marketing Commnications)

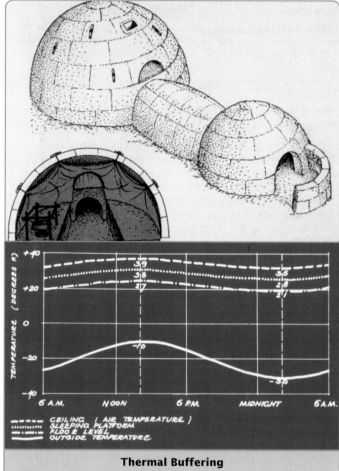

Thermal Buffering
Whilst the earth building described in Chapter 5 provides buffering against extremes of heat, the igloo provides buffering against extreme cold

Thermal response

Thermal response can be used to smooth out transient temperature variations. If a building is continually occupied or could be subject to high heat gains, it may benefit from being heavyweight. High thermal mass is especially valuable in reducing maximum summertime temperatures, thus avoiding or minimising the use of air-conditioning.

If an intermittent heating regime predominates, a thermally lightweight building would have shorter pre-heat periods and use less heating energy, provided that any tendency to overheat is well controlled.

Windows and glazing

The amount and type of glazing, and the shape, location and control of windows, is key to the effective control of heat losses and gains. When combined with good daylight it also provides architectural possibilities.

A robust solution is to use low-emissivity double glazing, with a heat loss equivalent to that of triple glazing and a light transmission of about 80%. Triple glazing is increasingly used as a selling point by developers, but to be justified it requires attention to build quality in other areas, such as airtightness.

Infiltration

Ventilation design is covered in a later chapter, but it is appropriate that infiltration – unwanted air leakage – is dealt with here. Infiltration is a priority area for all buildings. It has increased as a proportion of energy use as thermal insulation standards have improved.

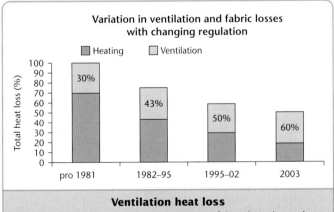

Variation in ventilation and fabric losses with changing regulation

Legend: ■ Heating □ Ventilation

Total heat loss (%)

- pro 1981: 30%
- 1982–95: 43%
- 1995–02: 50%
- 2003: 60%

Ventilation heat loss
With increasing regulatory attention to fabric heat loss, the proportion of heat loss due to ventilation has increased dramatically

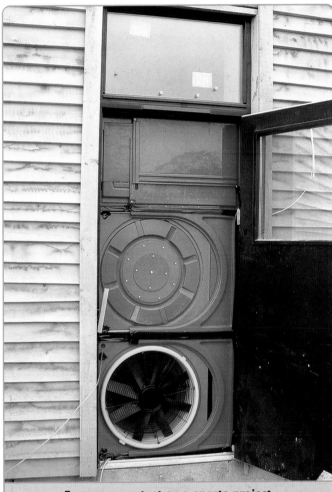

Fan pressure test on a sports project.
UK best requirements are almost a factor of ten more leaky than that required by the Swedish Body Heat Standard
(Photo: Paul Jennings)

Airtight construction is crucial to energy economy, building integrity and durability, but poor ventilation accounts for significant indoor environmental health concerns, so adequate ventilation to deal with moisture and indoor air pollutants is a vital aspect of design. Moisture travels in air and if air can reach surfaces within a structure at or below the dew point then it will condense, leading to problems of mould growth with the potential to adversely affect health.

A major development in Bergen is requiring 20% of houses to be built to a passive standard – known as the Swedish Body Heat Standard – such that no additional heat is required. This includes an airtightness standard of 0.4 air changes per hour at 50 Pa.

Case Study 7.1:

Okohaus, Frankfurt

Architects: Sambeth and Eble, 1992

The Okohaus cultural and business centre opened in May 1992. It is described by the architects Sambeth and Eble as *'an alternative example to Frankfurt's usual business premises, respecting ecological principles in its entirety and in its details, at costs not excessively above the usual'*. It is a modern design and uses traditional construction materials and methods.

It is situated near the centre of Frankfurt adjacent to a railway line. It is a 10 900 m² mixed use building built for a largely pre-existing mixed client group of 40 organisations, including a printer, doctor, dentist, various offices, restaurant and a kindergarten.

The building was conceived as a whole system in terms of building biology, heating/cooling, ventilation, water treatment, rainwater harvesting, air quality, etc. Care was taken in the material specification in order to scale down the services.

The basic construction is heavyweight, with 500 mm-thick solid brick walls and clay block floors, to reduce peak temperatures. The heavy mass building reduces peak temperatures. The glasshouse which encloses the south-facing aspect of the building captures passive solar energy, providing a bright circulation space. Reflective windows to the glasshouse reject solar energy from high angles. The heating consists of solar gain from the glasshouse and heat recovery from the printing works. The heat is distributed both via air circulation and through a low-temperature central heating system, fed by a heat pump and a back-up condensing boiler. It uses two conservatories, one to the north and one to the south, which are connected to either pre-heat or cool incoming air to the building as required.

The facilities manager reported the heat consumption as 70–80 kWh/m²/year and 25% of normal mains water consumption.

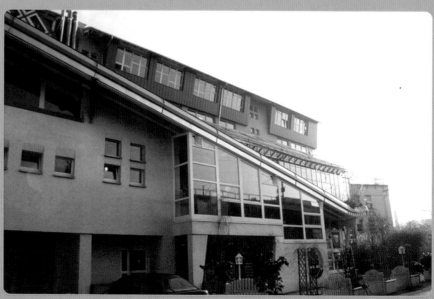

Photo: the author

Context – how a site can be exploited

Designs should avoid simply excluding the environment, but should respond to factors like weather and occupancy, and make good use of natural light, ventilation, solar gains and shading, in a beneficial way.

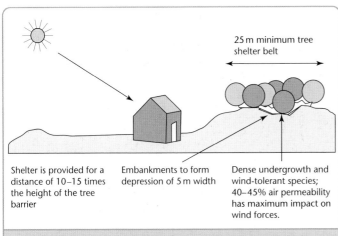

Shelter is provided for a distance of 10–15 times the height of the tree barrier	Embankments to form depression of 5 m width	Dense undergrowth and wind-tolerant species; 40–45% air permeability has maximum impact on wind forces.

Shelter provided by trees and topography
(From Liddell and Mackie, 1996)

Infrastructure

All major development is an opportunity for innovation in infrastructure. In a large development, reinvestigating the utility services to reduce demand for energy and power (and water and sewage) can reduce cost. A large development offers opportunities for district heating and to examine options for waste management and recycling, including using waste streams as fuel. Mixed use development is now recognised as good practice in many respects. It can significantly reduce travel times and increase social cohesion. Mixed use developments might also offer potential for energy outputs from one process to be used as inputs for another or provide flexibility in system selection, which is responsive to different patterns of occupancy than those of a single-use building. The chances to exploit the opportunities for sustainable resource use may increase.

Site selection

Site selection is a fundamental aspect of sustainable design. The nature of a site, its geography, topography, landscape, shelter, shading and surrounding buildings should influence the development of built form and services, sometimes in different ways on different façades. Issues include microclimate, orientation, protection from the prevailing wind, and optimum solar orientation to reduce energy requirements and to create outdoor spaces that are less exposed than they might otherwise be.

Local weather and microclimate

A building design should as far as possible respond to the local climate – for example, use local wind conditions to drive natural ventilation. Creation of a microclimate through the use of planted shelter belts and appropriate physical layouts can contribute savings of up to 15% on energy use and also improve amenity value by enhancing biodiversity, reducing the winds and the wind chill factor around buildings. It is difficult to assess in detail how wind will move through a site – but it can be modelled effectively at scale. It is reasonably commonplace in Scandinavia for models to be tested in a wind tunnel and minor adjustments to the massing of buildings to be made based on the findings. Matters such as the distance apart and the scale and density of trees in courtyards and adjacent to houses to lift wind can be dealt with at this point, and layouts optimised.

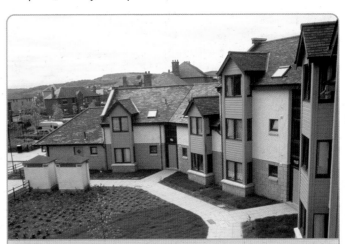

Affordable Housing, Leslie Court, Fairfield, Perthshire
Modern solar design – solar energy is a driver of massing, form and layout, and space planning for individual and groups of buildings, but not to the detriment of urban design
(Architects: Gaia Architects; photo: Michael Wolshover)

Case Study 7.2:

Grünberg House, Ullapool

Architects: Gaia Architects, 1996

The building has a timber-frame structure, and all windows, doors and finishes are in timber. A combination of wind and hydropower was supposed to give the building self-sufficiency in energy, whilst the design makes optimum use of passive solar warmth through a curving sun-trap form.

A composting toilet was pioneered and the building employs local and natural materials such as Scottish timber and slate, and has vapour transfusive construction and healthy internal finishes.

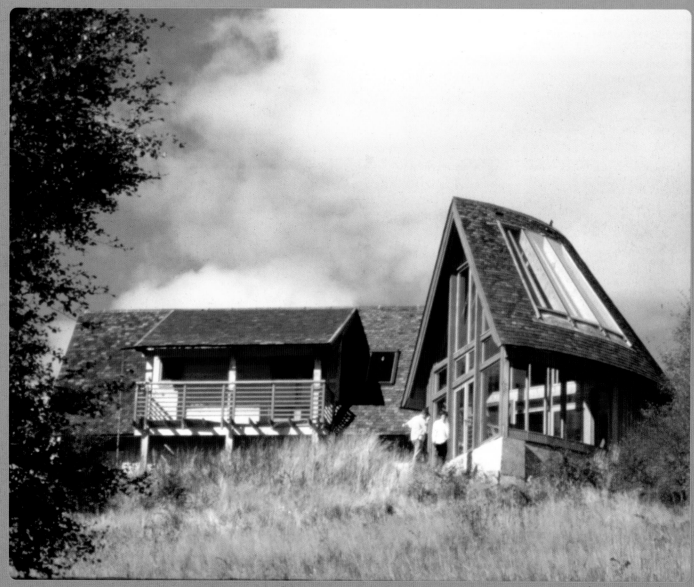

Photo: Gaia Architects

Solar spaces

Good examples of passive solar atria and sun spaces can contribute to thermal efficiency if appropriately designed, orientated and then managed. If not, then they can lose more energy than they gain. The tradition in the UK is for solar spaces to be heated and used as an additional space all year round, whereas the European tradition is for seasonal use.

Designs should respond to weather and occupancy, and make good use of natural light, ventilation, solar gains and shading, in a beneficial way. In the school in Norway illustrated special attention was given to external comfort, with a south-facing sheltered play area.

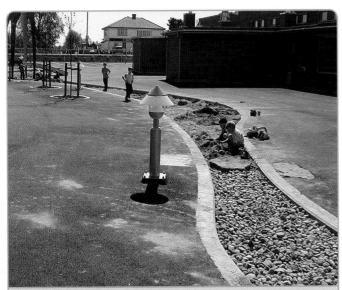

Sand river in sheltered playground, Øserod School, Norway
The plan was such that external comfort is maximised in the playground area and shielded to north, east and west by the classrooms (Photo: Howard Liddell)

Building orientation

Planning requirements, local and national by-laws, fire protection requirements, noise and air pollution may restrict the shape and orientation of a building, so as to adversely affect its energy performance. Notwithstanding any constraints, the designer should select the optimum orientation to meet the operational requirements – utilising winter solar gain when this is beneficial and minimising winter heat loss.

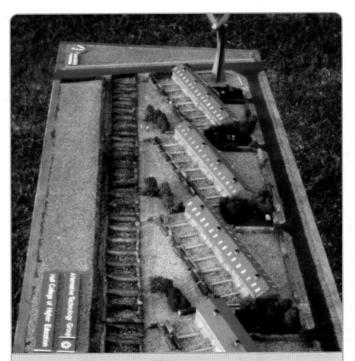

Hull Terraces
Project led by Howard Liddell at Hull School of Architecture in the 1970s to optimise building orientation
(Photo: Howard Liddell)

Massing and energy efficiency

Using compact building forms with relatively small exposed surface area for a given floor area can reduce the influence of weather and keep services distribution systems to a minimum.

Terraced housing and apartments are intrinsically more thermally efficient than detached dwellings, as they share walls. Theoretical studies and measured feedback have established the value of grouping buildings together for energy conservation, and this is common practice in most of Europe. In the UK, we build significantly more detached houses, in part because of unreliable acoustic performance, a problem that should be readily resolvable. Taller constructions can increase energy consumption due to greater exposure and the need for lifts. Many towns and cities are successfully developing the combination of high quality with high density.

However, the expectations of those moving to new housing may not concur with what might be emerging design solutions based on practical and technical sustainability criteria.

Case Study 7.3:

Elizabeth Fry Building, University of East Anglia

Architects: John Miller + Partners, 1995

The Elizabeth Fry Building at the University of East Anglia (occupied 1995) was only the second UK building to use the Swedish Termodeck ventilated floor slab system to provide year-round tempering of fresh air and enhanced levels of useful thermal capacity.

The building consists of 3130 m² of treated floor area over four floors with cellular offices, lecture and seminar rooms, and two dining rooms. The ceilings on all floors are constructed using the Termodeck hollow-core concrete slab.

The services strategy required:

- A good building envelope to provide stability and minimise heat losses and gains.
- Hollow-core, ventilated concrete floors slabs with exposed soffits to provide better radiant conditions in the room and heat transfer with the ventilating air.
- 'Trickle-charge' mechanical ventilation via the cores to achieve stable year-round internal conditions, with added heat if needed in winter and night cooling by outside air in summer. There is no mechanical refrigeration.

By using the building as a thermal flywheel and the ventilation system as a trickle charger, the designers felt no need to use perimeter heating. Further simplification and enhanced efficiency were achieved by using separate direct, gas-fired water heater for the kitchens and the main toilets, plus small electric immersion heaters for individual toilets.

The air temperature does not vary more than 0.5°C over the year, due to the thermal stability of the concrete slabs. Best practice recommendations for gas heating of naturally ventilated offices is 79 kWh/m²/year (97 kWh/m²/year for air-conditioned offices). The Elizabeth Fry Building has a gas consumption of only 30 kWh/m²/year.

With the use of heat recovery in the AHUs, the design heat loss fell to only 15 W/m², which is met with 50% standby/reserve capacity by three domestic, gas-fired condensing boilers.

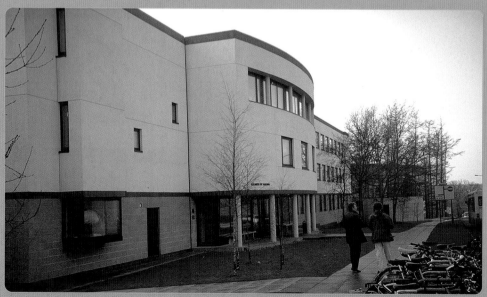

Photo: Bill Bordass, William Bordass Associates

Fuel – the least polluting sources of affordable energy

After attention has been directed to using form, fabric, good detailing, efficient construction and the local environment to full effect to minimise heat demand, then it is important to investigate the most appropriate fuel source for the residual space heating and domestic hot water demand.

Gas and oil produce lower emissions to the atmosphere for each unit of delivered energy than electricity, making electricity, in general, the least preferred option for heating. A zero-CO_2 emission option is to use active solar energy for hot water, wind energy and/or biofuels such as woodchip, waste, straw or paper. Renewable energy technologies are dealt with in Chapter 11.

Passive solar heating

Passive solar heating can contribute significantly to heating requirements, particularly when a building is designed with this in mind, although the economics require careful assessment.

Passive solar heating contributes to space heating requirements in a relatively small number of buildings in the UK. As a general principle, passive solar energy should be exploited wherever possible. It should be available to every house and make a contribution to heating needs in schools and other buildings as long as conflicts with overheating do not exist. For many buildings solar ingress has the additional appeal of excellent light quality and the connection to outdoor spaces.

In general, commercial and school buildings need to exploit solar heat in the winter but provide external shading in summer. This is due to improvements in fabric, which make overheating a major consideration. A major source of cooling demand in leaky 1980s offices is the unwanted ingress of external warm air.

Ground heat

The earth as well as the sky can be used as an energy source. The earth attains a constant temperature (the annual year-round air temperature) at only a small distance below the surface. Although inadequate in its own right to provide sufficient heat, this can provide insulation through berming or part building underground – the underground houses. Passing air through underground culverts can provide a source of pre-cooling in summer and pre-heating in winter.

Fossil fuels

Where heating demand cannot be met passively, or through renewable generation, then the environmental best practice is to use gas for heating where it is available in preference to grid electricity. This is now fully incorporated into the Building Regulations, which look to primary energy consumption. More options are also emerging to purchase electricity with a higher renewable context from the grid.

900	
1000	
1150	
1250	
1300	

Solar map (kWh/m²/year falling on the UK)

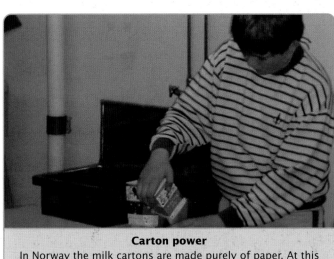

Carton power
In Norway the milk cartons are made purely of paper. At this school milk cartons are collected, folded to form neat bricks and delivered to the local energy plant in exchange for lottery tokens
(Photo: the author)

Case Study 7.4:

Hockerton Housing Project, Nottinghamshire

Architects: Brenda and Robert Vale, 1997

This terraced development comprises five earth-sheltered, single-storey houses, each 122 m², plus a conservatory area of 47 m². For much of the year, the conservatory is a habitable space. It is proportioned and glazed to maximise solar gains, and uses high levels of insulation and thermal mass to reduce heat loss and to store heat gains. The use of double and triple glazing is conventional by northern European standards. The strategy to bury the house in the ground – a client request – further insulates the house from annual exterior temperature swings.

Space heating was not provided and no energy, other than solar and casual gains, is used to provide thermal comfort. The high thermal mass construction stores and releases heat energy over a long period of time and maintains a stable internal temperature.

Two-hundred millimetre concrete block internal cross walls on a 300 mm concrete slab, a concrete beam-and-block roof and 500mm-thick external walls of two skins of concrete blockwork were used as formwork to contain mass concrete. Walls, slab and roof are insulated with 300 mm of polystyrene, with the mass on the inside of the insulation. The roof is covered with 400 mm of topsoil, and the north side and terrace ends are buried in the ground. Each house is 6 m deep with a 19m-long façade facing south. The rooms have 3m-high French windows, which are triple glazed with low-e glass and argon filling. All rooms open to the conservatory, which is glazed with double low-e glazing.

The thermal performance of the houses was monitored in year 1 of occupancy (Energy Efficiency New Practice Profile 119). Under normal occupancy the internal temperature has not dropped below 17°C. Typical temperatures in houses during winter are 18–20°C. There are minimal draughts and fabric temperatures are similar to that of air. Typical summer temperatures are 22–23°C, and the houses are kept relatively cool by the thermal mass and glazing, self-shading and use of passive ventilation in conservatories.

The residents generate their own clean energy, harvest their own water and recycle waste materials, causing minimal pollution, including CO_2 emissions. The houses are amongst the most energy-efficient, purpose-built dwellings in Europe, and use 25% of the energy of a new-build house.

The construction was managed by a professional builder whose expertise was an evident factor in the standards achieved in the building work and infrastructure. A small core of external workers were used to support project members, which ensured adequate understanding and training was provided for many elements of the build. However, relying on a limited pool of workers did result in some significant delays with the construction.

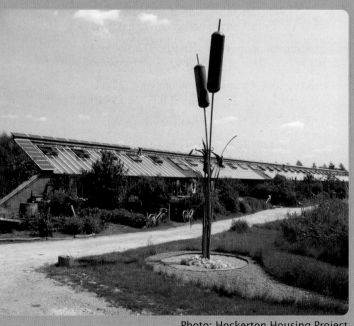

Photo: Hockerton Housing Project

System design – efficient and controllable equipment

After first and foremost reducing the heat demand, and then appraising the options with respect to fuel supply, it is necessary to consider the most appropriate and efficient technology with which to deliver the residual heating requirement. With efficient heat distribution systems and controls it becomes more cost-effective to choose low-carbon options, typically more expensive than traditional carbon fuels. A full option appraisal should consider all the possibilities, and focus on the most efficient, economic and practical combination.

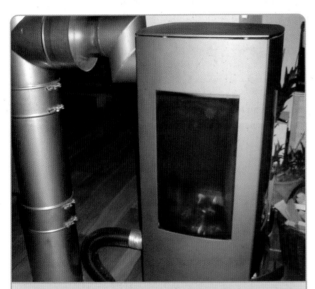

Meeting very low heating demand presents a real challenge to the design of heating systems. Europe is the best source of slow burn, low output biomass boilers that feature excellent turn-down ratios
(Photo: the author)

Recently, conflicts have become evident as designers reduce the heating demand of houses to levels at which central heating is not necessary and challenge social expectation. Also, at low levels of heat requirement alternatives to central heating can be more expensive in capital or maintenance costs, and heat distribution at low levels of overall demand is difficult. There are few small boilers. A small number of super-insulated buildings have incorporated a wood-burning stove as the heat source, but it is unlikely that this would be widely acceptable as a solution.

The use of ambient heat or heat recovery systems should be an early consideration but, if not well designed, these can shift loads to electrical consumption, which works well in a context of hydro-power – which is why this is more common in northern Europe – but less well with the UK fuel mix. Systems are discussed under renewable energy in Chapter 11.

Where buildings are designed with very low heating requirements using high insulation levels and good airtightness standards, then active renewables can become the major provider of heating. Waste incineration, biofuels, wind, wave bio-gas and hydroelectric schemes can all be considered at the design stage. Other possibilities include district heating schemes based on a renewable fuel such as waste or woodchip. A number of demonstration schemes have been supported in recent years and the possibilities of funding support, as well as genuine benefits from life-cycle costings, should be investigated.

Combined heat and power (CHP)

If heat demands are significant, then it is worth considering the potential for CHP to contribute to a solution. Typically, heat exchangers reclaim waste heat from exhaust gases and other sources during the electrical generation process, and this can then be used to provide hot water throughout the year and heating during the winter. It is possible to achieve efficiencies of 80% if a system is optimised. Economic viability is dependent on intensive use and the demand for heat. It is most attractive where electricity is expensive and gas is cheap, but maintenance has to be considered as a significant factor. CHP requires more maintenance than conventional boiler plants. Detailed energy demand profiles for both heat and electricity are fundamental to accurately sizing CHP and hence its viability.

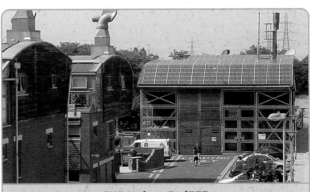

CHP Unit at BedZED
The housing at BedZed is built to need very low heating demand. This is supplied as a small coil from hot water storage
(Architect: Bill Dunster; photo: the author)

Equipment: boilers

European legislation (1997) forced manufacturers to increase efficiency of heating appliances.

There are roughly three categories of boiler:

- Basic (traditional) non-condensing: 77–80% efficient.

- High-efficiency non-condensing: 80–82% efficient – generally low water content and/or low thermal mass with improved heat exchangers and insulation.

- Condensing: 85–92% efficient (depends on system design) – generally gas fired and with an extra heat exchanger to extract heat from the products of combustion. In systems designed with low return water temperatures, such as underfloor heating, they can achieve year-round efficiencies of over 90% by taking heat out of the flue gases. This makes water condense out of the gases and also the gases are less buoyant. In standard radiator systems they can achieve seasonal efficiencies of 87–88% if controlled using weather compensation.

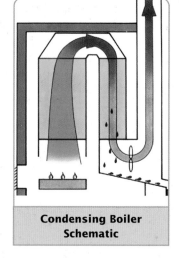

Condensing Boiler Schematic

Multiple boilers can improve energy efficiency and increase the options available for supplying heating and hot water. These may comprise an integrated package of modules or independent boilers, including CHP. A number of small boilers enable a good match between output and demand. They spend more time at full load, with improved seasonal efficiencies. Careful sequence control is fundamental.

Using condensing or high-efficiency boilers will reduce CO_2 emissions. They have good efficiencies at the part load conditions at which the heating plant operates for most of the time. They are typically 10–25% more expensive than traditional boilers. However, the energy savings often provide a payback within three to five years. They should be sized carefully as over-specifying will generally reduce seasonal efficiency and increase capital cost. Condensing and non-condensing boilers should be mixed to maximise efficiency at optimum capital cost. The most efficient plant takes the base load, with less efficient equipment taking the remainder and operating as standby.

Heat pumps

Heat pumps transform low-grade heat from water, the ground or waste into higher grade heat. They do this through the input of energy, usually electrical energy, at an efficiency referred to as the coefficient of performance (COP). They can produce high COPs when operating at low temperature differentials. They have found wide use in applications where low-grade heat is available – for example, where low-grade process heating is being dumped, or for ventilation extract heat recovery such as in swimming pools and supermarkets.

Ground source heat pumps and ground water heat pumps are becoming more common, particularly in rural applications, and are being considered for groups of housing.

When used to provide heating only, the COP of heat pumps does not usually compensate for the increased financial and environmental costs of using electricity to drive them, because the cost of electricity and its carbon content are three to four times that of gas that can be used directly. Where there is sometimes a need for cooling at different times of year – for example, in retail outlets with high heat gains – reversible heat pumps can be a cost-effective way of providing both cooling and heating.

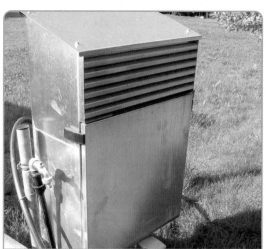

Inlet – Textile House, Austria
The inlet to the culvert for the textile house is 20 cm diameter, 25 m long, and embedded at least 1.2 metres deep with 40 cm sand around it.
The quality of the inlet air is important so the culvert slopes at a minimum of 2 degrees to allow cleaning (Architect: Unterrainer; Photo: the author)

Case Study 7.5:

Shettleton Housing Association, Glasgow

Architects: John Gilbert Architects, 1997

The L-shaped layout creates a safe access and semi-private children's play area in front of the south-facing, three-storey block of flats. The varied housing mix of one, two and three bedrooms includes convertible loft spaces, barrier-free standards and internal flexibility, and promotes the concept of lifetime housing.

It has high insulation standards (wall: 160 mm Warmcel cellulose; roof: 300 mm Warmcel cellulose; floor: 75 mm polystyrene).

The airtightness of the dwellings allows for pre-heated ventilation using a small fan, which pressurises the houses slightly. The air intake is through the void between the roof tiles and sarking, which reduces draughts as well as providing solar pre-heated fresh air using very simple and cheap technology. Draught lobbies are glazed and provided to the front and rear doors of the houses, creating additional amenity space as well as a thermal buffer to the main building.

Extensive planting and external structures around the buildings have been introduced to provide microclimate modification and thereby to minimise heat loss through the fabric by reducing wind velocities.

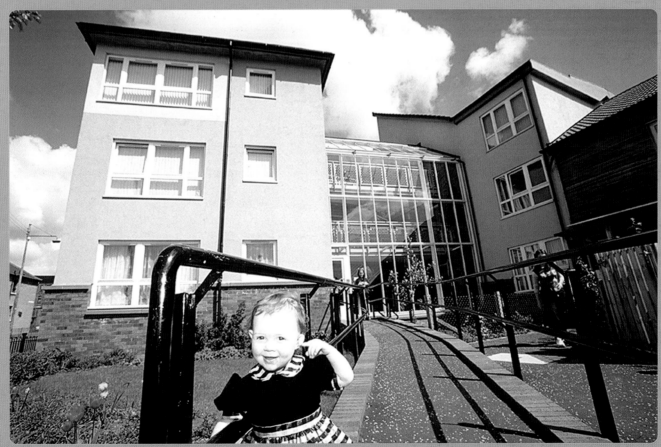

Photo: John Gilbert Architects

Controls – minimise heating and maintain comfort?

If adequate attention is not given to providing good controls, then it will not be possible to capitalise on the gains that result from good passive design and the selection of appropriate fuel and equipment to meet residual needs.

All heating systems should:

- have controls which operate systems efficiently, safely and economically
- allow individual occupants to alter their own comfort levels
- avoid systems defaulting to 'on'.

The key requirement is to provide heat and hot water only when and where it is needed, and at the right temperature.

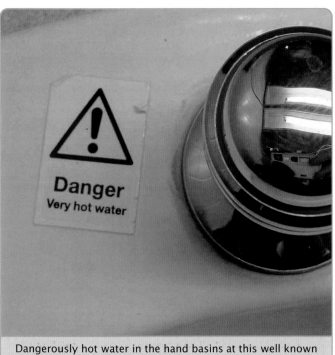

Dangerously hot water in the hand basins at this well known London society headquarters isn't just dangerous, it's a waste. Especially when there is an expensive wind turbine on the roof (Photo: the author)

Good circuit design

Good circuit design is fundamental to the efficient operation of controls. A constant water flow is normally required for modern boilers. As variable flow is created by the action of manual and automatic valves, most applications require a separately pumped secondary circuit with a common header or buffer vessel. This avoids interaction between circuits, enables the return temperature for the primary circuit to represent the load on the system and permits return temperature control of multiple boilers.

Boiler sequence control

Boiler sequence control is essential for maximising efficiency in multiple boiler installations. It matches the number of boilers firing to the load, minimises the number of boilers firing and avoids short cycling of burner operation.

Fixed time controls

A timeswitch provides a simple, robust and easily understood means of saving energy by turning heating off when not required. Weekday/weekend or seven-day timers are commonly available to allow different on/off times at weekends, etc.

Optimum start/stop controls

Optimum start/stop controls vary the heating system start-up time depending on the weather, so as to achieve a required temperature by a required time. Heat-up times are reduced during milder weather, saving energy. Optimum stop facilities turn boilers off when the resulting temperature fall-off will still allow the required temperature to be met at the end of occupancy. This means they close down earlier on mild days. The greatest energy savings are likely to be in lightweight buildings and with heating systems of low thermal capacity.

Temperature controls

Thermostats are a low-cost means of minimising consumption and maintaining comfort levels. Reducing room temperature by 1°C can reduce fuel use by 10%. This can be achieved using simple thermostats in many buildings, and only when buildings are complex will Building Energy Management Systems (BEMS) be required.

Weather compensation controls

Weather compensation controls provide a link to external temperature. In mild weather, a system operates at lower temperatures, thus saving energy. It is a standard form of control for condensing boilers, as it provides low return temperatures in mild weather and hence higher efficiency.

Night setback controls

Night setback controls reduce the temperature during a given time period and are often part of weather-compensating controls. They are particularly useful in continuously occupied buildings – for example, in elderly persons' homes – allowing a minimum temperature to be maintained and providing energy savings compared with continuous operation. Generally, it is more economical to switch the heating off at night with a low limit to bring it back on.

Zone controls

A successful control system allows independent time and temperature control on a zone-by-zone basis. Zone control is normally achieved using thermostatic radiator valves (TRVs) or motorised valves linked to room thermostats/timers. Larger buildings might have separate north and south zones.

TRVs

TRVs provide a low-cost method of local control of individual heat emitters, particularly where there are high incidental gains. TRVs are essential if solar gains are to be taken advantage of. They should preferably be used with variable-speed pumps to provide good control. Lockable tamper-proof heads are recommended in non-domestic situations. These can either be completely locked on one setting or provide a minimum level of control for occupants.

Motorised valves, room thermostats/timers

Motorised valves and room thermostats/timers provide independent temperature and/or time control of a zone – for example, by varying the room temperature at different times of the day. It is best used in areas with a small group of emitters, say totalling over 5 kW.

Sensing locations are better than TRVs and a wider range of emitters can be controlled. Programmable room thermostats are a convenient way of achieving this, as they combine the roles of timeswitch and electronic room thermostat. Larger zones should be weather compensated and have optimum start/stop controls, particularly to allow for differences in activity, internal gains and solar gains on different façades.

Management tools

One could argue that sustainable design is easy but sustainable management is more difficult. In truth, sustainable design cannot ensure optimal efficiencies, only seek to make these more difficult to undermine. As in many aspects of heating design, guidance is almost overwhelming.

Guidance is often sector based, with published indicators of energy performance broken down into elements such as heating and lighting. These can provide a basis for internal review and comparison, but in all aspects of environmental performance it is vital that an initial commitment is made at high level to review a company's facilities management and maintenance arrangements, school energy budgets or household energy consumption, and to establish options with regard to funding progress. Energy management can be, and often is, little more than tariff management. Care should be taken that decisions lead to real environmental and cost benefits. An environmental strategy for facilities management need not rely on a bureaucratic structure of high-calibre people. An initial impetus, generated perhaps through a review or audit mechanism, can establish a management and financial strategy for improvement based on life-cycle costs and environmental impact. In every case an initial review carried out by competent personnel will provide a good starting point and benchmark from which to progress.

Guidance documents like the *Environmental Code of Practice* and the *Green Guide to the Architect's Job Book* were written with a life-cycle approach to building management in mind. They provide a strategic framework and good indicators to best practice guidance in many areas, including heating.

Case Study 7.6:

Leith Academy Secondary School, Edinburgh

Architects: The City of Edinburgh Council, 1991

The design is planned with maximum flexibility and versatility in mind. It has a glazed main street, extensive planting, seats and a street café. There are community facilities and a swimming pool used by both school and community. Secondary streets, also glazed, run at right angles to the main street and provide independent access to each department. The blocks of accommodation between the streets have a clear span, with bays each side of a glazed barrel-vaulted spine at the apex above the 2.4-m-wide circulation zone. Sometimes this zone is incorporated within a room and sometimes it is a 'corridor', but all are well lit. Solar gain occurs and exposed solid, dense concrete blocks dampen the response of the fabric to thermal swings. To minimise overheating in summer, a series of additional ridge vents have been included in the streets. These are thermostatically controlled.

The main secondary streets have facing blockwork insulated cavity walls, roofed with patent glazing, which incorporates automatically opening sky-vents. Automatic opening louvres in secondary street doors allow the stack effect to operate to cool the streets. Windows have hardwood frames and are double-glazed. Intumescent foam in the main street glazing provides a fire barrier.

Dynamic energy simulation of the building was part of the in-house design process. Still-line natural convection units are supplemented by warm air ducted from the air-handling units located at high level in the main north–south street. The streets have partial underfloor heating, the residual heat from the overnight kindling of the coal-fired boilers. The heating and ventilation are controlled by a central BMS system linked to the Council's Department of Property Services. Fresh air supply rates can be reduced in the heating season. Fresh air can be used for free cooling in summer using the supply air fans. The swimming pool has CHP and a heat recovery system.

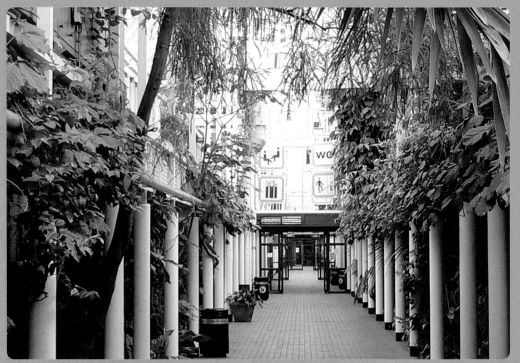

Photo: Howard Liddell

Heating rules of thumb

To architects, heating may appear to involve little more than heat emitters – more or less visible. To engineers, it can seem well-trodden territory with little creative opportunity. To quantity surveyors, perhaps, it is an area of early resolution and cost predictability. All of these perceptions are open to question.

Architectural design can have major implications on reducing heating demand without loss of comfort and with benefits to internal spaces. The challenges for engineers are significant, especially where they touch upon the work of other disciplines or the wider context. Lifecycle costing offers real opportunities to justify investment in effective long-term solutions. There is much to learn.

There are few universally applicable solutions, because of dependence on building type and context. However, what follows is intended to raise awareness of the issues and possible approaches that building professionals can use to improve sustainability in heating buildings.

- Decide whether it's strategic, specific, sectoral or solar guidance – or simply inspiration – you want and go find it!
- Do design the building structure and the building services as integrated functions.
- Try starting from an assumption of no heating and work backwards to find out what is really needed.
- Do design-out or minimise heating using high levels of insulation.
- Do not just assume the building regulation figures – take time to assess and calculate the real 'U' value and thermal response, and hence the space heating needs.
- Minimise air infiltration.
- Do use water-efficient fittings, such as spray taps and shower heads. Less water, less heat.
- Do make use of low water content plants. Less water, less fuel.
- Do look closely at hot water generation. Many systems are designed around large central storage with circulation. Can it be done more efficiently in another way? For large loads look at CHP.
- Do try and eliminate 'over-engineering just to be on the safe side'.

- If you've been in this business a while – be up to date.
- Formalise a complete and clear design brief to ensure that the operational needs are understood and can be taken into account at the outset. If designing an office, for instance, look at the level of free heat which can be offset against the total heating requirements.
- Do think about heat reclaim systems. Simple air-to-air heat exchangers can save energy if used in the right manner.
- Do make the client aware of how the system is expected to work, and how to use it correctly to meet real user needs.
- Do make clients aware that the system is designed to operate under set criteria and that, if neglected, these criteria change and the system becomes inefficient. Effective maintenance of the system is mostly forgotten.
- If possible, introduce self-certification of the energy efficiency of buildings on a three- to five-year period to show that the system and the efficiency are being maintained.
- Do look carefully at the possibility of buying energy that has been generated in a sustainable manner, such as wind, wood and geothermal sources. Can they be effectively used to provide all or part of the heating requirements?
- Do ensure that what is specified is what is installed, i.e. if you have specified a particular boiler on the grounds of its efficiency, then make sure the boiler installed is the same in all areas.
- Do not cut corners on quality – it costs.
- Watch out for operational anomalies, like summer heating.
- Consider using variable-speed drives in conjunction with TRVs to provide excellent control without the need for BMS systems.
- Use atria as a heat recovery/buffer space, e.g. pre-heating incoming fresh air or passing exhaust air through the atrium on its way out of the building.
- Do use condensing boilers where possible, particularly in low-temperature heating systems.
- Control the return temperature and ensure maximum condensing.
- Where there is a large base load demand for heat, then use CHP. This is the single biggest CO_2 reduction measure that can be achieved.
- Do use variable-speed pumps to match pump speed to demand.
- Ensure that time and temperature controls are installed with weather compensation and optimum start/stop controls where applicable.

Case Study 7.7:

Swimming baths, Ingolstadt, Germany

Swimming pools are unlike any other building type. They epitomise, in many respects, fundamental issues at the core of the sustainability agenda, which need to be balanced.

Most communities want easy and inexpensive access to a swimming pool bigger than they can sensibly afford. As they can make a significant contribution to the social adhesion and health of a community, they are highly desirable in a broad sense.

However, they are extraordinarily expensive to maintain and run, both in respect of the services systems but also the building fabric.

They are open most times of the year for long hours, require large amounts of warm water for pool water and washing, have high temperature (30°C air), and humid air which demands constant good ventilation.

Energy costs are consequently very high and to be sustainable a great deal of creative energy is required to make swimming facilities financially sustainable. As a consequence, there is a wealth of good-quality guidance on all types of energy-saving opportunities, including heat recovery, variable volume ventilation and the application of CHP, which, often in combination with boilers, is a cost-effective option and can deliver 35% savings in primary energy use.

Seventy per cent of the heat requirement of swimming baths is for warm air. The year round requirement for an air temperature of 30°C makes heating the air of the swimming baths an ideal situation for the active use of solar warm air heating.

The otherwise excess solar energy in summer can be used. Air collectors operate at any outside temperature, and heating air from 0 to 15°C in midwinter saves as much energy as heating from 20 to 35°C. At Ingolstadt, 350 m^2 of air collectors achieve a peak power of 235 kW and yearly efficiency of 67%. Measurements show energy production of 250 MWh for the heating periods 1991/92 until 93/94.

The cost of the system was about 200 000 DM, of which about 140 000 DM was for the collectors, 30 000 DM for the construction and 30 000 DM for peripherals. With a life expectancy of 25 years, the investment costs are 14 200 DM per year assuming an interest rate of 5%. The energy saved would have cost about 16 000 DM.

Solar radiation

Heated air

Building wall

Plenum

Outside air

Perforated absorber

Transpired collector

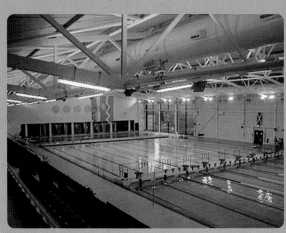

Photo: the author

Bibliography

There are thousands of publications covering aspects of heating for buildings. There are many imaginative approaches and an abundance of case study publications. The reader should also investigate the technical press for contemporary projects literature. The following bibliography includes a few documents that cover many of the important and interesting aspects.

Guidance and research output

Building Research Establishment – www.bre.co.uk.

Carbon Trust – www.thecarbontrust.co.uk.

Construction Information Service – http://products.ihs.com/cis.

Gaia Group – www.gaiagroup.org

PROBE Studies – www.usablebuildings.co.uk.

Background and case studies

Vale R. B. (1991) *Green Architecture – Design for a Sustainable Future*. Thames & Hudson.

GIR 38/39 (1996) *Review of Ultra-Low-Energy Homes*. BRECSU. Profiles of low-energy housing.

von Weizacher, E. and Lovins A. L. (1997) *Factor 4 – Doubling Wealth and Halving Resources*. Earthscan.

Stevenson, F. (2007) *Sustainable Housing Design Guide*. Scottish Homes. Coverage of housing-related issues, including heating.

Planning

Liddell, H. L. and Mackie, A. (1996) *Energy Conservation and Planning*. Scottish Office Central Research Unit. All aspects of physical planning from building layouts to microclimate and density.

Design – airtightness, BRE, SEDA

CARL (undated) *Energy and Environment in Non-Domestic Buildings*. Cambridge Architectural Research Ltd (www.carltd.com/pubs.asp). Coverage of passive design issues.

GPG 79 (1994) *Energy Efficiency in Housing*. BRECSU.

Halliday, S. P. (1994) *Environmental Code of Practice for Buildings and their Services*. BSRIA. Services-based process guidance on all aspects of building design from inception to demolition/or refurbishment.

CIBSE Guide (1998) *Energy Efficiency in Buildings*. CIBSE.

Equipment

BSRIA Technical Appraisal 1/90 (1990) *Condensing Boilers*. BSRIA.

GIR 40 (1996) *Heating Systems and their Control*. BRECSU.

GIR 41 (1996) *Variable Flow Control*. BRECSU.

GPG 176 (1996) *CHP in Buildings*. BRECSU.

CIBSE AM12 (1999) *CHP in Buildings*. CIBSE.

CIBSE Guide H (2000) *Building Control Systems*. CIBSE.

Energy management

CIBSE AM5 (1991) *Energy Audits and Surveys*. CIBSE.

EEO Econ 19 (1991) *Energy Efficiency in Offices*. BRECSU. The benchmark document on energy consumption in offices.

GIR 12 (1993) *Energy Management Guide*. BRECSU.

CIBSE TM22 (2006) *Energy Assessment and Reporting Methodology*. CIBSE. With benchmark data on energy consumption in some building types.

Refurbishment

Housing Façade Renovations – 10 New Overcoats. (undated) Danish Ministry of Housing and Building.

IEA (1997) *Solar Energy in Building*. James & James.

GIR 46 (1999) *Energy Efficiency in Scottish Housing Association Refurbishment Projects*. BRECSU.

Solar energy

Gould, J. R. et al. (1992) *Energy in Architecture: The European Passive Solar Handbook*.

DFEE (1994) *Passive Solar Design of Schools*. Building Bulletin 79. DFEE

IP5/01 (2001) *Solar Energy in Urban Areas*. BRE.

Hockerton Housing Project www.hockertonhousingproject.org.uk/

Chapter 8
Electrical installations

(with thanks to Clive Beggs, for his contribution to the original)

In which we investigate issues concerned with electrical energy and electrical equipment, and how careful design of electrical installations can contribute significantly to reduction in pollution of the local and global environment.

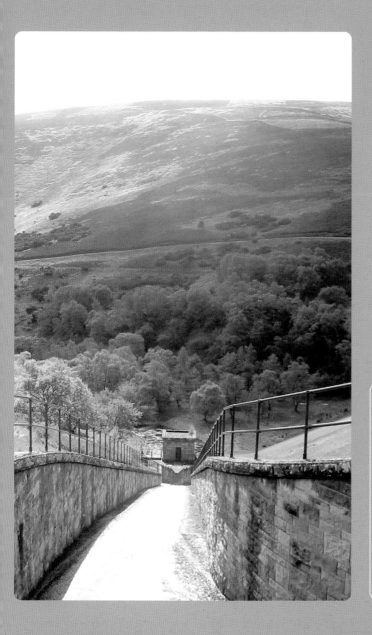

'For every six hours that a 20W energy-saving bulb is used in preference to a 100W bulb it saves its own weight in oil.'

From Factor 4 – Doubling Wealth and Halving Resources

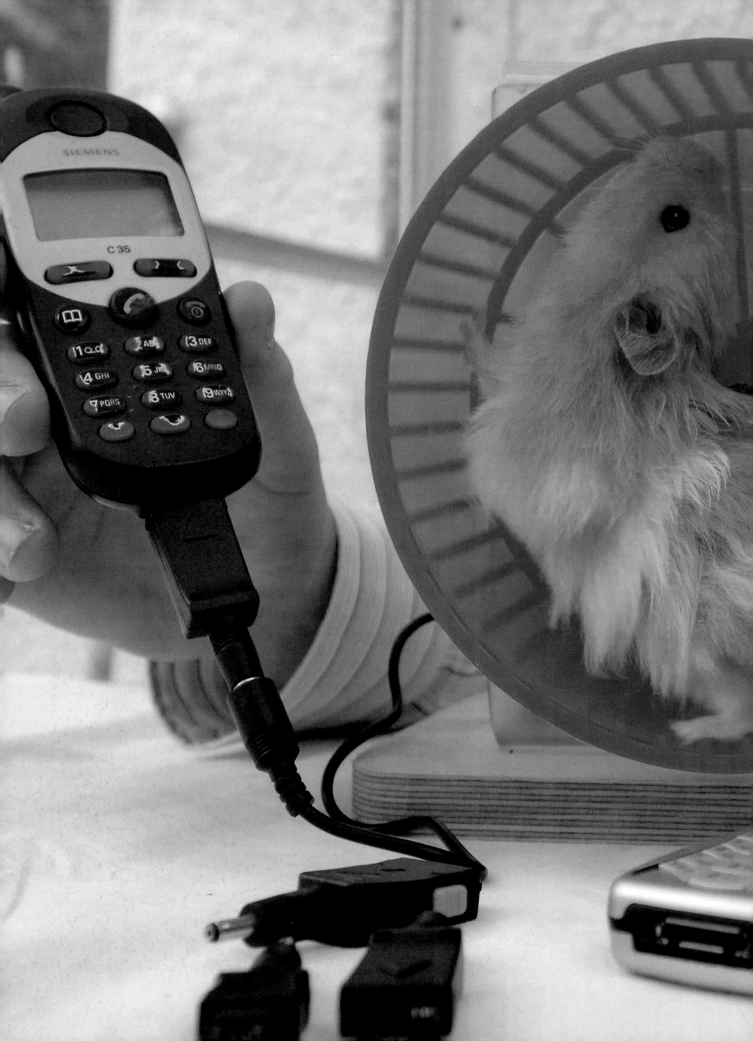

Contents

(Facing page)
**Elvis the hamster-powered
phone charger**
(© EMPICS)

(Previous page)
Hydro-electric scheme, Scotland
(Photo: the author)

Electrical installations

Introduction

Practically everybody, certainly every building design professional, is familiar with the idea that energy is an issue, and that we somehow need to control the way we use it to meet limits on environmental pollution that are subject to international obligations. There is real and justifiable concern about the rate at which we are utilising non-renewable fossil fuel resources to meet our electrical needs and generating pollution. There are also concerns about the alternatives, the unacceptable risks and cost of nuclear energy, and our ability to develop adequate sources of clean renewable technologies.

However, there is still far too little attention given to the simple techniques, appropriate behaviour and usage patterns that could deliver much needed and readily achievable efficiencies. There has been a lot of attention given to supply-side issues of renewable energy, but this is against a background of rising energy consumption, particularly electrical energy.

Environmental issues related to electrical energy are not restricted to CO_2 pollution. This chapter also looks at issues such as health, materials and transportation surrounding electrical generation, price, sourcing, equipment and control of pollution.

Other chapters deal with aspects of electricity: lighting (Chapter 9), ventilation and cooling (Chapter 10), renewable energy (Chapter 11) and some technologies are covered in heating (Chapter 7). However, electricity is of significant importance, and insufficient attention, to justify focus in its own right.

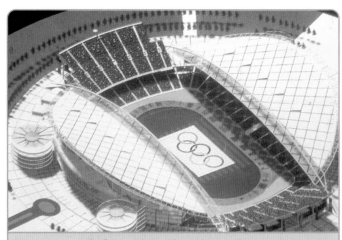

Sydney 2000 Olympic stadium
The multi-use arena had no PVC in the seating, cabling, floor coverings, wall finishes or plumbing

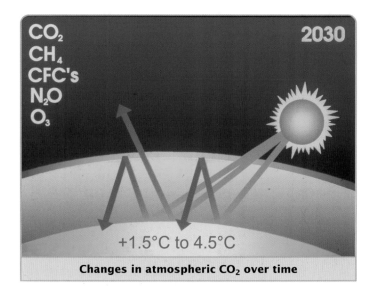

Changes in atmospheric CO_2 over time

Background

The thermal performance of buildings has been subjected to a good deal of study so that the energy used for heating can be minimised. Electricity in buildings, however, has received much less attention and yet it represents the major part of the carbon emissions from buildings and often a significant proportion of their running costs.

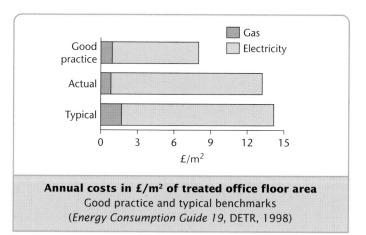

Annual costs in £/m² of treated office floor area
Good practice and typical benchmarks
(*Energy Consumption Guide 19*, DETR, 1998)

Electrical energy can be up to five times as expensive as the unit cost of heat, and significantly more polluting, yet much of it is needlessly wasted through neglect, standing losses, and poorly designed and maintained services, including controls. Increasingly, it is the electrical consumption that vastly exceeds design estimates because of lack of attention to fan power, pumps, IT and lighting controls.

Excessive use of electricity has implications for infrastructure, hence capital as well as running cost, and it also has visual implications. It is the demand for electricity that powers the debate over wind farms!

There are also significant end-of-life issues in relation to waste volumes and embodied pollution in electrical equipment, and there are significant and unresolved health implications in use. If it were not for the fact that it supplies many of our most basic needs and allows us to meet many of our aspirations, there would be little good to say. The question therefore is whether we can meet these needs and aspirations whilst minimising pollution, waste and health hazards. There is evidence of change.

Control of waste and pollution is increasingly embodied in European legislation, and concerns related to health impacts of electromagnetic fields (EMFs) have led to design solutions for those who wish to err on the side of caution for themselves or their clients. The growing interest in ecological impact means that there has been some diversification in product development, and greater opportunities now exist for benign material specification and more efficient appliances. Simple changes in behaviour and the selective use of a number of relatively simple controls and technologies, applied to motor drives and lighting, can greatly reduce costs and the adverse environmental impact of electrical installations.

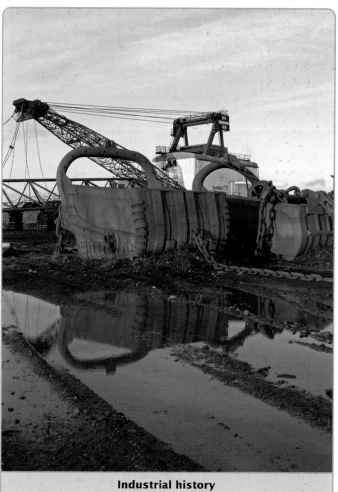

Industrial history
Our history of coal mining to feed our demand for power has left the marks of industrial heritage on the landscape
(Photo: Michael Wolshover)

Case Study 8.1:

Variable-speed drives (VSDs)

(after Clive Beggs)

One of the reasons why the energy consumption associated with fans and pumps is high in many buildings is the traditional approach to pipe and ductwork systems. Generally, they are oversized and then – at commissioning – valves and dampers are added to control the flow by increasing the system resistance. An alternative approach is to control the flow rate by using VSDs. These ensure that even if fans and pumps are oversized, energy consumption will not be greatly increased. But VSDs cost money.

As a first step in deciding whether a VSD installation is likely to be cost-effective, it is sufficient to calculate the simple payback period in years (Table 8.1).

If the simple payback look attractive it is worthwhile calculating payback in more detail.

Typical discount factors and predictions on energy pricing give an effective interest rate of about 15%. Assuming a life of 10 years gives a Present Worth Evaluation factor (PWE) of 5.0:

The Present Worth Evaluation factor (PWE)

PWE x PW x D x H = 5 x 0.05 x 5700 = 1430

for D = energy cost (£/kWh),

H = annual operating hours

NPV = Power x PWE = 30 x 1430 = £42 910

compared to a cost of £13 500

This makes the installation of a VSD one of the most cost-effective energy efficiency measures with payback of less than two years quite common.

Expected power saving	30 kW	
Annual operating period	5,700 hours	
Present electricity cost	5.0 p/kWh	
Annual financial saving	30 x 5,700 x 0.05	= £8,500
VSD installation	£13,500	
Payback period	£13,500/ £8,500	= 1.6 years

Table 8.1 Simple Payback Calculation

Basics

There is some misunderstanding about basic concepts in energy. In everyday language, the word 'energy' is used very loosely. Work, power, fuel, heat and energy are often used interchangeably and incorrectly. Energy can take a variety of forms: electrical energy, mechanical work and heat. It can be converted between these various forms. For example, a fossil fuel can be burnt to produce heat energy in a power station. The heat energy produced is then converted to mechanical energy by a turbine, which in turn produces electrical energy through a generator. Finally, the electricity is distributed to homes, offices and factories, where it can be converted to mechanical work using electric motors, heat via resistance elements and light using electric lamps. The losses in conversion and transmission are immense.

The difference between energy and power

In order that a machine can raise an object, it must expend energy. Whether the object is raised in one second or one day makes no difference to the energy required. But more power is required to raise an object quickly than to raise it slowly. Power, therefore, is the rate at which energy is expended or consumed. Energy is power multiplied by time. The kilowatt-hour (kWh) is commonly used as the unit of energy in the electricity supply industry. It refers to the amount of energy consumed in one hour by the operation of an appliance having a power rating of 1 kW (1000 W).

The difference between work and heat

1 Energy cannot be destroyed. You can exchange one kind of energy for another, but the energy inputs are always equal to the energy outputs.
2 Not all energy is the same.
3 Heat is one kind of energy.
4 Work is another kind of energy.

5 Work energy and heat energy are equivalent (first law of thermodynamics).
6 You can turn work energy completely into heat energy, but …
7 You cannot turn heat energy completely into work energy (second law of thermodynamics).
8 An unavoidable consequence of generating work as electricity is the creation of heat, which is mostly rejected as waste.
9 It is therefore generally agreed that electricity should not be used to provide heat which could be provided by burning a fuel directly.

The difference between voltage and current?

Water at high level will flow to the ground through a pipe. Similarly, electricity always flows from a higher voltage to earth (i.e. 0 V). Electrical current, measured in amps, is analogous to the flow rate of water in a pipe. The higher the voltage, the greater the flow of current. A large current requires a large-diameter electric cable, just as a large flow of water requires a large-diameter pipe. Multiplying voltage by current gives power.

The difference between three-phase and single-phase electricity

When electricity is generated in a power station, three separate alternating electrical currents are sent simultaneously down three separate conductors. Each of these separate currents is known as a phase and they are colour-coded red, yellow and blue. Due to the mechanics of the electrical generation process, the three separate currents are 120 degrees out of phase with each other. Many individual 240 V single-phase currents can be drawn from a single three-phase supply cable by 'tapping' into the respective conductors.

It is normal practice to supply small buildings with single-phase electricity cables whereas, for larger commercial and industrial buildings, three-phase cables are usually supplied because it is a more efficient means of distribution.

Case Study 8.2:

Water balance lift at Machynlleth

Centre for Alternative Technology

The entrance to The Centre for Alternative Technology in Machynlleth, sited as it is in a steep quarry, gave rise to issues of access. The traditional high-power requirements of a lift system were resolved by installing a water **balance lift. A pond at the site provides a focal point and a bio-diverse rich habitat. On demand it provides water to balance the weight of two funicular type trolleys which run on demand between the car park and the site.**

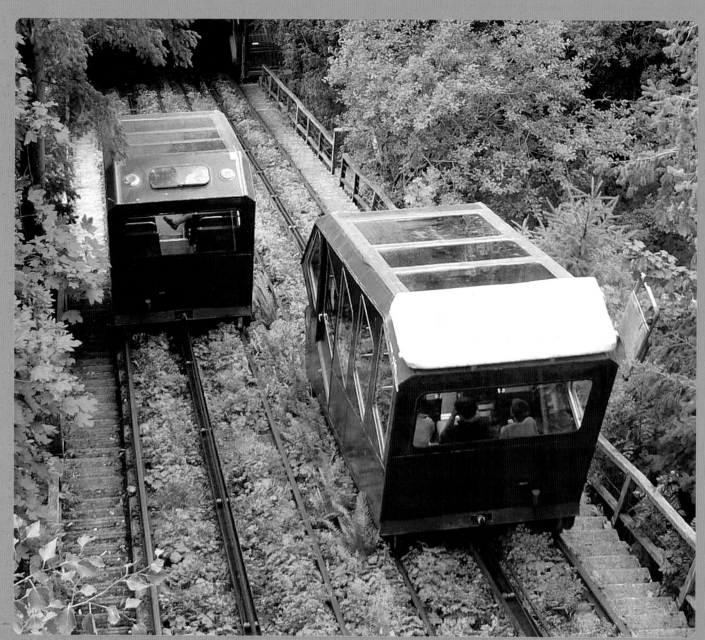

Photo: the author

Electrical generation

Electricity generation can utilise a wide variety of primary energy sources, including gas, oil, coal, nuclear, wind, wave, tide, sun and hydro.

The difference between primary and delivered energy is important. Electricity is often a secondary fuel, produced by inefficient conversion. For each unit of electricity delivered to a customer, several units of primary energy are consumed. This is reflected in the price, which must cover the primary fuel plus maintenance, transportation and management.

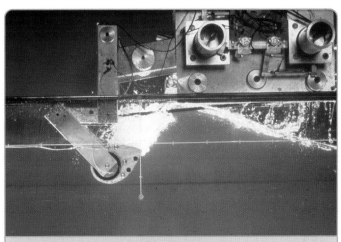

Wave Power
Small-scale model of the Edinburgh Duck, or Salter Duck, being tested in the narrow tank at the University of Edinburgh during the late 1970s
(Photo: Jamie Taylor, University of Edinburgh)

Fuel generation	Typical efficiency (%)	CO_2 produced (kg/kWh)	Special issues
Coal-fired power station	34	0.938	Produces sulphur emissions which are expensive to remove.
Oil-fired power station	36	0.819	Ditto
CCGT power station	43	0.431	Cheap to build, slightly more efficient and no sulphur emissions. However, it uses a premium fuel.
Nuclear power station	34	0.005	Huge life cycle costs & long term radiation & security problems.
Hydro-electric power station	90	0	Relies on geography.
Wind turbine	41	0	Good at large scale & increasingly seen as making a substantial contribution to the grid.

Table 8.2 Features of various common electricity generation technologies (2001) after Beggs

Microgeneration

Microgeneration is the production of electricity and/or heat, with low or zero carbon emissions, on a small scale. It represents a 'bottom-up', decentralised approach to energy consumption and presumes that generation is near to the point of use. It thereby removes the problem of loss incurred by the transportation of electricity over long distances. Grid connection – if available – allows for optimisation of size and cost with excess electricity exported and sold to the grid, or imported at times of peak demand.

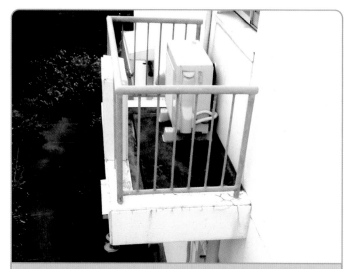

Overridden design intent
Every apartment in this same Japanese eco development has installed air-conditioning on the balcony (which was intended to be for airing clothes, as an energy efficiency and health measure)
(Photo: the author)

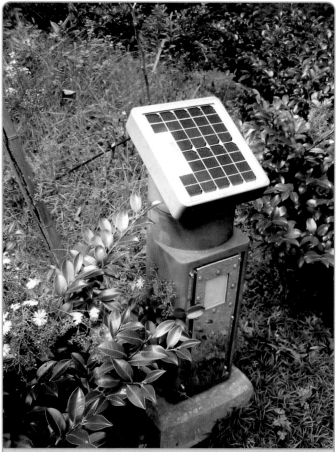

Eco-development Japan
Electricity generation from photovoltaic panels is still hard to justify commercially other than for small power in remote locations. Many examples are tokenist and cannot be justified against improvements in system efficiency
(Photo: the author)

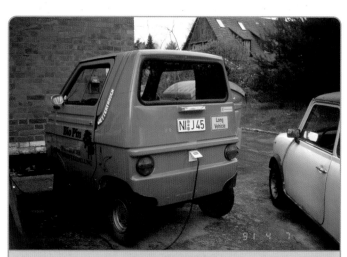

Electric Car
The 60-house eco-village of Lebensgarten at Steyerberg in north Germany has a fully integrated energy policy. The default output setting of the PV array is for charging the batteries in the village's shared electric car
(Photo: Howard Liddell)

Thermal generation

Most of our electricity is generated from conversion of primary fuel via thermal energy. A traditional thermal power station burns a fuel to heat water to make high-pressure steam, which turns a turbine and a generator to make electricity. The steam expands in the turbine and loses pressure as it cools, giving up energy to the turbine. It is a complex, wasteful and costly technique that involves the construction, operation and maintenance of large power stations. Interestingly, it is a result of legislation that was intended to ensure that converting heat into electricity was undertaken as efficiently as possible. Even so, most conventional thermal power stations have efficiencies of only 30–37%. The remaining two-thirds of the primary energy consumed is wasted, and dumped as heat, as the steam is condensed with cool water from a cooling tower.

Heat rejection

Heat rejected in cooling towers in the UK is about enough to provide for all our heating needs. Whilst this is a travesty, it is also not easy to resolve because demands for heat and electricity do not correlate. Very little heating is required during the summer, whereas the demand for electricity (particularly with increase in air-conditioning) produces a considerable amount of waste heat. In winter the electricity demand is not directly related to the outside temperature, whereas the heating demand is. Also, there are infrastructure problems in taking the heat is charged by electricity generation and using it directly.

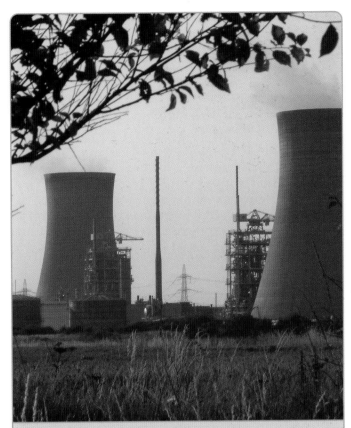

Thermal generation – Drax steam power station, Yorkshire, UK (Photo: Ian Franklin)

CCGT

The 'dash for gas' resulted from a new piece of technology, combined cycle gas turbines (CCGT), in which the energy in a flame at a very much higher temperature than the energy of steam could be used directly in a gas turbine to make electricity. But even with a gas turbine it is not possible to take all the heat out of the flame, and so the residual heat is used to make steam, to drive a turbine, and cooled down using cooling towers as before. The overall thermal efficiency of a CCGT power plant is still only about 43%. The introduction of CCGT has helped us to meet our Kyoto targets, but we are burning a premium fuel utterly inefficiently and then delivering further inefficiencies at every stage from transmission to end-use.

Case Study 8.3:

Westfield Biomass Plant, Fife

Billed as a waste disposal solution which has electricity as one of its main by-products, the plant is used to dispose of 110 000 tonnes of poultry litter per annum. It is the first plant in Scotland to generate electricity from biomass, and the first in the world to use advanced fluidised bed combustion technology for burning poultry litter.

The design of the boiler ensures complete combustion of the fuel and low emissions. The products of the plant are 10 MW of electricity and 11 000 tonnes of ash/per annum, which is sold as a fertiliser rich in phosphate and potash. The combustion process kills any pathogens that might have been present in the poultry litter, and which would normally have ended up on the land.

The Scottish Environmental Protection Agency (SEPA) has recently stepped up pressure to reduce the land spreading of poultry litter, and this plant plays a significant role in doing so. Electricity is sold under a Scottish Renewable Order (SRO1), with the plant providing a base load of renewable electricity to the grid, with enough capacity to supply over 20 000 homes.

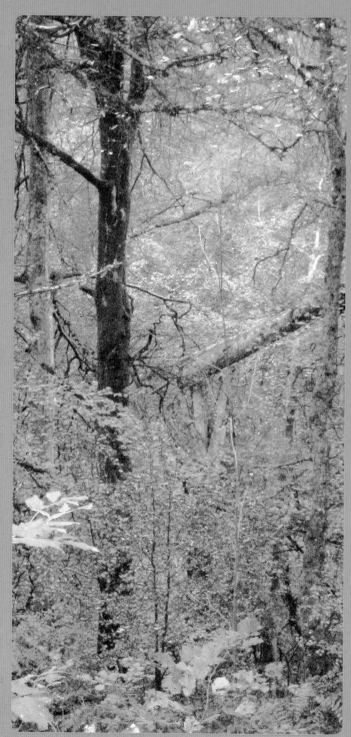

Photo: the author

Nuclear power

Nuclear power stations generate heat by controlled nuclear reaction to feed a steam turbine installation. The radiation control problems associated with nuclear power remain unresolved, with too frequent lapses. The storage issues remain uncertain, the security issues including transportation are self-evident and the life-cycle costs are so immense as to make privatisation non-practical. With such an immense combination of unanswered questions in respect of security, pollution, adverse effects on biodiversity, health risks and life-cycle management, it is hardly conceivable that nuclear technology can meet the requirements of a sustainable future.

Torness Nuclear Power Station
The decision to build a nuclear power station on the East Coast of Scotland led to huge protests in the 1960s, with protesters using straw bales to scale the construction work fence
(Photo: Howard Liddell)

Diesel engines

Diesel engines are interesting because the flame generates the pressure in a cylinder, which then expands and does work to generate electricity. Reciprocating engines are slightly more efficient because the metal is only exposed to the hottest flames for one stroke in four, so that a very high start temperature can be maintained.

Combined heat and power (CHP)

One way to avoid the waste associated with electrical generation is to collect and use the waste heat from the process. By combining the electrical generation and heat production processes it is possible to produce a highly efficient CHP, or co-generation, system which makes good use of primary energy.

CHP is normally rated on its electrical output (kWe). In most buildings the CHP plant is in packaged units – less than 500 kWe – run on natural gas, biogas or diesel. The high efficiencies, over 80%, are much greater than conventional power stations, reducing the amount of primary energy required to meet a heat and electrical load.

Economic viability is heavily dependent on the demand for heat and the price of electricity and gas, and has to be assessed on a project-by-project basis. In general, to achieve a simple payback of four to five years, a CHP unit must operate for 4500 hours per year or about 12–14 hours/day. As with condensing boilers, CHP should always operate as the lead boiler sized on the base load to maximise savings. A payback of three years would require operation at 6000 hours per year. Usually, these shorter paybacks can only be achieved where there is a significant demand for heating and hot water – for example, in hospitals, hotels or swimming pools. However, CHP can also be used to provide the heat source for absorption chillers to supply cooling and there have been a number of successful applications.

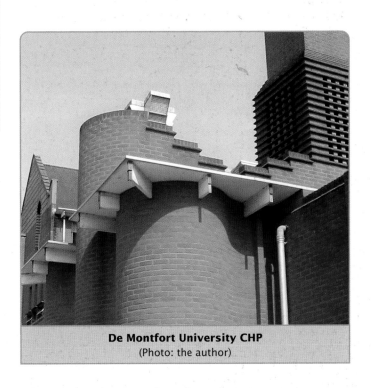

De Montfort University CHP
(Photo: the author)

Case Study 8.4:

Queen's Building, De Montfort University, Leicester

Architects: Short Ford Architects, 1994

The Queen's Building has academic facilities for about 100 staff and 1500 students in the School of Engineering and Manufacture at De Montfort University, Leicester. Occupied in 1993, it is of particular interest for its day lighting strategy and its innovative use of natural ventilation, with its distinctive ventilation stacks. The 9850 m² (gross) building has three distinct areas: the central building, the mechanical laboratories and the electrical laboratories.

The heating for the building comes from a 38 kW (electrical output) combined heat and power (CHP) unit, a condensing boiler and two high-efficiency boilers. The CHP unit has priority, so that it operates for as long as possible – maximising its effectiveness. The unit's installation was justified on the grounds of teaching demonstration and research.

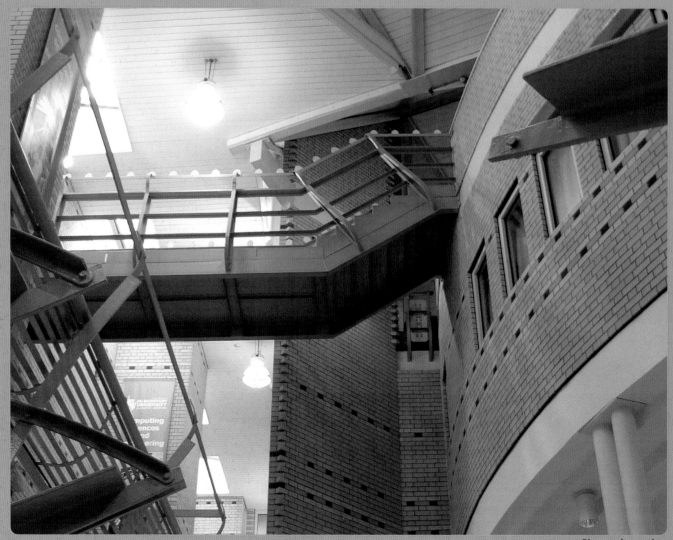

Photo: the author

Renewable generation

Renewable generation is in a phase of rapid expansion. Major investment is under way. The UK target is to achieve 5% of UK energy supply from renewables in 2003 and 10% by 2010. Scotland's current target is 18% by 2010.

A recent report identified a total renewable energy resource in Scotland of 59GW, three-quarters of the UK's total installed capacity. The report also concluded that all of it, including relatively expensive off-shore capacity, could be produced at less than 7p per unit by 2010 (excluding grid strengthening costs). Wind accounts for more than half of the potential, followed by wave and tidal power.

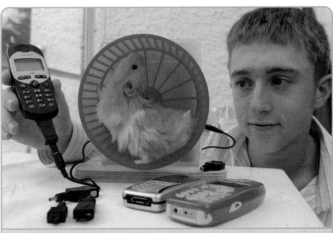

Elvis the hamster is the power source for these mobile phones (© EMPICS)

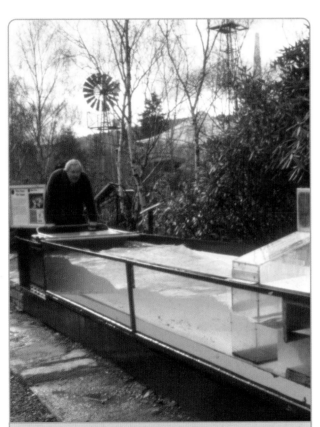

Miniature wave machine
The Centre for Alternative Technology has a wide range of practical demonstrations of renewable technologies and sustainable building techniques
(Photo: the author)

AC/DC

Increased generation of direct current (DC) electrical energy from renewable energy sources, such as photovoltaic cells, inevitably raises questions about the choices to be made between alternating current (AC) and DC systems and circuits in buildings. Grid connection of renewable energy, for storage, sales and much household equipment requires a conversion from DC to AC – called 'inverting' – and involves expense of extra equipment and inherent energy losses. Increasing numbers of electrical goods run off DC – phones, computers, radios – and require transformers in order to operate from AC supply. Converting back from AC to DC is called 'rectifying' – and involves blocking either the positive or negative portion of the waveform using a diode – and introduces further losses and cost.

Recent research into introducing DC low-voltage distribution systems into buildings concluded that appliances now work at a range of different voltages. Hence they are liable to need voltage conversion from AC or DC supply! Like the issue of standby, efficiency of AC/DC and DC/DC conversion appears to be a crucial area for joined-up delivery.

Case Study 8.5:

Withy Cottage, Herefordshire

Self-build: Nick Grant, Elemental Solutions, 2001

Withy Cottage is a low-energy, self-built house. As an experiment the occupants lived without mains electricity during the build period, which forced ultra-efficient use of electricity. Where possible these efficiency lessons have been transferred to the main building.

- PVC-free cables
- Minimised phantom loads
- Switched 5A sockets on lighting circuits
- Optimised lighting (fittings, location and room colours)
- DC extract fans
- DC wiring for LED accent lighting
- Efficient computer (iMac)
- Photovoltaic (PV)-powered solar thermal system
- No central heating
- No low-voltage halogen lights
- 'A'-rated white goods
- No answer machine – BT 1571 Call Minder.

Despite the attention-grabbing PV and wind, the owners are committed to an ecominimalist approach, with emphasis on efficiency and design. On the equipment side this means careful choice to minimise power, energy and phantom loads. On the design side the need for artificial lighting has been minimised by careful choice and placement of fixtures. Warm paint colours create a pleasant ambience with little light, despite the large open-plan living space. Switched 5A sockets allow task and standard lamps to be turned off with a single switch when leaving a room. Low-voltage halogen spotlights are banned.

Domestic solar hot water complements the wood stove for hot water and uses a PV powered pump. The washing machine is A-rated for energy and a switched spur above the worktop allows it to be switched off completely when not in use. The cooker is dual fuel and the cowl is a simple passive stack with manually controlled damper. Most cables are LSF but some flex and earthing are PVC, as these were stock items. The bathroom extract fan is a through-wall Baxi heat recovery model. It runs on 2 W standby and 20 W boost. The boost is switched by a thermostat on the hot water pipe to the shower. The design gives several minutes run-on, which can be adjusted by altering the amount of insulation around the thermostat. Electricity use for the first two months' occupancy (December and January) has averaged 3.9 kWh/day.

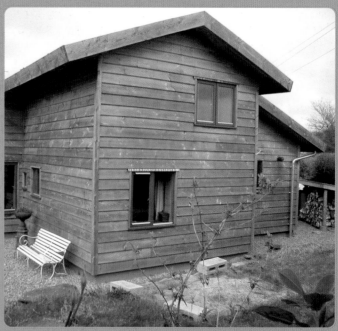

Photo: Nick Grant

Reducing use of electricity

What do we use electricity for?

Electricity is used to:

- power electrical equipment – computers, cookers, televisions, kettles, etc.
- provide artificial lighting
- power mechanical plants, such as fans, pumps and refrigeration compressors
- provide heating!

In many large buildings the electrical services are often provided by different specialists, yet decisions made by lighting designers and mechanical services designers heavily influence electrical energy consumption. If poorly designed, the knock-on effect of oversized fans, pumps and refrigeration chillers results in oversized electricity cables, distribution panels and transformers, and consequently high capital and operating costs. The specification of white goods is also an important consideration. There is an increasing range of opportunities to reduce energy and power at the design stage.

Standby power

Standby power for electrical equipment – sometimes called leaking electricity or phantom loads – is the electricity consumed by appliances when they are switched off or not performing their primary function. Standby power consumption is an increasing fraction of the world's energy use and is thought to account for between 5% and 15% of power used in homes in OECD countries.

A typical household in Britain is using the equivalent of 50Wh of standby electricity, with equipment in sleep mode using roughly 7TWh of energy and emitting around 800 000 tonnes of carbon. This is the equivalent of wasting around two power stations' worth of electricity each year by leaving TV sets and other gadgets on standby.

The issue of standby consumption, as with other demand-side issues, is rarely fully addressed. Yet designing buildings with photovoltaic installations without addressing widespread and avoidable standby losses (fax, cordless phone, hi-fi, photocopier, cooker clock, wall clock, answering machine, TV, computer) is common, very expensive and clearly misguided.

The International Energy Agency has received an award for its efforts to cut worldwide electricity losses from appliances in standby mode. Their campaign aims to guide government policy-makers and appliance manufacturers towards equipment that consumes no more than 1W when in standby mode.

However, many of the better ones have been forced off the market and typical standby consumption is now 5W.

Lighting

Designing efficient lighting and mechanical services installations will invariably reduce the costs associated with electrical services, and it should be a priority to reduce oversizing. Lighting installations based on low-wattage fittings and good controls are amongst the most cost-effective energy efficiency measures.

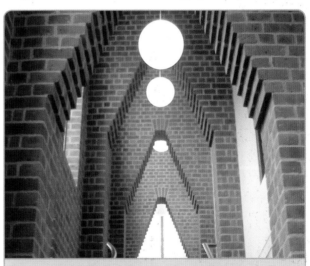

Good daylighting needs good control
Daylighting is one of the most cost-effective, energy-efficient measures when artificial lighting is controlled and integrated (Photo: the author)

Variable-speed drives (VSDs)

The traditional approach to pipe and ductwork systems has been to oversize pumps and fans at the design stage, and to correct this during commissioning using valves and dampers to control the flow by increasing the system resistance. While mechanical constrictions do control the flow, they increase the system resistance, which results in increased energy loss as well as unnecessary capital expenditure. This is one of the main reasons why the energy consumption associated with fans and pumps is high in many buildings.

An alternative approach to the use of valves and dampers is to control the flow rate by varying the speed of fan and pump motors. VSDs ensure that even if fans and pumps are oversized, energy consumption will not be greatly increased. This makes the installation of VSDs one of the most cost-effective energy efficiency measures.

Minimising the use of ducted mechanical ventilation systems

The traditional approach to air-conditioning is to provide a ducted system in which fans operate at a constant speed throughout the year. It is generally the case that much larger volumes of air are required to cool spaces than for pure ventilation. So an all-air system has large fans and airhandling equipment, in large ceiling voids. The duct and fan sizes are determined by the peak summer condition, which may last only for a few hours. The rest of the time the fans push large volumes of air around needlessly, and electrical energy consumption on air handling is higher than it need be. A contemporary space- and cost-efficient alternative is to use a cold surface (chilled ceilings or beams) to perform the cooling, and to use a reduced size air system for the ventilation and latent cooling roles. By using low air velocities (1–2 m/s rather than 5–6 m/s), it is possible to achieve substantial reductions in fan energy consumption.

Power factor (the ratio of true power/apparent power)

Electrical equipment can broadly be divided into two categories: those which impose a resistive electrical load, such as heating elements and tungsten filament lamps; and those which impose a reactive load, such as induction motors and fluorescent lamps. With reactive loads the current and voltage are out of phase, and the apparent power consumed is always greater than the true power that they can use. To differentiate between true and apparent power, true power is measured in watts (W) or kilowatts (kW), and apparent power is measured in volt amps (VA) or kilovolt amps (kVA).

Much of the electrical equipment found in buildings is reactive and hence buildings often have low power factors (PFs). Values of 0.7 or less are common. This means additional running costs, and oversizing of generators, switchgear, cables and transformers is necessary because of the need to draw a larger current than would be anticipated. It is therefore beneficial to ensure a PF as close to 1 as possible. Induction motors are used to drive fans and pumps, and cannot be avoided, but they should be selected with care. The PFs of smaller motors are not as good as those of larger ones but, because the PF varies with the motor loading, it is usually better to use a smaller motor than to under-load a large motor. It is possible to correct a poor PF by installing capacitors in a central bank before the main distribution panel, or on individual items of equipment. The latter is generally preferred, except in large installations, as this reduces the current and the losses in all the wiring leading to the item of equipment. It is possible to use banks of capacitors which automatically switch on and off in order to maintain an optimum PF.

Heating

To be avoided unless there is very good reason, such as local renewable generation or health issues like those associated with products of combustion.

Management in use

Regular auditing is a crucial element in improving electrical efficiencies. The high cost of electricity means that it is often an obvious first target for energy conservation. Tools such as the energy assessment and reporting methodology (EARM) can be used to quickly identify major opportunities for improvement, but even a simple walk-through can identify wastage. There are guidance documents on setting up energy management frameworks.

Transmission and distribution

Transmission is the process whereby electricity is transported over long distances through a grid. Transmission grids operate at very high voltages (e.g. 400 kV) to minimise energy wastage. They are expensive items of infrastructure, which may extend for thousands of miles, sometimes over very inhospitable terrain. At various points along the grid, electricity is 'siphoned' off into local distribution networks/regional grids that operate at a lower voltage (e.g. 132 and 33 kV), and the voltage is stepped down (through the use of substations) to the voltage required by the consumers (e.g. 240, 415 V or 11 kV). During the transmission and distribution, energy is always lost.

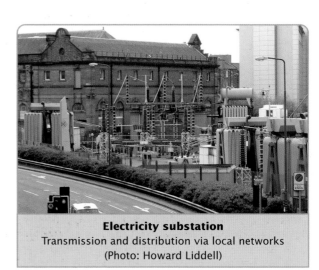

Electricity substation
Transmission and distribution via local networks
(Photo: Howard Liddell)

Electricity tariffs

There are certain generic costs, common throughout the world, that must be recovered from the end-user. These can be summarised as:

- The cost of purchasing the primary energy and converting it to electricity
- The cost of transporting electricity around a region or country
- The cost of distributing electricity to the customer
- The costs of selling to the customer (i.e. meter reading, billing and managing accounts).

Utility companies are sometimes obliged to bear the cost of supplying new buildings with electricity. This may involve laying new cable, constructing a transformer and substation, or even reinforcing the local electrical distribution network. So charges are often levied to discourage designers from oversizing electrical installations.

Peak demand

Because electricity cannot be stored, the size, and hence cost, of the supporting infrastructure is governed by the maximum instantaneous load on the system and not the amount of energy that is consumed. Generation, transmission and distribution infrastructure must be sized to cope with this peak demand and maintained ready for use. In the UK, this occurs at around 5.00 p.m. during the winter months. During this peak, if the infrastructure is not large enough, then the system will fail and power cuts will occur. However, for most of the day and most of the year, demand is considerably less than the peak, so transmission and distribution power grids are under-utilised and a considerable amount of generating capacity is idle. Suppliers try to balance out the load on the system by using a 'maximum demand tariff ', which levies high charges during periods of peak demand (i.e. during the winter in the UK), and encourages off-peak use.

Similarly, electrical installations in buildings (cables, switchgear and transformers) must be sized to meet the peak demand, which in the case of air-conditioned buildings often occurs during the summer. Designers should therefore seek every opportunity to minimise peak electrical demand, as this will minimise energy costs and reduce capital expenditure on the installation.

Green electricity

When the energy market was opened up to competition in 1998, it became possible and easy to switch to a supplier using green energy.

Call your chosen supplier and fill in an application form. The new supplier reads your meter and that's it. The website (www.foe.org.uk) details the green tariffs available in your area, what the different tariffs offer, what they cost and how 'green' they really are, so that you can make an informed choice with minimum hassle. It even provides phone numbers.

Signing up to a green tariff helps to increase the proportion of green electricity in the supply mix. There are different types of tariff:

- Energy – conditions vary. The supplier may ensure that for every unit of electricity you use, the same amount of green electricity is generated. Or they may promise to buy renewable energy to match some of your electricity usage and/or sell green energy to other suppliers.
- Fund. The electricity company takes the extra that you pay and invests in new renewable energy projects.
- Other tariffs may combine both or purport to offer some other benefits.

Friends of the Earth did produce a green electricity league table which advised buying energy-based tariffs. The service is now available at www.green electricity.org. It lets you look at all the available green tariffs and sign up to them online in the same way that FoE used to. Switching is easy. Choose your preferred supplier from the available options. Call them with your old bill to hand, fill in an application form and the switch from dirty power to a cleaner, greener power happens after the new supplier has read your meter.

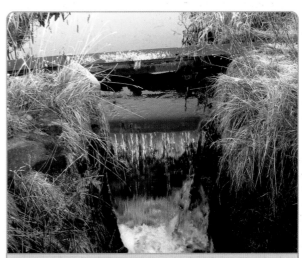

The weir is a traditional means of microgeneration for projects near to rivers
(Photo: the author)

Waste and health issues

The IT industry and eco-efficiency

Hardware, software, data processing and telecommunications sectors continue to expand at a greater rate than any industry of a comparable scale. They involve rapid obsolescence with consequent environmental damage, pollution and resource use. They have also had a major impact on building design, both because of the design pressures they place on buildings (new and refurbishment) and evolving issues such as design for homeworking. The concept of eco-efficiency was seen as a way for the industry to address sustainable development seriously. The aim of eco-efficiency was the delivery of competitively priced goods and services that satisfy human needs and bring quality of life, while progressively reducing adverse ecological impacts and resource intensity throughout the life cycle to a level at least in line with the earth's estimated carrying capacity. Movement towards agreed targets was slow and legislation is now being introduced to promote change.

Pollution

Dioxins, furans and polychlorinated biphenyls are compounds that are resistant to metabolic and environmental degradation, and so persist in the environment. They have been found in the fatty tissues of animals and toxic responses include carcinogenicity, immunotoxicity, dermal toxicity, and malfunction of reproductive and endocrine activity. This has led to unease about the possible human health risks and damage to biodiversity. They can be formed as by-product contaminants in production of pesticides, solvents and some plastics.

It has been suggested that disposal of sewage sludge and solid waste to landfill may be a route by which contaminated products enter the environment.

They can also be formed in combustion processes such as municipal solid waste (MSW) combustion; incineration of clinical waste; industrial coal burning; sintering; iron and steel production. Brominated dioxins and furans are chemical compounds formed during the burning of materials (printed circuit boards, plastic-encapsulated integrated circuits and certain thermoplastic housing materials) which have been treated with certain flame retardants.

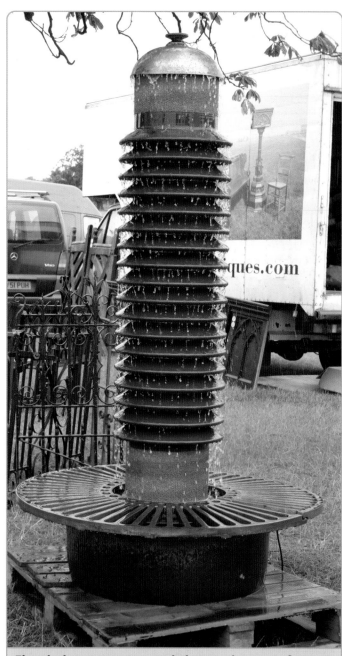

Electrical components recycled as garden water features
(Photo: Thornton Kaye – Salvo, www.salvo.co.uk)

PVC

Over 50% of PVC is used in construction, in pipelines, wiring, siding, flooring and wallpaper, replacing materials such as wood, concrete and clay. It has high environmental impacts.

From manufacture to its disposal, PVC can emit toxic compounds. During the manufacture pollutants are emitted into the air, water and land, presenting health hazards. During use, PVC products can leach toxic additives – for example, flooring can release softeners called phthalates. When PVC reaches the end of its useful life, it can be landfilled, where it leaches toxic additives, or incinerated, again emitting dioxins and heavy metals. When PVC burns in accidental fires, hydrogen chloride gas and dioxins are formed. For virtually all PVC applications, alternatives exist, using more sustainable, traditional materials.

Greenpeace host an international database intended to help anyone to track down alternatives to PVC products. The Greenpeace International PVC Alternatives Database can be searched by product or country to locate suitable suppliers (http://www.greenpeace.org.au/pvc/).

All the alternative cable types have better properties than PVC in the event of a fire. They generate less smoke, do not release hydro-chloric acid or dioxins and have fire-resistant qualities which match or outstrip PVC. All PVC-free cables cost more at present.

The use of PVC-free electrical cables is growing, particularly in the transportation sector where safety is critical. Many underground railway systems (Vienna, Berlin, Dusseldorf, Bilbao and London) use PVC-free cables (also known as low-smoke, zero-halogen or LSOH cables), and Eurotunnel, Deutsche Bahn, P & O Cruises and the US Navy all specify PVC-free cables.

Manufacturers have already developed and marketed several halogen-free alternatives to PVC cable as a result of concern over combustion emissions. When cable is designated halogen-free, this means it cannot contain PVC or any other organochlorine-based chemicals. The main alternative power cables use polyethylene as an insulation and sheathing material.

Rubber-sheathed cables are also available. There are alternatives to PVC for fittings, ducts and trunking.

WEEE Directive

Over 6 million tonnes of electrical and electronic equipment is disposed of every year in the European Union. This amount is set to increase. The Waste Electrical and Electronic Equipment (WEEE) Directive is an EU Directive, first proposed in 1988, designed to deal with the issue of disposal of electrical and electronic equipment. It also encourages the design of new equipment that will be simple to repair, reuse or recycle. Hazardous materials, such as lead, mercury, cadmium, hexavalent chromium, PBBs and PBDEs, and flame retardants were to be phased out by 1 January 2004. Systems of collection of waste electrical and electronic equipment are to be established so that private households, end-users and distributors can return them. For private households it is intended that this service is to be free, with the costs being borne by the manufacturers. Systems for treating waste equipment are also to be set up by the producers. The aim is to achieve a minimum rate of separate collection of 4 kg per inhabitant per year of waste equipment. The recovery of energy from waste electrical and electronic equipment is also being promoted, and producers are encouraged to incorporate recycled or used material in new products. Items covered by the WEEE Directive:

- Large household appliances
- Small household appliances
- IT equipment
- Telecommunications
- Radio, television, electro-acoustic musical instruments
- Lighting equipment
- Medical equipment systems
- Monitoring and control systems
- Toys
- Electrical and electronic tools
- Automatic dispensers.

Case Study 8.6:

McLaren Leisure Centre, Callander

Architects: Gaia Architects, 1998

The McLaren Centre achieved a saving on its electrical wiring due to a change in specification from the norm of PVC to non-PVC LSF (low smoke and fumes) wiring. The Centre has dynamic insulation in all of its main spaces: sports hall, swimming pool, squash courts and bowling hall. Because of the requirement for an airtight roof void, it is through the control membrane to a minimum. This meant that the wiring to the lighting, fire alarms, etc. was placed below the ceiling membrane but above the suspended ceiling finish. This meant two things:

1 **The wiring had to be of a higher specification for fire resistance.**

2 **Suspended lay-in cable trays were no longer needed (i.e. the LSF wiring was both accessible and supported by the ceiling).**

This resulted in a net saving.

The innovative nature of the ventilation strategy meant that the building was subject to a two-year monitoring exercise. The Energy and Reporting Methodology (EARM) was used in undertaking a preliminary audit and this identified a number of areas where radical savings could be made, in particular through modifications to control strategies.

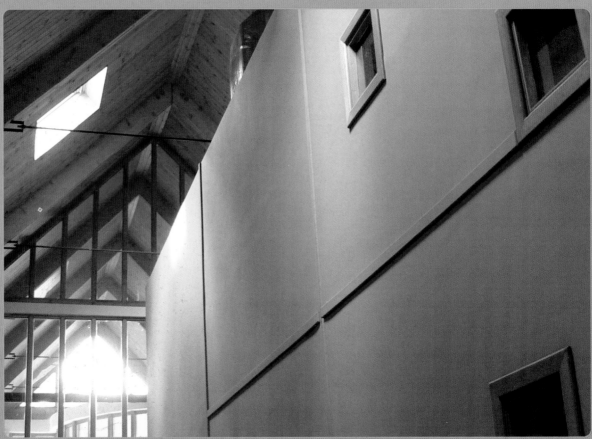

Photo: the author

Case Study 8.7:

Findhorn Ecological Village Project, Forres

Designer and engineer: John Talbot, 1995

Findhorn has been concerned about the effects of EMFs (electromagnetic fields) on the human body, and follows the principles of 'Baubiologie' (building biology) to reduce perceived effects from EMFs. The Foundation understands that the damage EMFs might present to the body are still to be fully understood and recommends that people should not become overly worried about EMFs. Instead, they say, take steps to learn more about the problem and determine whether you want to alter your particular situation.

Shielded cables were investigated for use in homes, but at the time there was no commercially available cable that would

properly shield EMFs. Other cables were investigated but found to be too expensive. Instead, they opted for demand switches which are connected to the main circuit distribution board.

A 4 V DC control circuit is used to sense when there is a demand for power. When no power is required, the electricity supply to the cable is switched off, stopping all EMFs. Careful planning is required (spur circuits instead of ring mains) to ensure that essential items, such as fridges, are left running. Their wiring should be kept away from sleeping areas.

Chlorine-free (LSF) cables are also now being used as an alternative to PVC wiring.

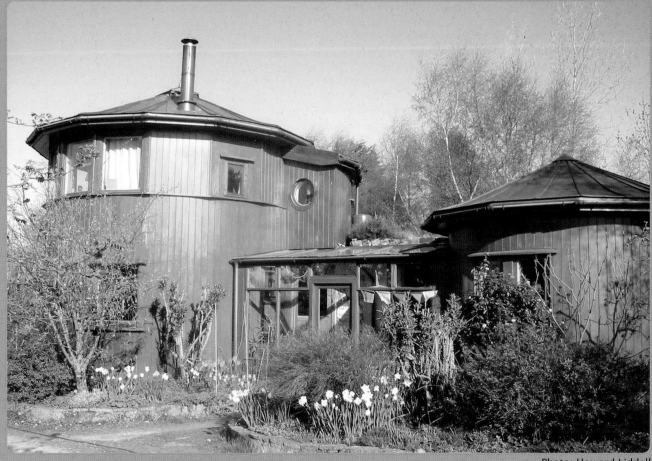

Photo: Howard Liddell

Electromagnetic fields (EMFs)

Electric fields are present in all equipment connected to a power supply, such as power lines, cables, appliances, mobile phones, base stations, and TV and radio transmitters. When an electrical appliance is switched on, a current flows and generates an electro-magnetic field.

EMFs are associated with high blood pressure, disturbed sleep, headaches, allergy sensitivity and nausea. Concern about the possible role of EMFs in ill-health has its origin in a study carried out in 1979 in the USA. A correlation between the incidence of childhood leukaemia and proximity to electricity supply wiring was demonstrated. Overhead power lines in particular are suspected of being harmful to people living underneath them, but no firm evidence has yet been produced.

There is a great deal of dispute about the harmful effects of EMFs and particularly weaker fields. There is wide variation in guidance and even between guidelines in different countries.

Recently, concerns have been raised that use of mobile phones has increased dramatically without sufficient understanding of the potential adverse health effects of the electromagnetic fields produced by the phones and their base stations. The most recently published reviews of the literature have concluded that whilst there are small physiological effects caused at levels within the existing guidelines, there are no definite adverse health effects from mobile phones or their base stations. However, all the main professional organisations have called for more research to be conducted since the possibility that radio-frequency radiation may cause adverse effects cannot be ruled out. Clearly there are large gaps in existing knowledge.

There are excellent sources of information for those who wish to know more, but like other disputed areas your own judgement is required. Good design guidance is available on how to minimise their effects for those who want to take a precautionary approach. EMFs are measurable. Any environment can be examined for them and rewiring or replacement options explored. The strength of the field is measured in relation to the voltage strength and the distance from the source. The fields associated with appliances and cables are not stopped by normal building floors and fabric, and so fridges, light fittings, etc. can have effects on adjacent rooms. To reduce exposure the Institute of Electrical Engineers (IEE) suggest that clock-radios and electric blankets are not used. Additional precautions for sensitive areas such as bedrooms, where we spend most time, include the use of shielded cable or automatic circuit breakers that provide only on demand, and eliminate all static fields and EMFs. It may be that a separate supply is required for items needing continuous power, and consideration can be given to siting these away from sleeping areas. Spur circuits rather than ring mains allow occupants to know what is on and off.

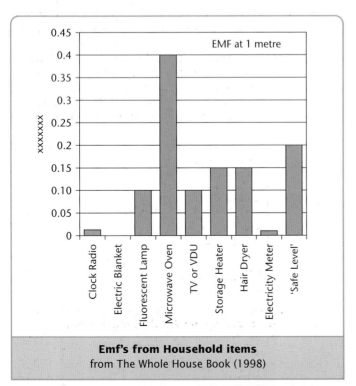

Emf's from Household items
from The Whole House Book (1998)

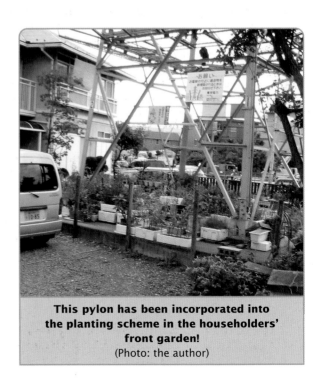

This pylon has been incorporated into the planting scheme in the householders' front garden!
(Photo: the author)

Policy aimed at reversing unsustainable energy use

Carbon trading

The carbon trading scheme was designed to allow countries to buy and sell their quotas for CO_2 emissions. It is similar to a system for limiting emissions of sulphur dioxide that has been operational and successful in the USA for some time. Organisations can volunteer to reduce emissions in return for a financial incentive.

Participants need to establish a baseline. If organisations over-achieve they can either sell the excess allowances or bank the excess for subsequent years. Underachievement means they have to buy the requisite allowances.

The bidding process is termed a 'descending clock' auction, whereby the auctioneer (i.e. the government) states a bid price in £ per tonne of CO_2. The participants submit their five year offer and if the price multiplied by quantity bid exceeds the money available, the auction begins again with a lower price, with revised offers invited until the total quantity of emissions reduction bids, multiplied by the price, is equal to the total financial incentive available.

There is a direct financial gain both from the incentive money on offer and the savings that will accrue from reducing emissions. The incentive money could make a project that had been previously rejected in simple payback terms more acceptable. However, the concept of carbon trading relies on a network of policing that may not be deliverable. The Kyoto trading scheme does not start until 2008, but the EU Emissions Trading Scheme came into action on 1 January 2005. There is significant ongoing negotiation about quotas. The fourth year (2005) results for the UK Emissions Trading Scheme, set up in 2002, show that direct participants have achieved emissions reductions of over 7 million tonnes of CO_2 against their baselines since the start of the scheme (http://www.defra.gov.uk/environment/climatechange/trading/uk/reports.htm#2005).

At the Kyoto summit of 1997, the United Nations set targets for developed countries to reduce their greenhouse gas emissions. Britain agreed to a reduction of 12% by 2010. The UK non-binding, domestic objective is 20% by 2010 and 60% by 2050.

Climate Change Levy

The UK introduced an energy tax, the Climate Change Levy, which, as of April 2001, added an average of 12% to business energy costs. It applies to energy used in industry, commerce and the public sector. Electricity (except large-scale hydro power) and heat produced from renewables are exempt, and so businesses who sign up to a green tariff avoid paying it. CHP has to be independently verified as good quality before receiving exemption.

The aim is to provide an incentive for business to opt for 'green' electricity. Revenue from the levy is recycled to business via a 0.5% reduction in employers' National Insurance Contributions and extra support for energy efficiency measures.

Having replaced much of the coal generation by gas in the 1980s and 1990s, the UK is in a strong position under the Kyoto protocol to meet its CO_2 targets and expects an ample surplus of carbon credits. It could earn up to £1 billion by selling its surplus quota to other developed countries. The collapse of economies in the former Soviet Union means Russia is also expected to join those able to sell.

EU energy efficiency labelling scheme

The EU labelling system was introduced in 1995 and now covers most domestic white goods. Labels must be displayed and range from 'A' for the most energy efficient to 'G' for the least efficient.

The aim is to make it easy to make like-for-like comparisons in energy consumption when choosing white goods. The scheme is based solely on self-assessment by manufacturers. It falls within existing consumer protection legislation, dealing with the description of goods by those selling them, and enforcement is dealt with in the same way as for other retail complaints. The scheme was introduced to deal with domestic appliances and there is no scheme for commercial appliances. The labelling scheme has recently been extended to cover public buildings.

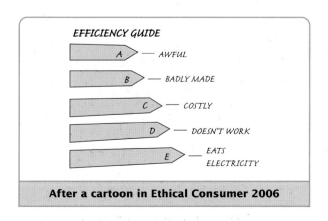

EFFICIENCY GUIDE

A — AWFUL
B — BADLY MADE
C — COSTLY
D — DOESN'T WORK
E — EATS ELECTRICITY

After a cartoon in Ethical Consumer 2006

Handy hints and tips

- Comply with European legislation to control waste and pollution from electrical equipment.
- Reduce demand by improving personal and automatic controls, and by providing good information.
- Look to the future, when carbon trading may become an option even for small businesses.
- Minimise the presence of electromagnetic fields within the home and the working environment to ensure minimum negative health effects.
- Incorporate benign material specification, avoiding PVC.
- Specify the most efficient appliances.
- Reduce standby power for electrical equipment to a bare minimum.
- Only purchase equipment that consumes no more than 1 W when in standby mode.
- Conserve energy so as to be better able to provide the requirement from renewable sources wherever possible.
- Minimise peak electrical demand wherever possible.
- Undertake life-cycle costing on lighting, controls and other energy-efficient items to support specification.
- Investigate green energy purchasing.
- Promote recycling on site.
- Put in place audit techniques in all buildings to reduce electrical power and energy demand.
- Only specify energy-efficient lighting indoors and outdoors.

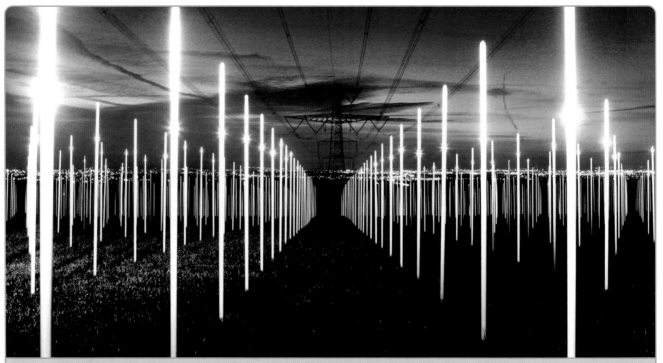

Art installation – electricity pylons and 1301 fluorescent tubes
The tubes were not connected to a conventional power source but are lit up by the electric field that is created between the cables and the ground. The installation highlights the power loss resulting from long-distance transmission and also raises questions about the potential health hazards of electromagnetic smog. By Richard Box, artist in residence at Bristol University Department of Physics
(Photo: SWNS)

Bibliography

Finding independent, concise, cogent and robust sources of information on electricity and sustainable design issues that are beyond the trivial yet still comprehensible is difficult. The issues are diverse and an integrated joined-up view is rare. The main recommended texts and principle sources of reference for this module are as follows.

General

Flavin, C. and Lenssen, N. (1995) *Power Surge*. Earthscan.

Hill, R., O'Keefe, P. and Snape, C. (1995) *The Future of Energy Use*. Earthscan.

von Weizacher, E. and Lovins A. L. (1997) *Factor 4 – Doubling Wealth and Halving Resources*. Earthscan.

DETR (1998) *Energy Consumption Guide 19*. HMSO.

Beggs, C. B. (2002) *Energy: Management, Supply and Conservation*. Butterworth-Heinemann.

TM22 (2006) *Energy Assessment and Reporting Methodology*. CIBSE.

European Biology and Bioelectromagnetics – www.ebab.eu.com.

Standby Power Use and the IEA "1-watt Plan"
www.iea.org/textbase/subjectqueries/standby.asp

Materials, health and waste

Coghill, R (1987) *The Dark Side of the Brain*. Element Books Explores the effects of subtle energies on the brain. Now out of print but available on CD-ROM from www.galonga.co.uk

BMA (1991) *Hazardous Waste and Human Health*. BMA, Oxford. Background info on a range of potential toxic waste hazards.

HMIP (1995) *A Review of Dioxin Emissions in the UK*. Report No. DoE/HMIP/RR/95/027. The Stationery Office.

DoE (1997) *A Review of Dioxin Releases to Land and Water in the UK*. DoE, London. AEA Technology plc.

Borer, P. and Harris, C. (1998) *The Whole House Book*. Centre for Alternative Technology Publications.

IEA (2000) *Things That Go Blip in the Night* IEA Publications www.iea.org/textbase/nppdf/free/2000/blipinthenight01.pdf

Chapter 9
Lighting and daylighting

In which we mainly aim to excite interest in, and bring to wider attention, the range of good-quality tools and guidance already available on lighting and daylighting, and to highlight crucial issues and priorities affecting the design of places, buildings and services.

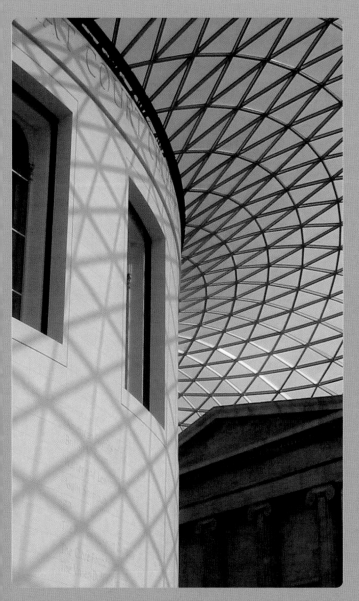

'One study found that in classrooms with the most daylighting, students' learning progressed 20% faster in mathematics and 26% faster in reading than similar students in classrooms with the least daylighting.'

Greg Kats, *The Costs and Financial Benefits of Green Buildings*

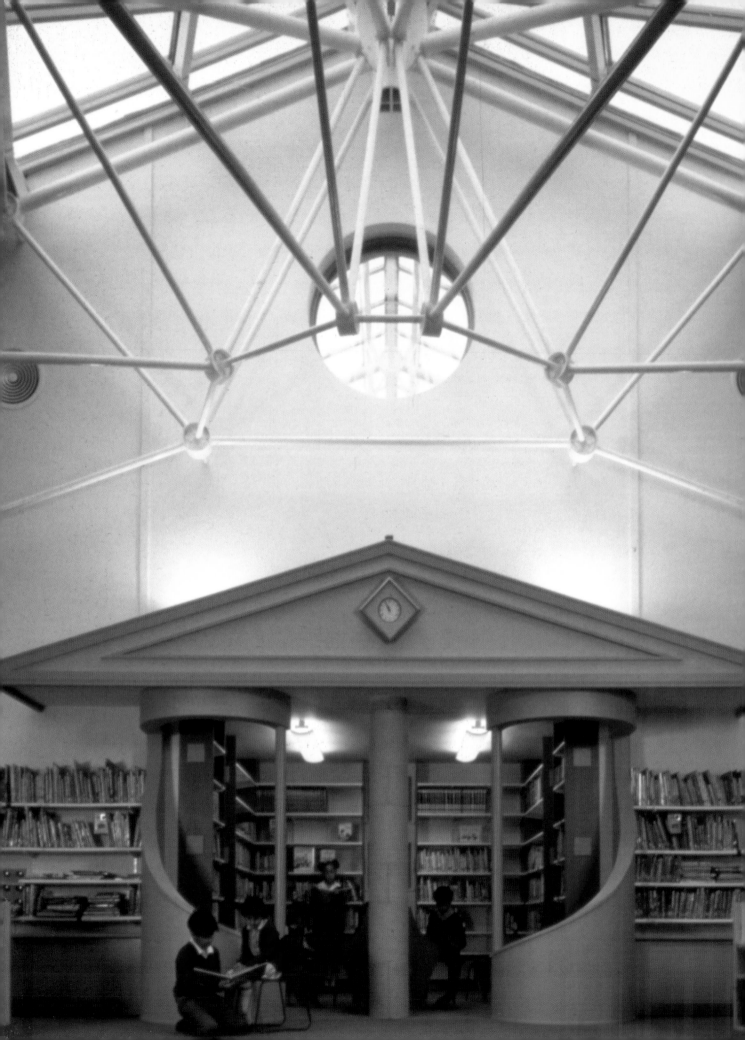

Contents

(Facing page)
Daylit library at Grove Road School, Hounslow
(Architects: Plinke Leaman Browning; photo: Paddy Boyle, (paddy.boyle@tiscali.co.uk) reproduced with permission from Plinke Leaman Browning)

(Previous page)
Great Court of the British Museum, London
(Architects: Norman Foster; photo: the author)

Lighting and daylighting

Introduction

Lighting is a major factor in determining the way in which people experience the internal environment, how they experience buildings and how they are able to respond to certain tasks. People like daylight, and the contribution it can make to the quality of internal spaces is increasingly being reintegrated into buildings, following a period when it was largely devalued by artificial alternatives. It is now accepted that daylight, when available, should be the predominant form of lighting in most types of building.

If appropriately designed and integrated, it can contribute significantly to distinctive and attractive architecture, and to occupants' sense of well-being. Indeed, there is evidence from Canada and Sweden that daylighting has an important role in health and in mental development.

Daylight, if properly designed into a building and well controlled, also offsets the energy consumption associated with artificial lighting. This is often a very significant proportion of the overall energy consumption of buildings. Hence we need to explore best practice in lighting, in and around buildings, which is intrinsically energy efficient and optimises the use of natural lighting.

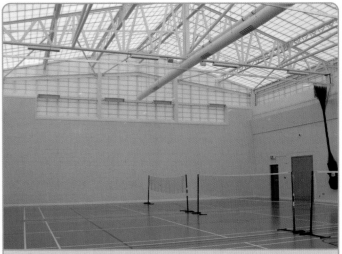

Jock Stein Centre, East Kilbride
Sport Scotland have promoted integration of daylighting into sports halls because people like daylighting and it encourages access by a wide range of users
(Architects: South Lanarkshire Council; photo: the author)

The design issues are complex. Optimising natural daylight and integrating it with well-designed electric light requires that the form, fabric, internal layout and systems of a building are considered holistically. Problems are real. Variations in light quality and quantity can be enlivening or they can be unmanageable and uncomfortable. Fenestration can provide welcome visual relief or it can lead to unwelcome distractions.

Lighting is important to the outside of buildings also. Appropriate orientation, overhangs and shading can optimise the opportunities for external comfort and energy efficiency.

Care is required to ensure that inappropriate natural lighting and/or poor control does not give rise to thermal discomfort, and increase the need for compensatory heating or cooling. Also, window openings are more expensive than solid walls and roofs, and any life-cycle cost, environmental, quality and amenity benefits need to be communicated to clients and funders. Last but not least, good control is absolutely essential if cost benefits are to be achieved.

It is not possible or necessary to give comprehensive coverage here. There is already extensive good-quality guidance and this is listed in the Bibliography. A number of free publications provide excellent information and many of the more expensive ones are a pleasure. These, along with a good reference book, will be necessary reading to achieve a good grounding in the subject.

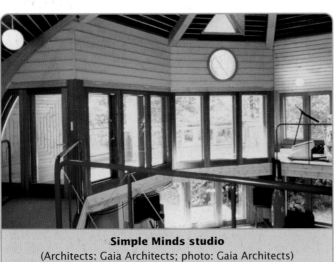

Simple Minds studio
(Architects: Gaia Architects; photo: Gaia Architects)

Principals of lighting design

Quality

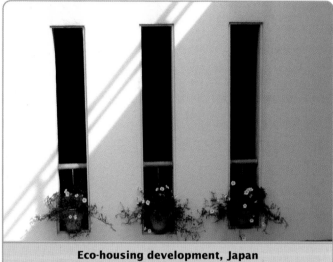

Eco-housing development, Japan
(Photo: the author)

Good lighting enhances the quality of a space and is a significant contributor to creating an appropriate atmosphere. Both artificial and natural light has to be of a high standard if occupants are to be satisfied. Colour and brightness of lighting, its interaction with surface colours, patterns and reflectances are all important aspects.

People enjoy daylight in particular, but only if it does not distract from what they are doing. Daylight can supplement artificial lighting to add quality and if properly controlled it can replace artificial lighting with savings in cost and energy.

When daylighting is well designed it is an aid to effective working and/or enjoyment of a space, and its directional qualities can assist occupants in discerning details.

However, care is required as it can be a nuisance if it is obtrusive, and occupants feel unable to control it. In particular, glare from the sky, artificial lighting and reflections, for example from computer screens, should be avoided as this can create eye strain, discomfort or worse. Flickering lights are a source of discomfort and are now commonly avoided by the use of high-frequency ballasts in fluorescent lighting systems.

Researchers in Sweden monitored behaviour, health and cortisol (a stress hormone) levels in 90 primary schoolchildren over the period of a year in four classrooms with varying levels of daylight. The results indicated that work in classrooms without daylight may upset the basic hormone pattern and this in turn may influence the children's ability to concentrate or cooperate, and also eventually may have an impact on annual body growth and absenteeism. In Canada, the Alberta Department of Education compared, over a two-year period, primary schoolchildren attending schools with full-spectrum light (daylight or artificial light sources simulating daylight) with children attending primary schools with conventional mixed artificial and natural lighting. (See NREL, 2000)

The results showed that the pupils subjected to the full-spectrum light were healthier, had fewer days off school, more positive moods and better scholastic performance. In addition, it was found that the use of daylight in school libraries resulted in significantly reduced noise levels, due to improved concentration levels among the children.

One study found that in classrooms with the highest levels of daylighting, students' learning progressed 20% faster in mathematics and 26% faster in reading than similar students in classrooms with the least daylighting. The apparent significance of daylighting quality surprised some of those involved and, to ensure the study's validity, California's Public Interest Energy Research (PIER) programme, administered by the CEC, funded a follow-up study, employing an independent technical advisory group to re-analyse the data. The re-analysis confirmed the initial study's findings with a 99.9% confidence level. (Kats, 2003)

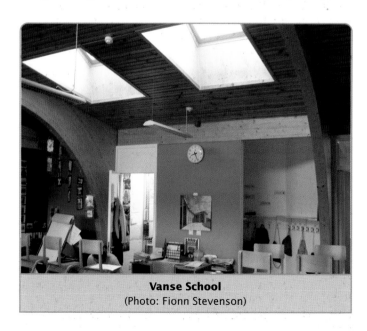

Vanse School
(Photo: Fionn Stevenson)

Energy efficiency, capital and running costs

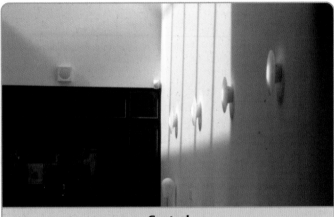

Control
These lights are on despite the incorporation of daylighting.
Energy savings from daylighting come from appropriate
behaviour as well as design!
(Photo: the author)

Energy-efficient lighting depends on the interplay of an extensive number of effects. These include: availability of usable natural light; how a building is used and managed; choice of lamp and luminaire; maintenance and cleaning regimes of lamps, luminaires and surfaces; heat gains and losses through glazed areas; and the extent of personal and overriding control, particularly glare management. It is no small issue for all to be considered and resolved if the potential significant benefits in economic and environmental terms are to be maximised. It is worth noting that good controls are amongst the most cost-effective energy measures, and are vital to both energy efficiency and amenity.

A number of tools are available for use during the early design stages. Most designers learn how to predict average daylight factors, back-of-room gloom and the role of sunpaths. These and others should be investigated to determine which is best suited to a situation. The lighting and thermal (LT) method is a simple tool that can assist in designing the building form and glazing distribution to minimise energy consumed by heating and lighting; also, various computer methods allow experimentation with different kinds of lighting. It is an area in which observation of existing buildings, combined with experimentation with design tools and modelling facilities, will be rewarded by better buildings.

Studies at the design stage should compare strategies on a life-cycle basis. Electricity is more expensive during the day and

so daytime savings are particularly economic. However, capital costs to incorporate daylighting can be two to three times that of a plain wall or roof. Build quality and maintenance costs need to be considered. Daylighting can therefore be difficult to justify purely on the grounds of energy economy. However, there is significant evidence emerging of the amenity benefits, including occupant satisfaction and productivity, that add weight to arguments for energy efficiency.

External lighting can be a significant element of the energy costs of buildings, yet often functionless and a source of 'night erosion'. It is important to make sure that it is efficient and well controlled without adversely affecting safety. It is a significant aspect of the waste of energy associated with buildings, but we need to consolidate responses to safety and security with good design in order to come to a solution.

Light quantity

The design illuminance (or maintained illuminance) is the minimum that should be available for a particular task. The artificial lighting needs to provide this. Advice on illuminance for specific tasks is available in the CIBSE *Code for Interior Lighting* and publications on specific building types. For example:

- Corridors and changing rooms – 100 lux
- Libraries and sports halls – 300 lux
- Chain stores and drawing offices – 750 lux
- Microelectronics – 2000 lux.

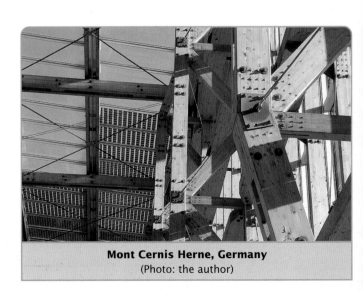

Mont Cernis Herne, Germany
(Photo: the author)

Case Study 9.1:

National Museum of Scotland, Edinburgh

Architects: Benson & Forsyth, 1998

The New Museum is constructed from concrete, with untreated plaster rendering, sandstone and timber internally. Daylighting plays an important role in the relationship of the various rooms and the experience of the visitor.

The main feature is a large atrium, which is lit from the top and either end by large expanses of intricately shaped glazing. Another space, the industrial revolution hall, is lit by clerestories under an inverted barrel vault. The curve of the ceiling and its white finish help the ingress of daylight and avoid any shadows being cast upon it.

Other spaces feature novel and wide-ranging types of window and shading designs to intrigue the visitor and successfully light the various rooms. Daylight is controlled mainly by the shape of the building, fixed louvres and the window orientation.

A sophisticated and fully adjustable spotlighting system for the exhibits is augmented with fluorescent luminaires and other specialised exhibit lights, such as optic fibre. Artificial lighting is computer controlled.

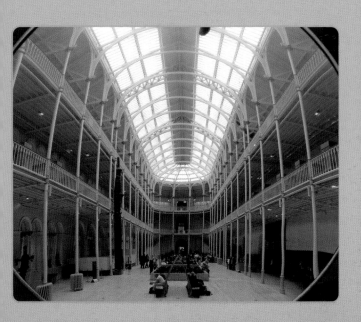

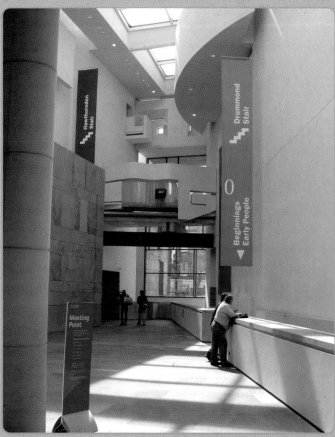

Photos: Howard Liddell

Integration

If a lighting scheme is to work (aesthetically, functionally and in terms of energy efficiency), then the natural lighting and artificial lighting have to be well integrated. This relies on consideration at an early stage of a large range of factors, including:

- window location and design
- how the building will be used, maintained and managed
- the shape and orientation of spaces in relation to activities
- surface finishes
- choice of lamps, luminaires, switches and controls.

It is important to consider the changing effects during the day, from partial to full daylight, and also the requirements at night. Blending the transition between daylight and artificial light can be achieved by using lamps of similar colour temperature to daylight.

A room needs to be visually bright if it is to be successfully daylit. All surfaces should receive some light, but some variations in illuminance are appreciated. Too much light coming from a single source, a bright light or small window in a large room, will cause glare and make a room appear gloomy, even if it is lit to the correct level.

> **Sunlight is the direct beam of the sun after it has been diffused by the atmosphere. It is welcome in some buildings and intermediate spaces because it provides interest and pleasure, and because it is an energy source. In some spaces it can cause problems. In offices, and sometimes schools, it is a major cause of occupant dissatisfaction, and frequently leads to discomfort, disability glare and overheating.**
>
> **Skylight is light from the sky, which excludes direct sunlight. It is the accepted description for daylight.**

Maintenance

All lighting is subject to diminishing output because of ageing and dirt on lamps and luminaires. It is important to understand the maintenance needs at the outset and to communicate these to those responsible.

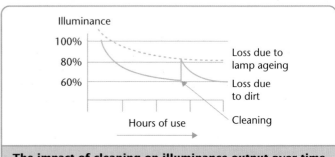

The impact of cleaning on illuminance output over time

Interestingly, old inefficient tungsten filament lamps almost invariably burnt out before anyone notices a drop-off in output. The introduction of longer-lasting, low-energy compact fluorescents lamps means that even in the domestic situation it may be necessary to change them before the end of their life – because of degradation – or to replace them and move them to areas where less light is needed. Maintenance factors and guidelines can be found in Tregenza and Loe (1998), and the CIBSE *Code* and lighting guides.

Elert Sund School, Norway
Integration of daylight into the circulation spaces brings these to life and helps to give the building a real sense of urban intervention
(Photo: the author)

Natural lighting

Daylight should always be the first choice for illuminating a space during the day, unless the function specifically excludes it. It is beneficial because of its zero energy consumption, directionality, variability, intensity and colour. None of these elements can be completely reproduced by electric lighting, although the extent of research itself is sufficient to highlight the relevance. People are tolerant of the variability of light levels if they know that the light is daylight. However, it can become a source of annoyance and/or give rise to a need for compensatory heating or cooling and therefore has to be balanced against excessive heat loss, or unwanted solar gain or glare. Natural light must therefore be considered alongside the view, the layout of spaces and the activities.

Windows

Windows may have many roles – providing daylight, orientation, views, ventilation, insulation, containment, means of escape, a sound barrier and/or glare protection. They affect the internal acoustics, energy consumption and ambience. Openings need to be adequately designed and controlled to prevent rain penetration and external noise may be a problem. Windows may also present a problem for theft, vandalism and safety.

All these factors inevitably lead to conflicts in managing the orientation of window openings. Attention to cleaning, maintenance, and operation of windows and blinds is also vitally important if a design is not to result in a building operating with blinds down and lights on.

The design team need to address the window design in an interdisciplinary manner and will inevitably struggle to reconcile all the conflicts to a fully satisfactory solution. If, as frequently happens, the window design is inadequately addressed by the design team, this leads to missed opportunities and worse.

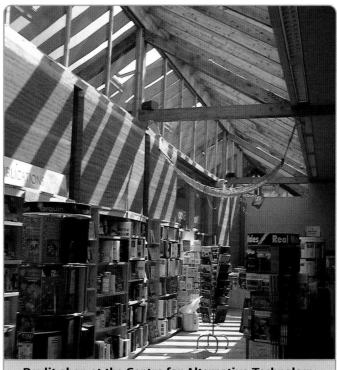

Daylit shop at the Centre for Alternative Technology
(Photo: Howard Liddell)

Location

- Borrowed light. A window or opening in a daylit corridor or atrium can contribute light to areas remote from an external window and also provide a visual connection. Noise, other distractions and thermal affects need consideration if the area from which light is borrowed is not to become a source of problems.
- Side windows. Windows provide views to outside if sills, transoms and internal heights are appropriate. Care needs to be taken that outside objects do not cause obstruction or reflected light, leading to glare.
- Clerestories and rooflights. Rooflights – including sunpipes – are effective because they provide light from the zenith, the brightest part of the sky, deep into a space. However, both clerestories and rooflights are potential sources of glare. Light-coloured surrounds and reveals are recommended to help to minimise this. Rooflights do provide a more even distribution of daylight than clerestories, but can be a maintenance problem.

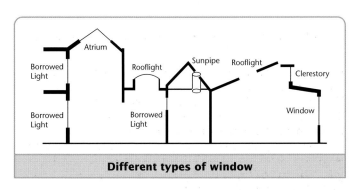

Different types of window

Orientation

Windows provide a link to outside which occupants appreciate, but orientation needs to be considered in relation to solar penetration at all times of day and year.

- Low-altitude morning and evening sun is commonly associated with glare. This should be considered in the design of shading in east and west orientations. Some opportunity for adjustment will often be required to exclude the low-altitude sun, but allow for beneficial daylighting at other times of the day.
- North-facing windows are least vulnerable to glare problems and can provide useful quality light, but they can be a source of local cooling, leading to heat loss and down-draughts. Heat balance and comfort are the principal considerations.
- South-facing windows are prone to creating a wide range of problems, unless adequate and well-controlled shading is provided. The best solution often requires some form of permanent shading and/or movable blinds to deal with particular times of day or year. If blinds are internal then solar heat will penetrate the building and have to be managed.

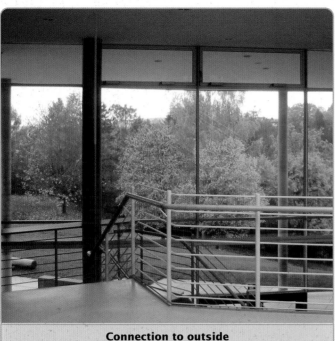

Connection to outside
The view out of a window is an important consideration for building occupants
(Photo: the author)

Control

Buildings should utilise daylight as much as possible because it provides amenity and aesthetic value. In general, there should not be any difficulty in providing adequate daylight factors of 2–5%. Smaller amounts of daylight may be inadequate to prevent use of artificial lights, and hence energy and running cost savings. However, high levels of daylight alone do not deliver energy efficiency. Good control is essential. Electric lighting will usually be required in the morning, on dull days and at night, and without proper control will be left on when daylight is adequate.

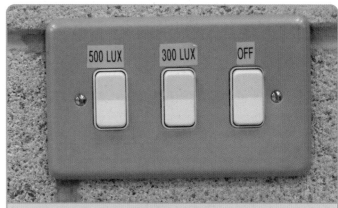

Simple controls
Building users will respond to good information on how to control lighting and energy consumption
(Photo: the author)

Location of light switches and zoning to take into account the variations in daylighting should be considered. Where possible, lighting should be zoned to enable fewer lights to be used, with intermediate daylighting strategies for different conditions. If lights can be switched in rows, parallel to windows, either automatically or using clearly marked switches, then this will allow best use of daylight.

It is best to avoid banks of switches that can all be turned on simultaneously and then tend to be left on.

The required flexibility will depend on the type of space and the way in which it is used, and should be discussed at the design stage. A school, for example, may need to suit a variety of moods in a single day and the lighting design will need to respond to this. A sports facility requires zoning to respond the to use of individual courts and play areas. An office environment or gallery may have a very fixed space plan, but all will require consideration of the varying occupancy patterns, including cleaning regimes.

Case Study 9.2:

Sainsbury's Supermarket, Greenwich

Architects: Chetwood Associates, 1999

The building achieves energy savings of up to 50% compared to a standard supermarket design, by using a combination of novel and best practice sustainable construction methods. It scored the maximum BREEAM rating of 31 points for energy efficiency. Low ambient artificial lighting levels mean that fewer luminaires are installed at ceiling level. The localised merchandise lighting is economical to install and operate.

The building has a series of high-angled, north-facing windows that sweep across the roof, at 6.5 m above floor level, which admit sunshine-free light. This gives an average daylight factor of 5% and has enabled the daytime ambient lighting load to drop to only 3.5 W/m², at 200 lux. The windows are sealed and incorporate external motorised aluminium louvres. These are computer controlled and can close to reduce glare inside or to prevent light leakage and some heat losses at night.

Ceilings are white-painted steel and the floor has been specifically designed to have a high reflectivity, ensuring even illumination and reduced daylight asymmetry.

Artificial lighting is provided by T5 fluorescent tubes in Urbis fittings. These are located in the steel trusses between each row of rooflights. The combined ambient light levels in the store achieve 200 lux. Lighting for product shelving is localised and suspended around the perimeter of the merchandise gondolas. This provides localised (task) light levels of 1000 lux, without enduring the energy penalties of lighting the whole store to this level.

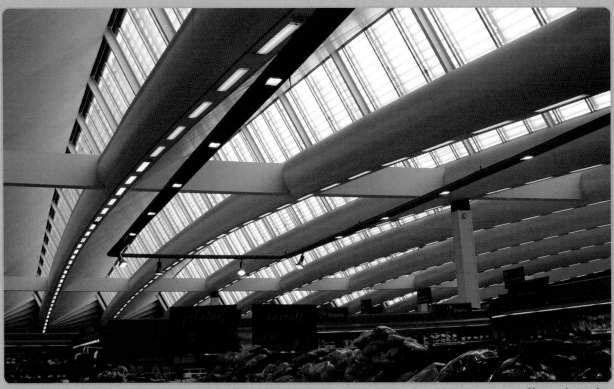

Photo: the author

Case Study 9.3:

Dyfi Eco-Park, Machynlleth

Architects: Acanthus Holden Architects, 1996

Located in Machynlleth, Wales, this small office and industrial unit development was designed in 1996. The units range in size from 500 to 2000 m². Daylighting features extensively in the building, both in the ground-floor industrial unit and the first-floor office space.

Daylighting was a major aspect in determining the form and orientation of the building. Average daylight factor calculations were used to calculate the window areas in order to ensure sufficient daylight levels to meet most daytime needs. The ground-floor industrial unit has a DFave of 2% whilst the office space has a value of 5% or higher.

Daylight and the white internal walls contribute to the bright and stimulating interior. Passive solar gains are also exploited, through the use of glazed gables. Solar shading was designed to reduce glare and overheating. Solar control was achieved by using timber slat brise soleil and roof overhangs. Post-occupancy residual measures have been required. Translucent cloths in front of the windows reduce glare.

The lights are high-frequency fluorescent. Simple on/off switches are provided for localised control. Automatic lighting control was avoided.

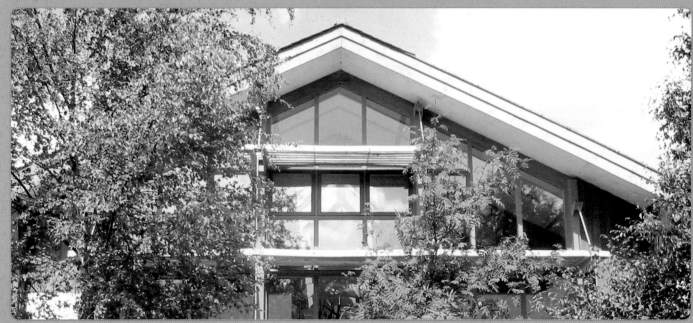

Photo: the author

Daylight factor

One of the simplest ways of beginning to develop an understanding of daylight in buildings is to become familiar with the daylight factor (DF). It defines a constant relationship of the daylight available at an unobstructed place outside, which is received at a point inside a space. For most spaces, the optimum DF_{ave} is in the range 2–5%.

Average daylight can be found from summing the daylight available:

$$DF_{ave} = \frac{T_1 A_{w1} q_1 M_1 + T_2 A_{w2} q_2 M_2 + ...}{A (1 - R_2)}$$

T= diffuse transmittance of glazing
M = maintenance factor for glazing
A_w = window area, excluding area of frame
q = angle of visible sky above the horizon from centre of window
A = combined area of walls, floor and ceiling, including windows
R = average reflectivity of room surfaces

The concept is best understood by practical experience. It is worthwhile taking time to calculate the DF_{ave} in a number of rooms, and then to compare your calculations with measurements using illuminance meters. This will provide an opportunity to get a sense of the numbers involved.

Daylight factors vary throughout a space. They tend to be high near the windows or directly below roof openings and rapidly decrease further away. The average daylight factor (DF_{ave}) is often used to give an approximation of the available daylight in a space. Approximate measurement of the daylight factor involves taking simultaneous readings – on a horizontal plane – of light levels in a space and at an unobstructed place outside. Taking readings on a grid enables a map to be drawn of the daylight available in a space and this can be averaged to provide the average daylight factor (DF_{ave}).

A quick calculation can give an approximation of available daylight in a space. It involves estimating DFave across the horizontal plane based on the window areas, their light transmission properties and factors such as room size. This gives a useful prediction of the brightness of a daylit interior and guidance on whether the window area is excessive or insufficient. It should be noted that successful daylighting requires qualitative as well as quantitative assessment. neither will be adequate alone.

Diffuse transmittance of clean glazing – T (approx)
Clear single glazing 0.8
Clear double glazing 0.7
Low-e double glazing 0.65
This should be multiplied by the appropriate maintenance factor. Values of T for other glazing systems and M can be found in the CIBSE *Daylighting and Window Design Guide Code* and from manufacturers.

Reflectivity
Reflectivity of surfaces affects distribution of light within a room. Low reflectivities and dark colours reduce the amount of available daylight.
A perfect black surface, R = 0, absorbs all light. If all incident light is reflected, R = 1.
It is found by weighting the reflectance of each surface. An estimate of 0.5 is often used for light surfaces.

In reverse, the equation can be used to estimate the area of glazing for a required DF_{ave}. That is, by assuming a value of, say, 2–5%, the equation can be used to provide a first estimate of total window size for a particular space.

It is not adequate as an indicator of light quality when used alone, because it is only quantitative. However, it is a useful measure when used together with other methods that deal with variability, brightness, glare, uniformity, gloom and solar gain.

There is also a need to consider optimum glazing ratios in relation to solar gains or heat loss. The lighting and thermal (LT) method, described below, provides a way of estimating this optimum.

Estimating DF_{ave} – In the early stage of designing a three-court badminton hall (18m x 27m x 7.6m), a double-glazed clerestory to the north is proposed of 2m x 27m where the angle of visible sky is 70°. The place is to have light internal finishes (R = 0.5) and is in a clean environment. The first approximation gives:

$$DF_{ave} = \frac{T \times M \times \sum \text{Window Area} \times \text{sky angle}}{\sum \text{Room surface areas} (1 - R^2)}$$

$$= \frac{0.7 \times 0.9 \times 54 \times 70}{1656 \times 0.75} = 1.9\%$$

This value is on the low side and further glazing would be recommended.

Available daylight

Having calculated the daylight factor or designed a space to a required level, it is then possible to determine how much daylight a space will receive. The published graphical data assumes a base standard – the standard overcast, unobstructed sky – which is defined as having an illuminance of 5000 lux. The graphs indicate how often this is exceeded.

In the UK, 5000 lux will be exceeded for about 83% of the year between 09.00 and 17.00. Therefore, a space with a DF_{ave} of 5% will have 250 lux (0.05 x 5000 lux) of interior daylighting under a standard overcast, unobstructed sky and this 250 lux will be exceeded for 83% of the typical working day.

In much of the UK the external illuminance exceeds 10 000 lux for 60% of daylight hours and this can make a significant contribution to lighting needs. It means that a room with 5% daylight factor, even on a cloudy day with white clouds and sunlight nearly breaking, provides a horizontal illuminance of about 12 000 lux. On a sunny summer day, with white clouds, the outdoor illuminance can be as much as 100 000 lux. The graphs and tables are available in the CIBSE *Daylighting and Window Design Guide*: LG10.

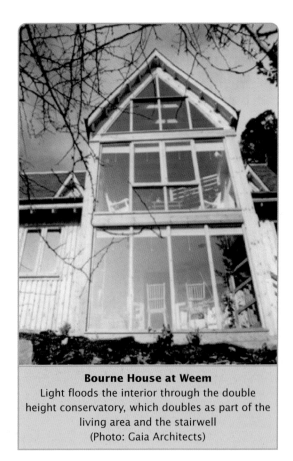

Bourne House at Weem
Light floods the interior through the double height conservatory, which doubles as part of the living area and the stairwell
(Photo: Gaia Architects)

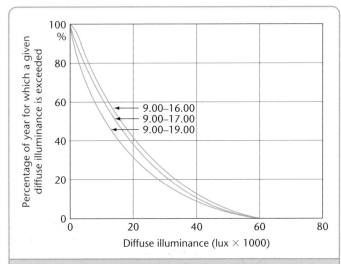

Daylight hours
Once the daylight factor has been calculated published graphs are used to determine how often the required illuminance is achieved or exceeded

Effect of DF$_{ave}$

Less than 2% – a room appears gloomy under daylight alone. Full electric lighting is often needed during daytime and dominates the daytime appearance. Sensitive spaces, such as art galleries, may require low DF_{ave}, but generally it is preferred to aim higher.

From 2% to 5% is usually the optimum range of daylighting for overall energy use. Rooms have a predominantly daylit appearance but supplementary electric lighting is needed away from windows and during dull weather. Most room types benefit from this range of DF_{ave}, such as offices, shops, sports halls, warehouses and factories. Above 5% – a room is strongly daylit and daytime electric lighting is rarely needed except perhaps to balance illuminance in dark recesses with the general light level, to avoid glare problems. High values of DF_{ave} tend to be found in atria, conservatories and other large, glazed spaces. In other buildings, with a DF_{ave} of 5% or more, unwanted thermal and acoustic effects may arise due to large window areas.

Sun paths

Sun path diagrams provide information on the path of the sun for particular times of year and day. These are necessary in order to estimate the depth of solar penetration into a space and for designing appropriate overhangs and louvres.

Care must be taken that control features – such as brise soleil and blinds – do not fall victim to cost-cutting, despite being fundamental to a design. Simplicity helps.

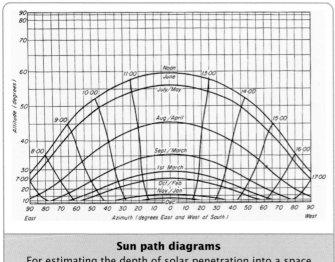

Sun path diagrams
For estimating the depth of solar penetration into a space

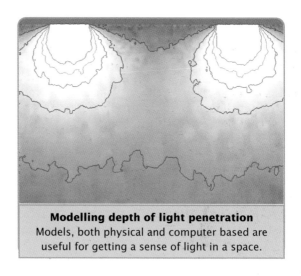

Modelling depth of light penetration
Models, both physical and computer based are useful for getting a sense of light in a space.

Optimising glazed areas

It is important to consider efficiency gains from daylighting, through increasing window area, against the thermal losses due to glazing. The lighting and thermal (LT) method provides a way of estimating the optimum for a particular set of criteria during the initial design stages. It is therefore an easy route to comparing scenarios.

No sky line

The no sky line is the point beyond which no direct light from the sky reaches. Supplementary lighting is usually required unless light can be introduced from more than one direction. It affects the design of window size, shape and location in relation to the room dimensions and the desired daylighting effect, depending on the direct skylight.

Uniformity ratio

The uniformity ratio gives an indication of the variation in light levels throughout a room. It is the minimum DF divided by the DFave. Uniformities of 0.7 are preferable in most situations, as complete uniformity creates a bland appearance, whereas excessive variation can be distracting and have a risk of glare.

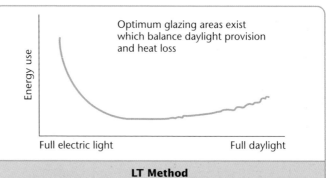

LT Method
There is a balance to be achieved between efficiency gains from daylighting and thermal losses

Case Study 9.4:

Acharacle Primary School, Ardnamurchan

Architects: Gaia Architects, 2007

Amongst the criteria stipulated in the model brief for a sustainable school – written by Gaia – was a requirement for excellent lighting and daylighting. To achieve the optimum daylight factor in each classroom the lighting system combines a south-facing horizontal window at the front with skylights at the back of each room. Skylights provide a more intense quality of light because the sunlight is direct and uninterrupted by buildings or vegetation. Direct sunlight – and hence heat gains – are avoided and diffuse daylight is maximised. A combination of large windows and smaller skylights provides an even distribution of daylight.

South-facing windows are made up of two layers with a 500 mm cavity, which helps prevent solar heat gains to the classrooms by trapping warm air and extracting at high level by natural convection. They are protected from summer solar gains by a roof overhang, which allows maximum light infiltration in the winter when the angle of the sun in the sky is lower. The entrance hall is lit by a large glass skylight in the centre of the roof and has glazed external walls to the east and west.

As the space is more dynamic and not used as a study area, there is less need for the daylight factors to be so onerous.

The main hall has a capacity of 300 and is used by both the school and community. It is lit by a series of low-level windows facing east and a clerestory strip window to the west. This orientation also allows for natural ventilation to the space.

The school's resource centre is situated in the corridor of the school wing that links the classrooms; skylights ensure adequate working light levels in this area.

Most of the remaining rooms in the building are cellular and not used constantly; they are lit by a combination of windows and skylighting. Internal windows between the office and staffroom to the entrance hall allow extra light into these spaces.

Artificial lighting controls (a combination of daylight-linked dimming, occupancy sensing, key switching and manual switching) combine with a careful selection of luminaires to provide efficient additional lighting whenever natural daylight levels are not sufficient.

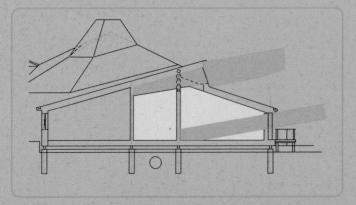

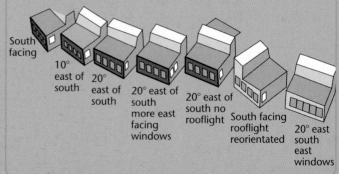

Images: Arup, Edinburgh

Glare from daylighting

Glare is a common problem in many daylit buildings. Problems with glare occur because one part of the visual field is significantly brighter than the larger part of the field to which the eye is adapted. It is a problem for significant parts of the year if windows have inadequate protection. It can be associated with any window orientation, although problems are most evident as a result of south-facing windows, and to east and west when the sun is at low altitude.

Rooflights can give rise to glare if the luminance of the sky is high and is visible to the line of sight of a task, which has a significantly lower illuminance. The contrast will make details difficult to see, cause inconvenience, discomfort, or make a task impossible or dangerous.

- Discomfort glare causes a person to have to squint, or to shield their eyes. It can cause headaches and eyestrain.
- Disability glare is used to describe a situation which prevents occupants from performing required tasks.

In specific cases, such as sports halls, disruption can be accentuated by the speed of movement of people or objects, and make it particularly difficult for the eye to adapt between different light levels. Solutions include ensuring that the contrast between a window and its surroundings is minimised by the use of light-coloured finishes on the wall and adjacent ceiling, light-coloured frames and splayed window reveals. Care must be taken with high-reflectance surfaces to ensure that they are not a source of glare.

Avoiding glare

- **Avoid point light sources**
- **Hide the source, light the walls**
- **Prevent occupants from seeing bright sources, directly or reflected**
- **Diffuse as much light within the space as possible**
- **Use colours that brighten the appearance of a room.**

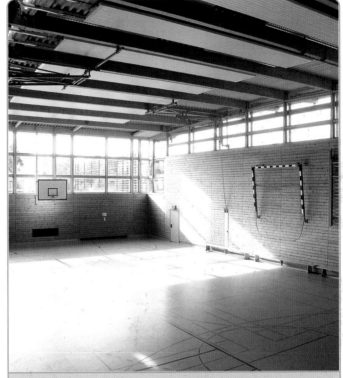

Sports hall lighting
Poor daylighting of sports halls has contributed to the tendency to enclose them as black boxes. Here, lights on undermines any energy efficiency benefits, and reflections and glare are distracting for players.
(Photo: the author)

Permanent features often exclude beneficial daylight in northern climates, and adjustable screens are therefore more desirable. However, they can introduce problems of maintenance, operation and cleaning. Diffusion can be counter-productive, as it significantly reduces both the amenity and energy benefits. Long-lasting, proven, quality solutions should be sought and some of these can be identified from case study buildings.

Modelling and simulation

To calculate and judge the effectiveness of any daylighting design strategy, it is necessary to perform some form of modelling exercise. Simple hand calculations of average daylight factors to the fully rendered computer images of simulation programs can be used. The simplest methods are sometimes the most effective, especially in the early stages.

A productive approach for many designers will be to observe and record the daylighting characteristics of existing buildings. Visual assessment of an interior, for glare and solar ingress, and measurement of light levels with an illuminance meter will provide a useful basis for daylighting design.

A scale model can reasonably accurately show the effect of light through windows. It is usually sufficient to construct a model no larger than a desktop. Surfaces should have the same reflectance and colours as in the completed space, and should be viewed under lighting conditions similar to the intended site. This can be done in an artificial sky or under a real sky.

Sensors mounted inside a model allow a designer to take readings and to assess the daylight factors when combined with

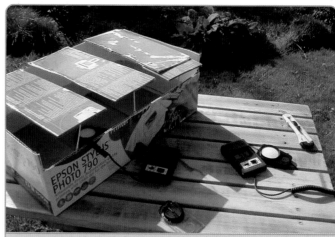

Modelling of daylighting need not be expensive or difficult
A simple scale model positioned at the proposed orientation and two light meters provides an impression of daylight levels through the space at different times of day (Photo: the author)

simultaneous unobstructed measurement using a second meter. The technique is useful for assessing lighting scenarios, comparative assessment of different shading or glazing combinations, and/or to verify calculations and computer simulations. Larger mock-ups are needed for complex lighting systems, but these can evolve from simple studies.

Other physical options are the use of a heliodon or artificial sky in which to model buildings, and again these are simple, relatively inexpensive processes requiring little training that can give simple assessments of the internal and external lighting. However, they are increasingly redundant because of the growth of desktop visualisation tools. Computer visualisation, shaded perspectives or model building will be more valuable once architects and engineers have an idea of the numbers and proportions involved.

Numerical analysis beyond daylight factors can be difficult and although some complex tools can be downloaded free from the Internet, their real cost comes in the length of the learning process.

Amongst the most commonly used design tools are *Radiance* for daylight, *Lightpro* for the lighting layout, *FlucsDL* for daylighting assessment and *FlucsPro* for lighting design. Many engineers are familiar with *Cymap*, which provides simple daylight factor modelling. The *Virtual Lighting Designer* is available on the web and *HyperLight* is a self-help encyclopedia.

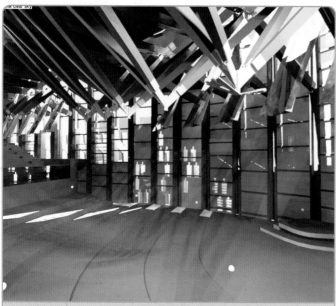

Computer modelling
This can provide excellent detailed daylight visualisation as here in the model of the Scottish Parliament.
(Image permission Scottish Energy Systems Group, University of Strathclyde)

Case Study 9.5:

BRE Environmental Building, Watford

Architects: Feilden Clegg, 1996

This office was designed as a model for future offices and a flagship for integrated passive design. The brief called for minimum use of artificial lighting and air-conditioning. It requires about 30% less energy than typical offices built at the time. The building is L-shaped in plan: a main, three-storey, open-plan office block for 100 staff and a smaller seminar block.

The narrow plan (13.5 m wide) and high ceilings (3.45 m) allows natural light to be exploited. There are large areas of glazing, in the form of opening windows. At occupancy level these are manually operated, while the high-level hopper windows are integral to the natural ventilation strategy and under the control of the building energy management system. The top floor incorporates clerestory windows, giving this floor much higher daylight levels than those below. DFave values above 2% are normal.

Daylight and solar gains are controlled by external, motorised, fritted-glass louvres mounted on the south façade. The louvres are normally automatically controlled, to follow the path of the sun. On overcast days they are moved so that sky luminance can be admitted.

The lighting uses a system of suspended fluorescent luminaires, with high-frequency ballasts. Some light is allowed to shine onto the floor soffit to increase the ceiling illuminance and so reduce glare problems and gloominess. There is also task lighting. Artificial lighting control is automatic, but can be overridden by the occupants.

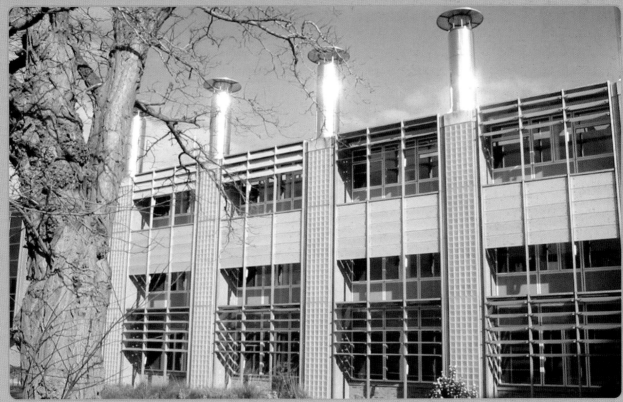

Photo: the author

Colour

Colour plays a very important part in the appearance, operation and ambience of a space, both internally and externally. The colour characteristic of lighting, both appearance and rendering, as well as surface colour and reflectance are the major considerations. However, a number of research studies highlight the importance of colour to how people feel and it is increasingly incorporated to support the architectural form. For example, at Pfennigäcker School in Germany, Barbara Eble – a colour specialist – uses colour externally: blue tones on towers and roofs connecting to the sky, and red and yellow to connect to the earth. These colours are gradually lightened in the common internal circulation spaces and are lightened again for the classrooms so that 'the children's personalities can have greater importance'. This use of colour in this way has a very strong basis in Goethean philosophy and tends to be most evident in Steiner Schools, particularly in Germany. Barbara Eble has produced many such colour schemes, including one for the Schafbrühl estate that takes into account solar orientation and the relationship of buildings to traffic and landscape.

Surface colour

The colour of surfaces is very important to the ambience of a space and to its functionality. The spread of daylight through a space is aided by internal reflections of walls, ceiling and floor.

Material	Reflectance (R)	Material	Reflectance (R)
White Paper	0.8	Wood (Medium)	0.2
Stainless Steel	0.4	Wood (Dark)	0.1
Cement Screed	0.4	Quarry Tiles	0.1
Carpet (Light)	0.4	Window Glass	0.1
Wood (Light)	0.4	Carpet (Dark)	0.1

Table 9.1 Typical reflectances of internal materials

Dark surfaces will reduce the effectiveness of natural and artificial lighting. Warm-coloured walls will give a cosy and relaxing atmosphere, whereas a white room can appear clinical.

Colour concepts
In much of Joachim Eble's work colour is incorporated as a fundamental aspect of putting buildings into their context. It is used to reflect the patterns of sunlight and shade and to brighten courtyards
(Colour design: Barbara Eble)

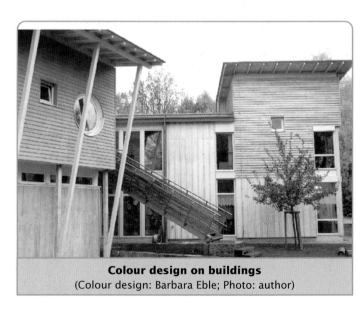

Colour design on buildings
(Colour design: Barbara Eble; Photo: author)

Artificial lighting

A good artificial lighting strategy has functional and amenity aspects, and will aim to be efficient and interesting. It will usually combine general, task and accent lighting with good daylighting. Issues to consider include colour, types of lamps and luminaires in relation to a wide range of factors, and problems such as glare, flicker and reflection.

Where artificial light and daylight are combined, then lamps should be screened from view to avoid glare and direct comparison between daylight and a bare lamp.

Colour appearance

The most commonly used light sources are classified according to their correlated colour temperature scale (CCT), measured in Kelvin (K). There are three main classifications: warm, 3300 K; intermediate, 3300–5300 K; cold, 5300 K.

Low-pressure sodium street lights and tungsten bulbs have a low CCT, which indicates a warm appearance. Fluorescent tubes get increasingly closer to daylight quality and have a high CCT. The colour temperature of daylight varies throughout the day. Strong midday sun has a higher CCT than sunset, which is warmer in appearance. A representative CCT for indoor daylight is normally taken as 6500 K. When daylight and electric light are to be integrated, a lamp of intermediate colour temperature is recommended.

Colour rendering

A light source affects the appearance of the surfaces it illuminates. This quality is quantified by the colour rendering index (CRI). It compares surfaces under a particular light to their appearance under a reference light. Good colour rendering equates to a high CRI, with a maximum of 100 indicating that the source renders all colours identical to the reference. Incandescent lamps have a CRI of very near 100. Low-pressure sodium lamps, such as those used for street lighting, have an extremely poor colour rendering quality, typically about 60. Fluorescent lamps are available in a wide range of colour rendering quality.

One of the problems to date with extending the use of high performance, high efficiency LEDs is that they in the very cool range and are not suitable for many applications. A "warm LED" has recently been launched that may see the start of a market transformation.

It is usually found that the higher the CRI of a lamp, the lower its efficacy, so a designer has to compromise between colour quality and energy consumption. The CIBSE *Interior Lighting Code* recommends minimum colour rendering qualities for different rooms.

Types of lamps and luminaires

Selection of luminaires and their installation requires careful consideration of layout, tasks, maintenance schedules, access, fittings and finishes, including flooring. Even the cleaning regime for surfaces, including windows, needs to be considered if the lighting strategy is to work as designed. These issues need to be considered at the outset.

> **Factors to consider in selecting lamps**
>
> - **Dim or stepped switching**
> - **Installed cost**
> - **Power consumption**
> - **Re-lamping cost**
> - **Lamp life**
> - **Colour quality**
> - **Colour stability**
> - **Frequency/strobe**
> - **Warm-up time**
> - **Presence detection**
> - **Emergency use**
> - **Black hole if lamp fails?**
> - **Perceived brightness**

Lamp characteristics include colour rendering, colour temperature, efficacy, life expectancy, control gear, lamp start-up, lamp restrike and dimming capabilities. It is useful to be familiar with these terms and the implications for design. A number of the referenced publications include good glossaries; the CIBSE *Code for Interior Lighting* and lighting manufacturers' catalogues provide much of this information.

A designer may wish to use a variety of different lamp types to create different moods. It is important in large organisations to try and minimise the potential confusion and perhaps also the implications for stock keeping.

Problems with artificial lighting

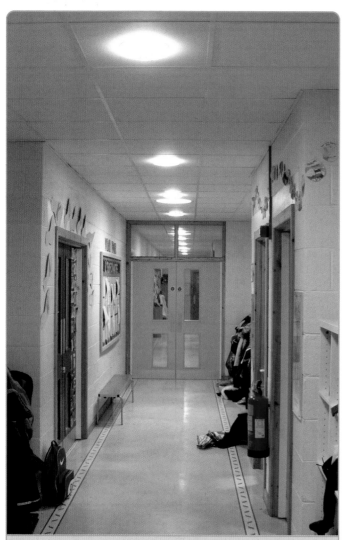

This corridor at a school in Tyne and Wear has alternate artificial lights and 'sunpipes'
As in many similar applications, the daylight is insufficient for the majority of the time to allow lights to be switched off. Consequently it is an expensive solution with minimal quality and cost-in-use benefits
(Photo: the author)

Glare

Glare problems should not be overlooked, even in general areas and circulation spaces. Electric lighting can give rise to discomfort glare and this can be disabling to the visually impaired and to those involved in specialist tasks. Light distribution is enhanced by the use of high surface reflectance from walls and floors, but gloss finishes will give rise to unwelcome specular reflections and glare, and will emphasise irregularities. The glare evaluation index combines the luminance and size of the source, its position in the field of view and the background luminance into a single figure, which should be below a specified limiting value if discomfort is to be avoided. Offices should be designed for a glare index of 19.

Flicker and high-frequency operation

Oscillations (perceived as flicker) in the output from discharge lamps can cause annoyance and may be dangerous, such as when using rotating machinery. High-frequency control gear raises the oscillation rate from 50 Hz to several thousand hertz, which is undetectable to humans and also increases the lamp efficiency by up to 30%.

Veiling reflections

Reflections can occur when a light source is reflected from shiny objects, computer screens or glossy finishes. It is recommended that matt surfaces and/or the layout are such that they are avoided.

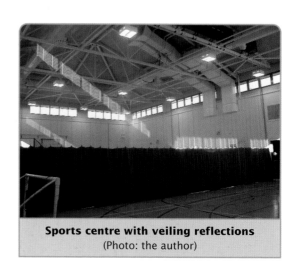

Sports centre with veiling reflections
(Photo: the author)

Lighting – rules of thumb

Process

- Have you approached the lighting strategy in an interdisciplinary manner to integrate the structure and other services?
- Does the built form and orientation optimise daylight whilst minimising problems such as noise and glare?
- Might the installation in future be adaptable to reuse?
- Have you considered passive design options with respect to other services, e.g. ventilation?

Windows

- Have you calculated the daylight factors and assessed the occurrence of solar penetration?
- Is the thermal insulation value of glazing sufficient to minimise any local cooling or heat loss problems associated with the daylighting?
- Is unwelcome solar gain minimised by appropriate shading or selection of heat-rejecting glazing?
- Is solar gain employed usefully where and when beneficial?
- Is the acoustic insulation value of glazing sufficient to minimise any problems associated with external noise?
- Does the daylight strategy constrain choice of window positions or prevent window opening?
- Has night glare from buildings and exterior lighting been minimised?

Management and affordability

- Have all the zones of the building (internal and external) been considered and incorporated in a control strategy?
- Have cost-in-use benefits been assessed?
- Has consideration been given to long life and low maintenance?
- Does the light quantity and quality, fittings and controls match user and management needs and requirements?
- Does the handover plan include for adequate training?
- Are the lighting controls ergonomically designed for ease of use and to take account of building operation?

Building services

- Are the selected lights and fittings energy efficient?
- Is unwelcome heat from luminaires minimised and/or dispersed efficiently?
- Has artificial and natural light been properly integrated?
- Have opportunities for integration of daylighting and other servicing strategies, such as ventilation and fire, been fully explored?
- Is wiring to luminaires compatible with other wired services, such as communications?
- Has care been taken to ensure that luminaires do not interfere with air flows for passive or active systems?

Health and safety

- Has attention been given to occupants' need?
- Can the installation be installed, cleaned and maintained easily and safely?
- Have the heavy metals and other materials harmful to users and the environment (in lamps, wiring, luminaires, etc.) been minimised?
- Have assurances been sought that lamps or luminaires that contain necessary materials which are harmful to the environment can be reused, recycled or disposed of safely?

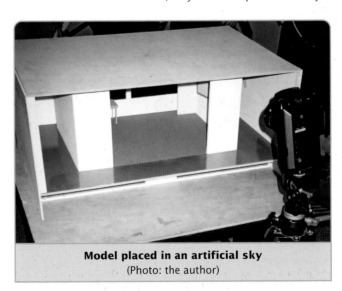

Model placed in an artificial sky
(Photo: the author)

Sources of technical information

Glossary of lighting terms

Bell and Burt.
CIBSE *Code for Interior Lighting*.
DFEE Building Bulletin 90.

Standard values of illuminance

BRE publications on specific building types.
CIBSE *Code for Interior Lighting*.

Detailed lamp and luminaire descriptions

Bell and Burt.
CIBSE Code for Interior Lighting.
DFEE Building Bulletin 90.
Manufacturers' information.

UK locations of artificial skies and heliodons

Commission of the European Communities, Daylighting in Architecture.

Point daylight factors, illuminance and luminance

CIBSE *Code for Interior Lighting*.
CIBSE LG10: Daylighting and Window Design.

Values for transmittance and dirt values

CIBSE *Code for Interior Lighting*.

Colour of surfaces, colour temperature (CCT) and colour rendering index (Ra)

BRE publications on specific building types.
CIBSE *Code for Interior Lighting*.

Glare and glare evaluation index

CIBSE TM10 *Calculation of Glare Indices*.

Sun path information

Bell and Burt.
CIBSE LG10: *Daylighting and Window Design*.

Modelling of lighting

The Bartlett School of Architecture www.bartlett.ucl.ac.uk
Scottish Energy Systems Group www.sesg.strath.ac.uk

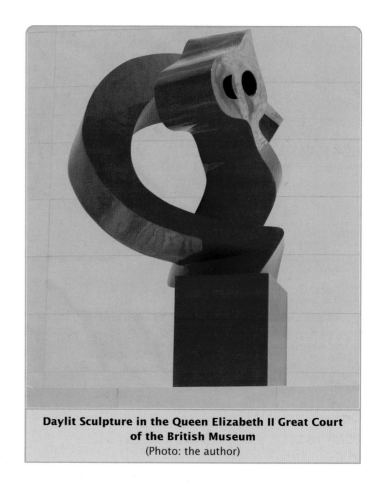

Daylit Sculpture in the Queen Elizabeth II Great Court of the British Museum
(Photo: the author)

Bibliography

CARL (undated) The LT Method: An energy design tool for non-domestic buildings. Cambridge Architectural Research Ltd (www.carl.co.uk). Understanding and designing optimum window areas.

CIBSE TM10 (1985) *Calculation of Glare Indices*.CIBSE

Crisp, V. et al. (1988) *Daylight as a Passive Solar Energy Option*. BRE.

CIBSE LG04 (1990) *Lighting Guide*. CIBSE.

EEO Econ 19 (1991) *Energy Efficiency in Offices*. BRECSU.

BRE Commission of the European Communities (1993) *Daylighting in Architecture: A European Reference Book*. BRE.

CIBSE (1994) *Code for Interior Lighting*. CIBSE.

Thermie (1994) *Daylighting in Buildings*. European Commission. Out of print. Copies from Energie on 0161 874 3636.

Bell, J. and Burt, W. (1996) *Designing Buildings for Daylight*. BRE. An excellent self-learning tool.

BRE IP 6 (1996) *People and Lighting Controls*. BRE.

Littlefair, P. J. (1996) *Designing with Innovative Daylighting*. BRE.

BRE (1998) *Environmental Design Guide for Naturally Ventilated and Daylit Offices*. Useful and free from BRECSU.

BRE IP 16 (1998) *Interior Lighting Calculations: A Guide to Computer Programs*. BRE.

DETR GPG 245 (1998) *Desktop Guide to Daylighting – for architects*. BRECSU.

Thermie (1998) *Energy Efficient Lighting in Offices*. Thermie.

Tregenza, P. and Loe, D. (1998) *The Design of Lighting*. E. & F. N. Spon.

BRE BR364 (1999) *Solar Shading of Buildings*. BRE.

BRE IP 2 (1999) *Photoelectric Control of Lighting: Design, Setup and Installation Issues*. BRE.

CIBSE LG10 (1999) *Daylighting and Window Design*. CIBSE.

DETR GPG 272 (1999) *Lighting for People, Energy Efficiency and Architecture*. BRECSU.

DfEE (1999) *Lighting Design for Schools*, Building Bulletin 90. HMSO. An indispensable guide to lighting of schools that provides a good basic grasp for adaptation to other building types.

Fontoynont, M. (1999) *Daylight Performance of Buildings*. James & James.

Littlefair, P. J. (2000) *Developments in Innovative Daylighting*. BRE.

Phillips, D. (2000) *Lighting Modern Buildings*. Architectural Press.

Plympton, P. et al. (2000) *Daylighting in Schools: Improving Student Performance and Health at a Price Schools Can Afford.* NREL www.deptplanetearth.com/nrel_student_performance.htm Just a starting point for research on daylight and health.

Baker, N. and Steemers, K. (2002) *Daylight Design of Buildings*. James & James.

Kats, G. (2003) *The Costs and Financial Benefits of Green Buildings*. California's Sustainable Building Task Force.

Gaia Group (2006) *Design and Construction of Sustainable Schools Vols 1 and 2*. Scottish Executive (www.gaiagroup.org).

Virtual lighting designer from GE Lighting Site (www.gelighting.com).

Chapter 10
Ventilation and cooling strategies

In which we look at strategies for ventilation and cooling that take into account moisture management, airtightness and materials selection as fundamental aspects. These contribute to the good indoor air quality, well-being, energy efficiency, cost savings and enjoyment that we expect from buildings.

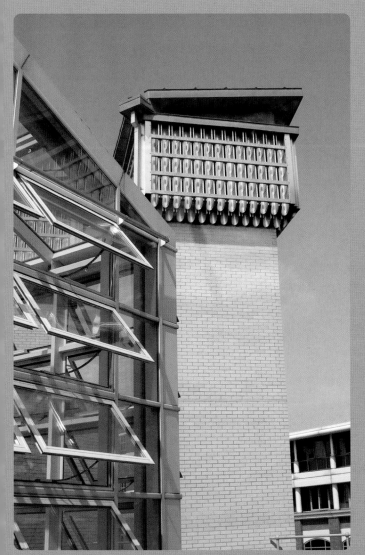

'Good indoor air quality is a human right.'

Dagfinn Jorgensen, engineer, Kjeldas School, Norway

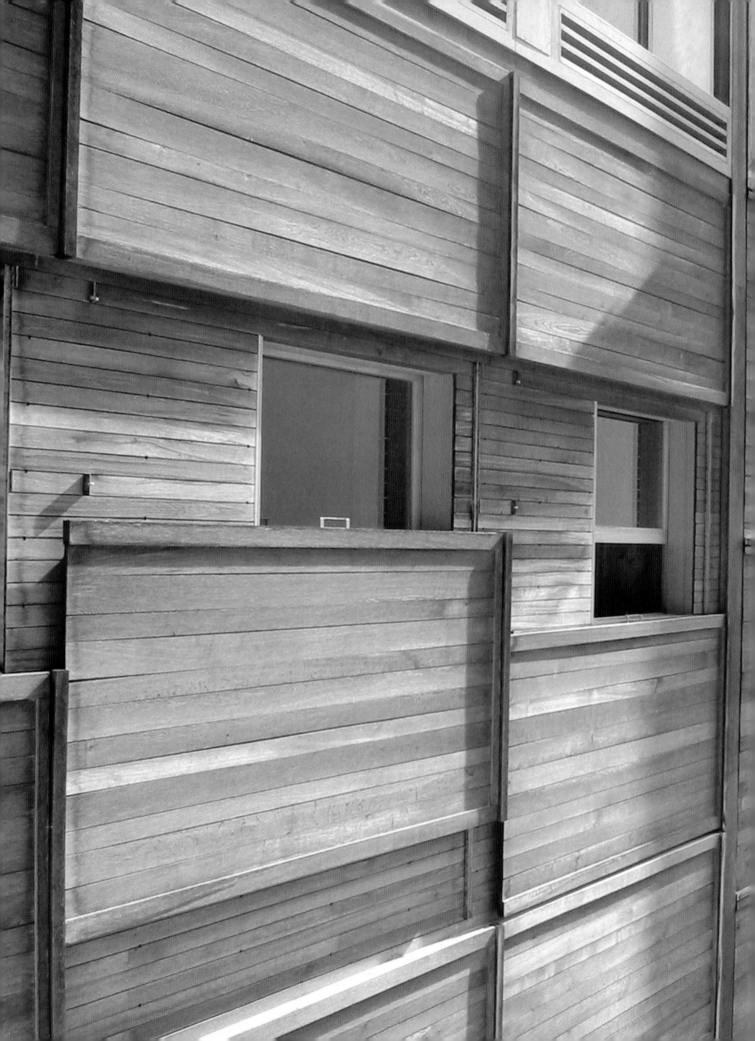

Contents

(Facing page)
**Background ventilation,
Biel-Bienne College, Switzerland**
(Architects: Meili and Peter;
photo: the author)

(Previous page)
Coventry University Library
(Architects: Alan Short Architects;
photo: the author)

Ventilation and cooling strategies

Introduction

There is plenty of guidance already available on ventilation and cooling. Arguably, no other design issue has been subject to as much controversy as a consequence of the requirements of sustainable building. However, many buildings remain less comfortable and less healthy than they might be, and they consume unnecessary energy for ventilation and cooling.

Increasing attention to energy efficiency in the 1970s led to a sealing up of domestic buildings and a fashion for close controlled commercial environments. It subsequently became clear that this was undertaken with inadequate consideration for moisture management and movement in buildings, pollution from mechanical ventilation systems and the effects of indoor materials. Notably at this time, synthetic materials were increasingly replacing natural ones. The resulting buildings often failed to address the worst problems of unhealthy buildings and undoubtedly contributed to creating new unhealthy indoor environments. This gave rise to a range of illnesses, which became known as sick building syndrome (SBS) and subsequently as building related ill-health, and to mould and moisture problems in housing, which have been the focus of remediation strategies.

The confusion that resulted still permeates design approaches and teaching methods, with seemingly an overriding assumption that both leaky and tight buildings are bad but necessary! A lot of information has been generated in the intervening period and

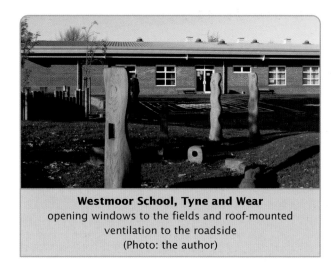

Westmoor School, Tyne and Wear
opening windows to the fields and roof-mounted ventilation to the roadside
(Photo: the author)

changes in attitudes are now being consolidated in good ventilation strategies that deliver healthy indoor environments with energy efficiency. There is therefore a need to bring the most contemporary information about cooling and ventilation in the design of buildings and services to wider attention. There is great variety and few absolutes.

Poorly controlled mechanical ventilation systems can use a great deal of energy to little effect, and if badly maintained be a source of pollution. Poorly controlled natural ventilation systems can also introduce external pollution, as well as lead to unnecessary waste of heat or to unacceptable variability in indoor temperature, air movement and humidity. Neither approach offers a panacea, hence the appearance in recent years of what has become known as 'mixed-mode' or hybrid strategies, which combine approaches rather than provide one fixed solution for everywhere. These are essentially a reminder of the need for designed ventilation and cooling to meet potentially very different requirements at different times and spaces within a building.

The transition of design thinking from fully managed mechanical design solutions and largely artificial indoor environments to a much greater flexibility, combined with understanding of context, natural processes and awareness of human factors, is well under way.

Simple solutions are preferable to more complex ones, especially systems, which are easier to clean, control, maintain and repair. A clear design strategy where manageability and control have been considered produces the best results.

Of the case studies selected, only one has no fans at all, three are referred to as naturally ventilated, at least three are hybrid/mixed-mode designs and no two use the same approach.

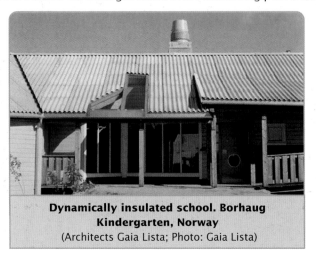

Dynamically insulated school. Borhaug Kindergarten, Norway
(Architects Gaia Lista; Photo: Gaia Lista)

Recent history

For many years design and regulatory effort to make buildings more sustainable and energy efficient focused on improving heating and insulation. Recently, ventilation and cooling have been recognised as fundamental issues, and have become the primary consideration in many types of building for many reasons:

- Health in buildings is often related to air quality
- The proportion of heat loss through air movement has increased as insulation standards have improved
- Uncontrolled air infiltration adversely affects comfort and energy efficiency
- Internal and solar heat gains have increased in many buildings
- However, the trend to lightweight construction makes them less able to store/lose heat
- The climate is getting warmer.

Approaches to domestic and commercial buildings differ. The trend in the 1970s to close control of commercial buildings combined with mechanical ventilation (MV) and cooling provision came under scrutiny when energy studies identified them as a very significant aspect of the global warming impact of many buildings, largely due to use of electrical energy. Also, studies identified them as a significant proportion of the initial and running costs of buildings and:

- ventilation systems were often associated with poor indoor air quality (IAQ)
- occupants were often dissatisfied with buildings that gave them little or no control over their environment
- ventilation systems were taking up the proportion of cost and space which in the past would have resulted in larger, taller rooms delivering similar performance.

Building related ill-health (BRI)

The impact of building related ill-health, which describes a collective adverse reaction to an indoor environment, in the 1980s, should not be underestimated. The phenomenon was associated largely, but not wholly, with tightly controlled and mechanically ventilated buildings. Symptoms included congested nasal passages, inflamed eyes, palate and pharynx, dry skin, headache, fatigue, and attention deficits. Despite significant research and identification of possible causes – including the correlation with volatile organic compounds (VOCs) and high temperatures – it proved difficult to identify either a specific cause or to predict affliction rates. However, the association with VOCs, tight control and mechanical ventilation stuck.

Many designers sought solutions in natural ventilation (NV), which also proved difficult. Ultimately, it has transpired that neither full air-conditioning nor NV is a panacea in terms of energy efficiency, health, comfort or manageability. Studies by Bordass and Leaman (see Usable Buildings Trust) compared air-conditioned, assisted NV, mixed-mode and NV buildings, and identified that occupant satisfaction was largely independent of the ventilation strategy.

It has become evident that the requirement is for spaces to be designed with more attention to detail in the early stages of design. At this stage, considering how spaces will be used is vitally important, as is attention to eliminating avoidable heat gains and pollutants.

Strategies need to be easy to understand and control by occupants and managers. Truly effective ventilation can only be achieved if it is designed to meet individual needs and to operate with minimal technical complications.

The correct strategy should be thought through from inception of a project, as it will depend on location, occupancy patterns, fit-out and management, and will influence all aspects of the design. Windows are crucial, whatever the strategy, because they have to meet a large number of requirements.

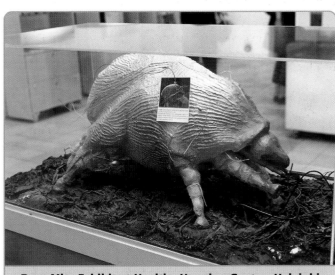

Dust Mite Exhibit at Healthy Housing Centre, Helsinki
(Photo: the author)

Why ventilate?

We ventilate buildings for a wide variety of reasons. Improving thermal comfort and indoor air quality through provision of fresh air is known to be vitally important to individuals' perception of a space, their health and well-being, and productivity. Any ventilation system should be flexible because it will need to work under a wide range of conditions:

1 To remove excess heat from people and equipment.
2 To remove moisture, smells and pollutants generated by people, pets and cooking, which can be unpleasant or hazardous to health and/or buildings.
3 To remove gaseous emissions from materials, furnishings, cleaning agents and, in affected areas, the products of radon.
4 To act as a carrier for heating, cooling and/or humidity control.
5 To provide oxygen for breathing, although the safe requirement is a tiny proportion compared to the other needs.

Whilst the concept of fresh air is not directly associated with CO_2, it is a useful indicator of adequate ventilation, how fresh the indoor environment is and hence how satisfied people are likely to be. In many situations, the airflow required for cooling

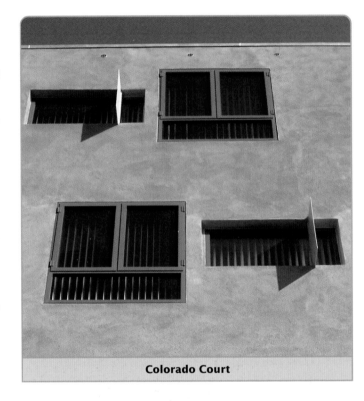

Colorado Court

is the major requirement, much higher than that for control of air quality.

How much ventilation is needed?

'Fresh air' has evaded definition, so ventilation standards must rely on rates of external air supply, which depend on how much heat, moisture and pollution it is necessary to remove. Odour is a determining factor. For sedentary people, typical rates of outdoor air supply are between 5 and 25 l/s/person. For normal office occupancy levels with little or no smoking, this equates to 1–2 l/s/m² of floor area, significantly less than was required in offices when smoking was common.

If cooling naturally, the hotter it gets the more ventilation is needed. Typical peak summer rates in offices suitable for natural ventilation are in the range 5–10 ac/h. Higher airflow blows papers around. Night cooling tends to operate at 2–5 ac/h. *GPG224 Improving Airtightness* and *GRG 21 Improving Ventilation* provide useful guidance for housing, but should be accompanied by an awareness of moisture management issues.

Units of measurement

Ventilation tends to be quoted in three sets of units:

- **litres/s/person (l/s/person)**
- **litres/s/m² of floor space (l/s/m²)**
- **air changes/h (ac/h).**

These can be converted to one another if occupancy densities and room heights are known. For example, typical office provision of 15 l/s/person:

- **at an occupant density of 10 m²/person is equal to 1.5 l/s/m² (i.e. 15 l/s/person divided by 10 m²/person)**
- **at a room height of 2.7m is equal to 2 ac/h (i.e. 15 l/s/person – 3600 s/h divided by 27 m³/person).**

Airtightness

A consequence of improvements in thermal performance of building fabric is that the percentage of heat loss due to infiltration increased dramatically. The response, now being wrapped into legislation, has been to construct more tightly sealed buildings. This has subsequently given rise to real and justified concerns about indoor health because of poorly designed and maintained mechanical systems. This is particularly evident in housing.

'Build tight – ventilate right'
Ventilation is airflow resulting from a designed intention.
Air infiltration is unintentional and uncontrollable leakage of air because of imperfections in detailing and construction.
It can be a significant heating or cooling load, and may be a pathway for noise and pollution.
Infiltration should be eliminated in favour of controlled ventilation when, where and in the quantity required.

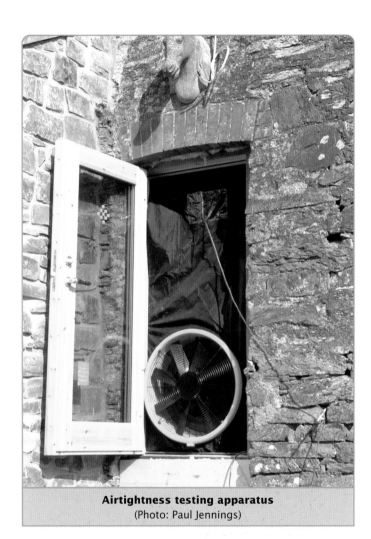

Airtightness testing apparatus
(Photo: Paul Jennings)

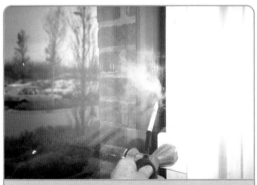

Simple leakage test using a smoke pencil
Smoke escapes through inadequately
sealed windows
(Photo: Bill Bordass)

The indoor environment

Air quality

The materials used in building have undergone perhaps greater changes than any other aspect of construction. At the beginning of the twentieth century, about 50 materials were used. Now, some 55 000 building materials are available, and of course many are synthetic. The change in materials specification has led to a significant increase in indoor pollutants and a change in the heat- and damp-retaining capacities of buildings. Fluctuations in moisture content are greater, as are the problems caused by moisture, which serves as a medium for chemical reactions and microbial growth. The value of investing in a better quality indoor climate is undisputed – an increase in productivity or reduction in absenteeism by 0.6% is sufficient to justify 60% increase in expenditure on indoor air quality. Ventilation systems themselves have increasingly been seen as part of the indoor air quality problem. In a study of 15 office construction projects in Copenhagen, Fanger found that only 12% of the pollution of the internal air originated in the occupant metabolism: 25% derived from smoking, 20% from materials and furnishings, and 42% from the ventilation equipment. Of these, the materials are the easiest to deal with and the ventilation perhaps the most difficult.

One OLF is the emission rate
of polluant from a
standard person,
defined as an average
sedentary adult
in thermal comport
with a hygenic standard
of 0.7 baths/day

Pollution from a standard person
The 'olf' was proposed as the unit of measurement of scent emission of people, objects and systems by P.O. Fanger and later adopted by ASHRAE

Thermal comfort

Design approaches, for a generation or more, were based on an objective criterion of comfort derived from laboratory experiments based on thermal models. Whilst initially intended as guidance, these standards were increasingly rigidly applied and even in mild climates it proved hard to meet the requirements other than mechanically. It was argued for many years that narrow definitions exaggerated the need for air-conditioning. It had, for instance, been known for decades that people's response to thermal comfort requirements differed in naturally ventilated and mechanically conditioned buildings.

Research in offices, schools and factories reinforced the inadequacy of rigid standards throughout the 1980s and 1990s, and relatively recently sufficient evidence has been obtained to allow good sense to prevail. It is now recognised that people will tolerate higher temperatures than previously thought, as long as they have some control over their environment.

A more sensitive and flexible approach is increasingly evident, with benefits in occupant satisfaction, comfort and productivity.

Draughts, in particular, are often a source of avoidable problems. At low temperatures we are less tolerant of air movement and it has a greater cooling effect. Better insulation and tighter construction can help to create higher and more constant surface temperatures, and hence reduce the uncontrolled internal air circulation which creates draughts.

Moisture management

Depending on factors such as insulation, materials, 'cold bridges' and air leakages, a building can cope with more or less moisture in the air. Hygroscopicity describes the ability of some materials to absorb moisture when the humidity rises and emit it when the air becomes dry. These materials stabilise the relative humidity (RH) and can help to prevent damp-related damage. Some porous materials can hold quite large quantities of moisture without any special risks of biological activity or degradation. Materials such as timber, plaster, earth and textiles have hygroscopic properties, so long as they are not given impervious coatings.

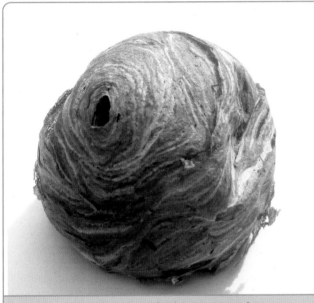

Moisture transfusive construction
Fabric is vitally important in many structures. In wasps' nests
the heat and moisture must be allowed to escape
(Photo: the author)

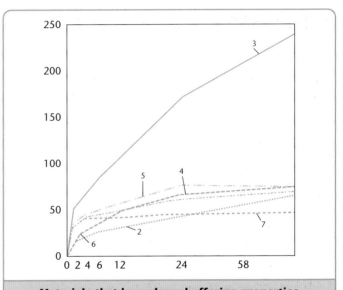

Materials that have damp-buffering properties
1 planed pine; 2 planed limba (tropical wood); 3 clay; 4 clay
render; 5 clay render with cocoa fibre; 6 lime cement render;
7 plaser. (Graph from Roalkvam)

Recent research undertaken in Finland indicates that materials
are more than nine times better at dealing with moisture than
mechanical ventilation.

Two people occupying a standard (15 m^2) bedroom overnight in
autumn, in which the materials are not hygroscopic, require
0.9 ac/h to keep the moisture less than or equal to 60% RH. With
hygroscopic materials, only 0.1 ac/h is needed to keep the
moisture < 60% RH.

This 0.1 ac/h is less than the leak in a very airtight building. It
means it is potentially as critical to design in the hygroscopic
materials as it is to put in the ventilation system. This provides
support for the experience from Toll House Gardens, Fairfield,
where the difference in moisture load between the buildings
with mechanical heat recovery, dynamic insulation and trickle
ventilation was much less than might have been expected. A
theory proposed was that the hygroscopic design implemented
throughout the housing was responsible for much of the
moisture management.

Spaces exposed to sudden changes in moisture loads, including
most wet rooms and schools, may have problems coping with
temporary loads. Films of moisture form on non-hygroscopic
surfaces. As nutrients dissolve in the moisture, micro-organisms
proliferate and then respond to the drying of the film, as the air
dries, with spore production, release of toxins and other
metabolites. Fluctuating conditions lead to the worst effects of
microbial activity. Hence, when the indoor atmosphere is likely
to be subjected to sudden moisture loads, the damp-buffering
capacity of materials becomes particularly important for
maintaining an acceptable RH. Thermal mass can also have an
impact on moisture management, as rapid cooling of buildings
gives rise to fluctuations in RH that are detrimental to both
building and occupants. Building materials can sustain very large
populations of micro-organisms – for example, plastic membranes,
glass fibre, etc. can have colonies of fungi and bacteria that are
1000–50 000 times greater than natural materials.

Emissions from building products

Concentrations of more than 35 VOCs (volatile organic compounds, including vinyl chloride, benzene, formaldehyde and toluene) are typically 10 times higher indoors than outdoors.

Many of these VOCs have been identified as emanating from building products and are associated with a wide range of detrimental health effects in humans and animals (including cancers, tumours, irritation and immune suppression). The higher the temperature, the more VOCs appear in the gaseous phase. It has also been shown that gaseous concentrations of many VOCs are indirectly proportional to air humidity (though this is not the case for formaldehyde). Information is available on sources of VOCs, the extent of emissions, and assessing emission rates and indoor air quality, although avoidance is the best strategy.

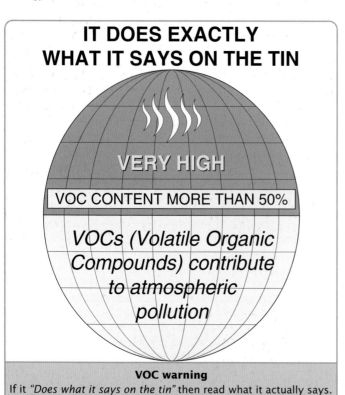

IT DOES EXACTLY WHAT IT SAYS ON THE TIN

VERY HIGH

VOC CONTENT MORE THAN 50%

VOCs (Volatile Organic Compounds) contribute to atmospheric pollution

VOC warning
If it *"Does what it says on the tin"* then read what it actually says.
"The contents of this tin are a risk to skin, eyes, lungs and the atmosphere"

Prevention is best

- **Build airtight**
- **Remove pollutants and unwanted heat at source**
- **Control internal gains**
- **Avoid deep plans and have:**
  - **Rooms high enough to allow stratification above the occupied zone**
  - **Solar control and shading**
  - **Appropriate glazing**
  - **Some thermal capacity in exposed ceilings.**

Appropriate choice of low-emission materials can reduce ventilation requirements and this is an accepted trade-off under the Norwegian building regulations. There is presently no limit for VOC emissions in the European Product Standard, although schemes exist in a number of countries.

Methods of ventilation

The unaided volume of airflow through a building depends on the number, position and orientation of openings, the difference in temperature between inside and outside, and the wind velocity. The wind creates pressure differences that drive air into a building on the windward side and out on the leeward side. Indoor activities create thermal gradients as warm air is 'lighter' than cold air and will tend to rise and leave at high level to be replaced by air entering at low level – the so-called 'stack effect'. These forces of wind pressure and gravity may act together or separately and can, if well understood and properly managed, be a driving force for NV. However, not all buildings, or parts of a building, will require the same approach, and strategies need to reflect outside air quality, orientation, location, seasonal effects and usage patterns, including temporary loads. Variability in wind regimes and uncontrolled pressure differentials mean that the task is non-trivial even in simple buildings. Corridors, stairs, lift shafts, and so on all impact upon airflows. Conflicts with fire containment strategies are likely. As a consequence, a range of techniques have been developed to assist and modify the flow and temperature of air, its speed and direction.of countries.

Case Study 10.1:

Toll House Gardens, Perth

Architects: Gaia Architects, 2001

Domestic environments are known to be a source of breathing-related problems, which can be exacerbated by poor construction and ventilation. One in seven children in Scotland suffers from asthma, and an affordable specification is a major step forward in barrier-free design and improved quality of life for a large number of sufferers and their families.

A commission for 14 houses and a small research grant provided an opportunity to create low-allergen/asthma-friendly buildings that extended the specification to barrier-free design for people with breathing disabilities. The overall aim was to give the same importance in building design to allergy/asthma as is presently the case for physical access and enable tenants with breathing-related problems to lead relatively normal lives.

Gaia developed an affordable low-allergy building specification to avoid, wherever possible, known and suspected building related-allergens and minimise the conditions in which they can have an adverse impact. The result is the attractive and award winning one- and two-storey development at Toll House Gardens.

The specification paid attention to the global environmental condition; moisture management through fabric, ventilation and air tightness; no/low-emission materials; and reducing the areas where dust mites might readily populate. Materials with hygroscopic properties were used throughout to maintain relative humidity at acceptable levels and to minimise the conditions that provide a host environment to dust mites and mould. Sensitisation is associated with a number of chemicals and these were avoided.

The ventilation strategies are of particular interest in respect of their efficacy, affordability and energy efficiency.

Dynamic insulation was used in five houses, and this allowed comparison with Baxi Whole House ventilation systems in five houses and standard

provision in the other houses. The houses were monitored for known triggers and the ability of the environment to resist their build up. Operational factors such as pet ownership and cleaning regimes were taken into account. A notable aspect of the results was the extent of moisture management in all the properties, regardless of the ventilation system.

The traditional expectation is that mechanical systems perform much better than naturally ventilated properties in moisture control. The results at Fairfield appear to accord with the recently published Finnish research that the extent of hygroscopic materials was having a effect greater than the mechanical systems. However, the number of properties involved meant that the results were never going to be statistically significant.

Projects like this are at the core of a discussion on sustainable housing because instead of stating that sustainability involves economic, environmental and social aspects, they seek to prove it and generate the momentum for change. This specification of benign materials and high-performance housing has clear environmental benefits in pollution prevention; it provided social benefits with improvements in occupants' health.

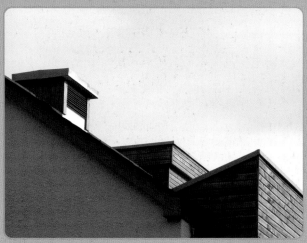

Photo: Michael Wolshover

Natural ventilation

In natural ventilation (NV) systems the driving forces are small (normally less than 50 Pa). An advantage of low pressure gradients, low airflow and absence of fans is that NV has the potential to be more efficient and quieter than mechanical systems, as long as airflow is well controlled and noise into and within a building is given careful consideration.

Because pressure differences are low, it is also important to minimise resistances to airflow. There is a limit to the amount of heat that NV can reject because, at peak demand, the difference between indoor and outdoor temperatures is too small to be useful and can be counter-productive. This limited cooling capacity makes it vital to minimise thermal and pollutant loads, and so building form, fabric and fit-out must play a part.

Rooms should be high enough to allow polluted air to rise above the occupied zone and be removed through high-placed vents without air movement generated by people and equipment stirring the outflow air. Close temperature control is not possible, but is no longer believed to be necessary, provided that occupants can make adjustments if required.

Natural ventilation strategies

- **Opening windows:**
  - **high level – cross-ventilation**
  - **low level – local ventilation**
  - **trickle ventilation – winter**
  - **large openings – summer**
- **Night cooling**
- **Passive stack**
- **Atria**
- **Wind scoops**
- **Ducted or underfloor.**

Opening windows

When relying on natural ventilation it is important that all ventilated areas are within designed distances of an opening. As a rule of thumb, the plan width should be less than five times the floor-to-ceiling height. The benefits of such an approach are that it can also aid other aspects known to be important to occupant satisfaction, namely daylighting and provision of external views. In multi-storey buildings with internal stack effect ventilation (e.g. atria), openings need to be larger and higher up in order to get similar ventilation rates on each floor.

It is important to do calculations or modelling to ensure that the air really does follow the right arrows and to make sure that excessive amounts of air are not introduced during the heating season!

- Single-sided, single-opening ventilation is effective to a depth of about two times the floor-to-ceiling height
- Single-sided, double-opening ventilation is effective to a depth of about 2.5 times the floor-to-ceiling height
- Cross-ventilation is effective to a depth up to five times the floor-to-ceiling height.

It is vitally important with window design that the whole design team thinks through what they (and ventilators) will be required to do (the different modes of ventilation, as well as light and shade and view) and how they could be used in practice, in order to select an appropriate solution. Real care is required if windows are to meet trickle ventilation requirements in winter and higher summer requirements without excessive draught or blowing about (of papers and frames!).

Passive stack

Stack ventilation is the designed use of gravitational force, perhaps enhanced by chimneys and/or by having outflows into zones of negative pressure, where the effect will be enhanced. Care has to be taken to position and insulate chimneys to ensure that the air cannot cool below the temperature of the ambient air, as it will lose buoyancy and reverse flow will occur. Modern roof-mounted vents have multiple openings which automatically close on windward and open on leeward sides. These and wind-driven centrifugal ventilators can aid the flow of air.

Solar gains can be used to promote buoyancy of the air; again, care is required. Airflow can be enhanced by use of an extract fan in the event that flow is insufficient, but the fan should default to off and should not prevent significant resistance to the flow of air under passive operation. Vented double façades are forms of stack effect.

Case Study 10.2:

Borhaug Kindergarten, Norway

Gaia Lista, 1999

The nursery in Borhaug is very well sited and has a very healthy indoor climate. In keeping with Gaia's philosophy it is sensitive and responsive to its exposed micro-climate.

The micro-climatic design includes both outdoor and indoor comfort whilst delivering a building with a low energy demand. The building incorporates both a culvert ventilation pre-heat system and ceilings with dynamic insulation.

The incoming air is delivered through the insulation in the roof and is introduced into the room through a perforated ceiling finish. The dynamic insulation proved to be so efficient that the culvert has not been needed.

There is extensive use of natural materials, from the dry-stone walls and untreated external timber through to the non-toxic materials and finishes internally. The wall construction is also moisture transfusive (a breathing wall), by virtue of its untreated finishes and environmentally sound components.

The exterior areas have been given an equal amount of detailed attention as the indoor areas. The building relates on all its façades to the outdoor climate, creating sheltered areas to the leeward side and turning its back to the prevailing wind.

The outdoor areas are also varied. There are at least three different kinds of 'place' within the small field in which the building sits so that different parts of the playground are optimal according to the weather.

The design is simple and has a flexible layout internally. The whole approach of the design is that it is orientated towards the child and is effectively a large playhouse, with windows at a 3 year-old child's eye level. The ethos of the school is set down in a set of explicit principles, which were derived together with the children and which are located on the wall in large letters at the entrance.

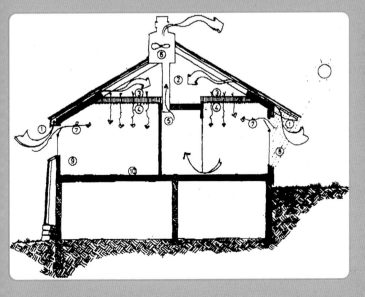

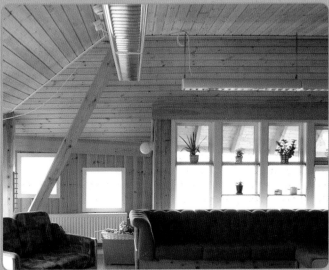

Photo and Image: Gaia Lista

Atria

Atria operate in the same way as chimneys, but as they have a number of potential roles and added benefits they may not always be exploited to their optimum for ventilation. They can increase the effective depth of a building by drawing air from all sides into a central space. A 15 m floor plan is probably the limit for a cross-ventilation strategy using an atrium. It is important that, if they are to be useful amenity spaces, the temperature in the highest occupied zone of atria does not exceed that required for comfort. A rule of thumb is that an effective exhaust atrium should be 3 m above the heads of standing people on the floor.

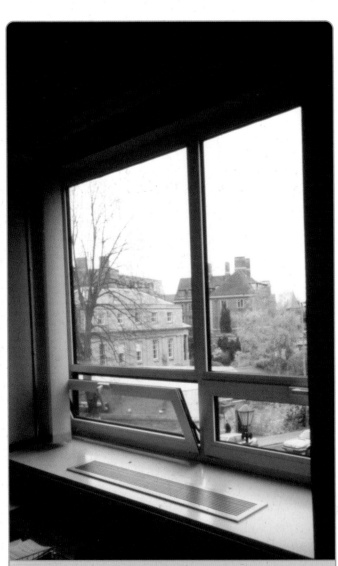

Oxford County Hall
In a refurbishment project in the early 1990s, workers in Oxford County Hall decided that natural ventilation with local control was preferable to the existing air-conditioning. This was despite concerns about the noise and pollution ingress in the city centre site. The project illustrated the change in design responses to thermal comfort, advances in glazing technology and the impact of setting long-term strategies for the built environment including traffic management
(Photo: the author)

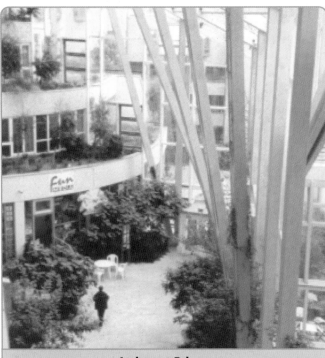

Atrium at Prisma
Architect: Joachim Eble Architects
(Photo: Joachim Eble Architects)

Ducted/underfloor

Ducts can be used to supply air from one side of a building without it being contaminated. A range of examples can be found in CIBSE AM10: *Natural Ventilation in Non-Domestic Buildings*.

Case Study 10.3:

Coventry University Library

Architects: Alan Short Architects, 2000

Coventry University's Library site was compact, noisy and enclosed. However, the University specified that the new building be 'maintenance free' and super energy-efficient.

It was evident that the size of the site would force a deep-plan approach and that noise from the nearby elevated roads would not allow reliance on opening windows for ventilation. A highly heat-efficient 50m square plan was selected, with vertical wells punched through for natural light and air supply and removal, supplemented by perimeter ventilation stacks. This still left a lot to do to make it all work, as this building was billed as the biggest naturally ventilated building of its type in the world. The overall stack head available (4 Pa) has required considerable attention to limit the pressure losses in the total airflow path from inlet via plenum, heater battery, inlet dampers, room exhaust dampers and exhaust dampers/louvres.

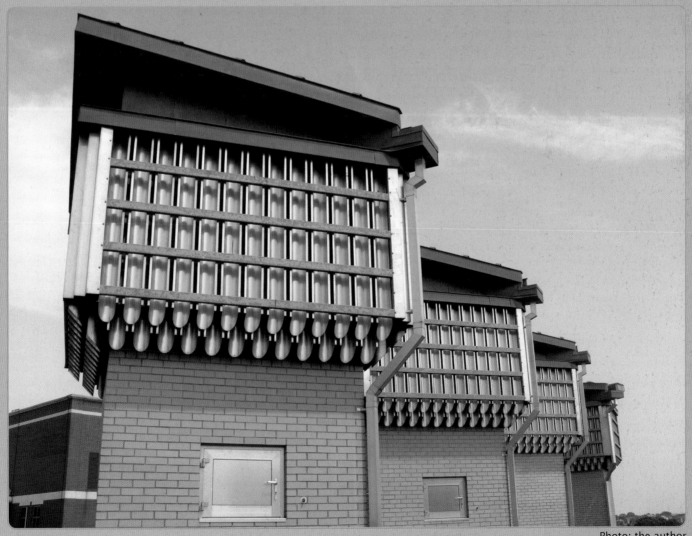

Photo: the author

Mechanical ventilation

Mechanical ventilation (MV) involves forced air movements, with pressure differences typically 100–1000 Pa. It may be required when there is a perceived need for closer temperature control, where internal heat gains or pollutant levels are too great, where plan depth, external noise or air pollution restricts the use of NV, for all or part of the time, or where security or physical restrictors preclude adequately sized natural openings. Complete MV which denies occupants the opportunity to open windows is known to be unpopular, and hybrid (mixed-mode) solutions in which MV is used in combination with opening windows is increasingly common. Clearly, care must be taken to design both strategies so that they can work to assist the preferred flow of air and do not undermine each other or the overall efficiency. GIR 56 Mixed mode buildings and systems is essential reading.

There are essentially three types of MV: supply, extract and balanced.

Supply-only pressurises a building to resist the inflow of uncontrolled infiltration. It is important that designed exhaust vents are provided and that the structure is airtight if interstitial condensation is to be avoided.

Extract-only is applicable to spaces with localised pollution, moisture and odour problems, and is used for extracting pollutants close to the source – bathrooms, kitchens and densely occupied spaces such as meeting rooms. Heat recovery is often an option. However, if the building is not airtight, and designed openings are not provided, then infiltration air will give rise to draughts and inefficiency.

Balanced ventilation involves both controlled input and extract and provides opportunity for heat recovery between them but unless it is well designed and controlled, the energy advantages may not be sufficient to offset the energy and capital cost of fan power and two ducted systems. Also, balanced ventilation has the same potential interstitial condensation risks as supply ventilation. If this is a hazard then the extract rate should be made to exceed the supply, an energy cost to offset a health risk.

Design issues

Fan power

The principal source of energy consumption, which can be 5–15% of overall running costs of a building, is in the fan power. Fans consume energy and heat up the air passing across them, especially if inefficient fans are chosen. The lower the ventilation rate specified, the lower will be the resulting energy consumption. Energy efficiency can be dramatically improved if the pressure drop in the system can be reduced, efficient fans are used and excess air supply is avoided. It is important not to oversize systems because of energy, cost and space implications.

The size and cost of many installations now exceeds that which might be incurred with natural systems.

The measure of system efficiency commonly used is SFP (specific fan power), which is a measure of energy required to move a certain quantity of air. The lower the SFP, the better the system efficiency. High efficiency is an SFP <1.5 kW/(m^3/s).

Ventilation effectiveness

Air may be introduced in a variety of ways and ventilation effectiveness is a measure of the extent to which occupants can experience fresh air. It is not adequate to simply add a quantity of fresh air to a space – extracts too close to intakes will cause short circuits and be ineffective. The shape of the room and the positioning of heat sources, thermal gradients between warmer and cooler surfaces, the relative temperature of the incoming and room air, and the sizes of ventilation openings all have an effect.

Displacement ventilation aims to introduce slow-moving fresh air at low levels where and in the quantity required so that draughts are avoided. If the incoming air is at too high a temperature compared to the room, then the buoyancy will also lead to short circuits and ineffectiveness.

Pore ventilation (also called dynamic insulation) is a means of introducing air into a building through a designed façade. It relies on maintaining a constant pressure by natural or mechanical means.

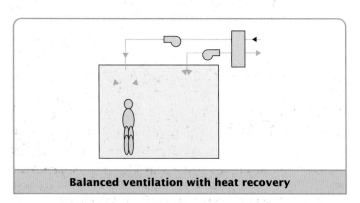

Balanced ventilation with heat recovery

generation is also important, particularly if large openings are disruptive to the environment, such as other classrooms, meeting places or where there is noise outdoors.

Controls

Good control is important if buildings are to operate as designed and if occupants are to be satisfied with a space. The design of good control requires that attention is given to how a building, and the different spaces within it, are to be used and how the controls might respond to how that use may change with time. All controls should be readily understood by whoever is to use them. In terms of overall operation, appropriate sensors can determine how much ventilation is required, but overrides should be provided and they should default to low-energy operation.

Control should not be seen as the domain of building management alone and separate controls should be designed which allow building occupants to manage their own environments without adversely affecting the strategy – that is, causing air to flow in the wrong direction. Controls should be readily accessible and be self-explanatory in terms of what they control and how. Controls and inlets and outlets should not blocked from view or placed where they may become so as a consequence of changes. Feedback that indicates that change will happen is appreciated. Some level of personal control, the ability to open a window or turn on a fan, is preferred by occupants.

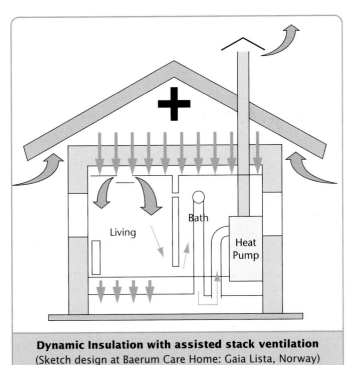

Dynamic Insulation with assisted stack ventilation
(Sketch design at Baerum Care Home: Gaia Lista, Norway)

Zoning

Good zoning will make the task of ventilation easier. Zones should be hierarchically arranged with the highest temperatures, odour, moisture and pollution levels (kitchen, bathrooms) closest to the outflow zone. Good organisation can be crucial for the effective use of natural and low-pressure systems. Proper layout means that heat is conserved, the need for ducting is reduced and there is more flexibility for indoor planning. Zoning of noise

Controls should:

- **be territorial**
- **be intuitive**
- **be obvious and unobscured**
- **be robust and flexible**
- **have simple overrides**
- **be understandable**
- **have low-energy default**
- **turn unneeded systems off.**

(From GIR 31.)

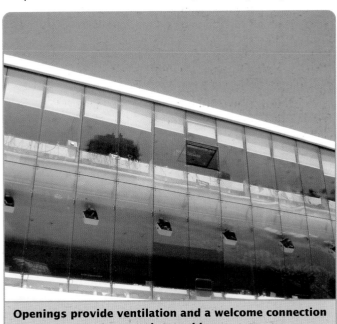

Openings provide ventilation and a welcome connection to the outside
(Architects: Future Systems. Photo: the author)

Case Study 10.4:

The Great Court of the British Museum, London

Architects: Norman Foster Architects, 2000

The Great Court was opened in September 2000 and was designed to open up the centre of the British Museum to the public for easier circulation. The space created by the demolition of book stacks from the old library allowed a 6700 m² courtyard to be created around the famous round reading room of the old library, which has been retained and restored. The court is now glazed over by a curved lattice, glass and steel shell, to provide a space for public circulation, meeting, shops, restaurants and access to new underground education facilities.

Ventilation to the Great Court and associated spaces involved the creation of four new plant rooms, tunnels and shafts within the surrounding museum buildings. The new development requires 45 m³ of air/s, ranging from full air-conditioning of exhibition spaces to the tempered environment in the Great Court. Of particular interest is the ventilation for the Great Court itself.

A bespoke displacement ventilation system was developed to keep peak summer temperatures at acceptable levels. This is supplemented by the ability to cool the floor slabs of the court and the upstairs restaurant area during the night. The cooling is performed by conventional chillers. Natural ventilation is possible by opening high-level vents under the roof perimeter and underground ducts, which allow fresh air to flow in from outside the museum. The air comes in through the same inlets as the mechanically supplied displacement air, and is used whenever the outdoor air temperature is suitable to cool the interior.

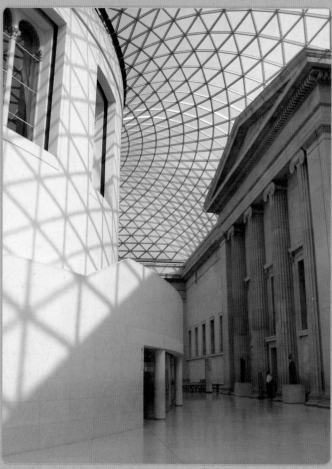

Photo: the author

Case Study 10.5:

McLaren Community Leisure Centre, Callander

Stirlingshire, Scotland. Architects: Gaia Architects, 1998

The centre opened in 1998. It has accommodation on two floors, a 25 m swimming pool, sports hall, squash courts, changing rooms, fitness suite, four-lane bowling hall, snack bar, meeting rooms and climbing wall.

The centre uses a pore ventilation system – also known as dynamic insulation, due to its ability to dynamically alter the U-value of the insulation. It is the first time that such a system has been used for ventilation in a pool hall.

The ventilation system is based on a variety of small air-handling units, supplying the swimming pool, sports hall, squash courts and bowls hall. The roof voids in the dry sports areas are pressurised to 10 Pa, while the swimming pool roof is pressurised up to 25 Pa. A 100 mm layer of cellulose fibre insulation is laid over a perforated polythene sheet, which is located above a permeable ceiling of timber slats or Heraklith boards

such that ventilation air enters through the whole ceiling.

Air is extracted at low and medium level in the pool hall and wet changing area, and is then passed over the evaporator of a heat pump, which is used to heat the pool water.

Air from the bowls hall passes into the street and out through the kitchen extract fan. The sports hall air is extracted via first the dry and then the wet changing areas.

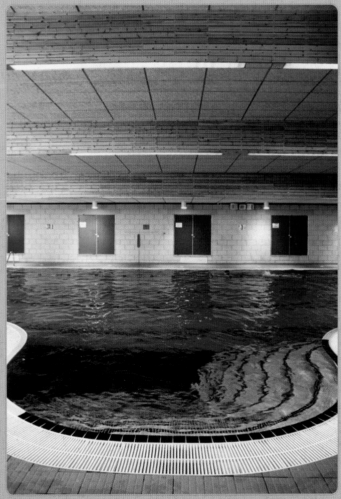

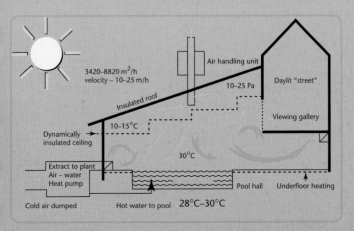

Methods of cooling

The primary means of indoor climate control should be the building envelope, minimising solar gain and using energy-efficient lighting and equipment. Dealing with these issues at an early stage can deliver space, capital and running cost savings. *GIR 31 Avoiding or minimising the use of air-conditioning* gives excellent guidance on how this can be achieved and includes a number of case studies. If cooling is required, then in many situations maximum opportunity should be made of passive cooling strategies, as the sole means of providing cooling or to reduce the times that a mechanical cooling system is in operation.

Passive cooling strategies

Passive cooling strategies include:

- Natural ventilation
- Structural thermal mass to absorb daytime heat loads
- Night cooling so that the structure can take up heat during the day
- Culvert ventilation to take up ground cooling

However, passive cooling has limitations:

- It is not possible to maintain specific thermal conditions, so flexibility and some high temperatures must be acceptable.
- Only cooling loads up to about 40 W/m^2 can normally be handled passively, then mechanical systems are required.

When it is necessary to provide tighter control of room temperatures and humidity – for example, manufacturing processes and museums – a mechanical cooling system will often be required. This can be achieved using a variety of benign low-energy mechanical techniques.

Mechanical cooling strategies

Mechanical cooling strategies are as follows:
- Absorption cooling, using waste heat from a process or renewable source
- Night cooling
- Culvert cooling
- Evaporative cooling by spraying water into extract air
- Refrigerative cooling using benign refrigerants
- Groundwater cooling
- Chilled ceilings, floors or beams in association with displacement ventilation or desiccant cooling
- Desiccant cooling can be powered by waste heat from a process, or renewable source.

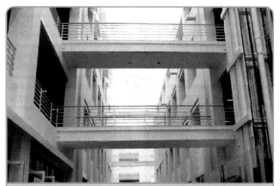

Barclaycard HQ, Northampton
Ventilation is provided through floor-mounted swirl diffusers. There is no mechanical extract, recirculation or heat recovery. Peak summer cooling for the 6000 chilled beams and ventilation is from two ammonia chillers; waste heat is dumped to a nearby lake. For the rest of the year the 'coolth' from the lake is supplied to the chilled water circuit through heat exchangers, with occasional supplement from the chillers (see Probe study, Building Services Journal, Jan. 2000, pp. 37–42) (Photo: Bill Bordass, William Bordass Associates)

Absorption cooling

In a conventional (MVC) chiller, refrigerant evaporates at low pressure, taking in heat, is compressed mechanically and then gives heat off as it condenses. Absorption chillers allow cooling to be produced from heat, rather than electricity. They have chemical absorbers and generators, namely water and lithium bromide or water and ammonia. Heat is required to separate the chemical solutions and required changes in pressure are achieved by a pump which uses less energy than a compressor. Conventional electric chillers and gas-fired absorption chillers are energy intensive. Absorption chilling begins to make sense environmentally and economically if heat for the absorption process would otherwise be wasted, hence its possible use with CHP or any other waste heat.

Evaporative cooling

This decreases the dry bulb temperature by adding water, either directly into the air stream (with risk of health problems – for example, legionella) or indirectly into a second air stream which cools the first.

Night cooling

If a building has high intermittent gains and enough thermal capacity to store heat during the day, then allowing cool air to flow through it and across designed surfaces at night is an established technique. The higher temperature differences at night can allow more heat to be rejected than daytime temperate differences allow. It needs good understanding and control if it is to operate efficiently and effectively. Attention is required to security and to opening, and window orientation and design. Coupling a building to an underground culvert can enable cool air to be introduced at night.

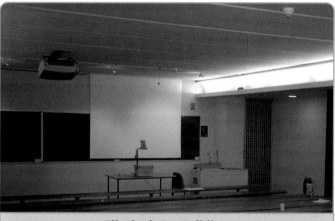

Elizabeth Fry Building
Cooling, when required, is achieved by running the AHUs during the day and after 10 pm on full fresh air. A comparison between the night-cooling fan power consumption and a conventional cooling system has indicated that the coefficient of performance (heat removed divided by electricity supplied to the fans) is estimated to be 5.8, which is at least twice as good as most chiller-based cooling systems (Photo: Bill Bordass)

Ground cooling

This uses water from aquifers or lakes to avoid the need for refrigeration. Chilled ceilings/beams supplied by groundwater or lakes are now a mature technology. Design and operating strategies have largely resolved earlier concerns about condensation risks. They are often used in combination with displacement ventilation or desiccant systems, and allow the latent and sensible cooling to be separate.

Culvert systems

These are designed to provide pre-cooled air in summer and pre-heated air in winter by adding extensive underground systems. They often requires some mechanical assistance but have been designed to operate entirely passively and in combination with heat recovery.

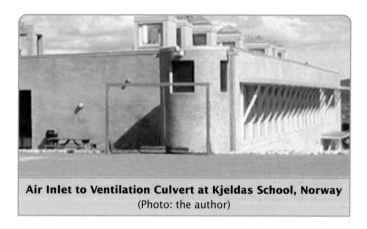

Air Inlet to Ventilation Culvert at Kjeldas School, Norway
(Photo: the author)

Desiccant cooling

This operates without refrigerants, and electrical compression has developed rapidly since the phasing out of ozone-depleting refrigerants. Fans are used to drive external air through a cycle of dehumidification, heat exchange and humidification to provide air at the right temperature. Heat is required for the regeneration process but this can be provided by any low-temperature source. The overall system can be used for heating and cooling, and provides a cost-competitive solution for large installations.

Controls are:

- **People**
- **Moisture sensors**
- **CO_2 sensors**
- **Particle sensors**
- **Occupancy sensors**
- **Mixed gas sensors.**

Case Study 10.6:

Vanse School, Norway

Architects: Gaia Lista, 2003

The 530 m² kindergarten building is designed for 120 people. The air intake is via an automatic damper through a culvert underneath the building, where the regulated underground temperature provides pre-heating in winter and pre-cooling in summer. Classroom windows open inwards and are hinged at the bottom. Underfloor low-temperature heating is used.

A ridge-level opening is designed to assist the stack effect by drawing air upward through the driving effect of the wind – the Bernoulli effect – and is controlled by an extract damper in each classroom. These are opened by teachers in response to the internal conditions and all close automatically at the end of the day. Night cooling is an option but the building is unoccupied during the warmest months, and heavy thermal mass in combination with a shape and orientation to minimise solar gain, and high-frequency lighting to reduce internal gains, maximise passive cooling. The building has no fans.

Internal moisture control is through the use of hygroscopic materials, including wood surfaces and moisture open-paint finishes. No outdoor clothes or shoes are permitted.

Information on this and other Norwegian natural and hybrid ventilation projects can be found at www.byggforsk.no/prosjeckte/hybvent/Norske_bygninger.htm.

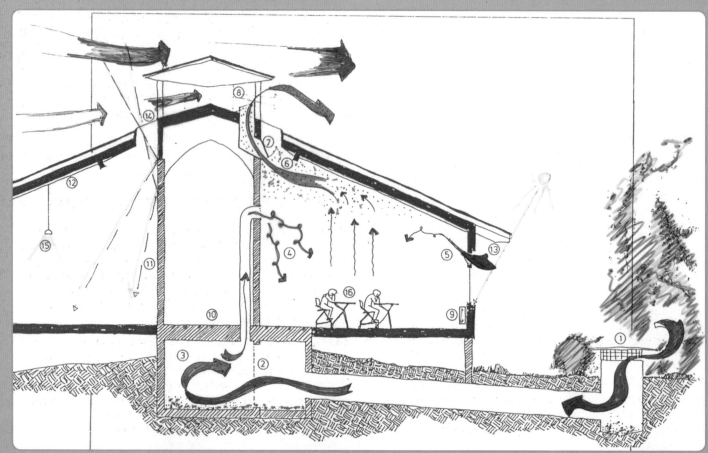

Image: Gaia Lista

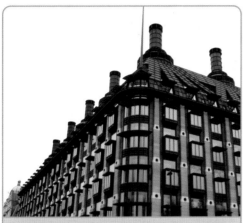

Portcullis House, Westminster, London
Architects: Michael Hopkins and Partners,
2001 Cooling is assisted by the thermal
capacity of the room structures. When external
air temperatures exceed 19ºC, water from
boreholes, at 14ºC, is pumped through the
air-handling units to cool the supply air down
to room temperature
(Photo: the author)

Plants

In recent years there has been much investigation into the role of plants in microclimate, VOCs and acoustic control of the indoor environment. Field identified that indoor environments with plants – both with and without full-spectrum lighting – reduce discomfort.

Humidification by transpiration of evergreen plants could be useful in winter when RH can be low, and could potentially replace humidification provided by expensive and energy-intensive mechanical processes.

In order to raise humidity, plants require light for photosynthesis. Simple models to quantify the cooling and humidification attributes of plants are available. Among a number of interesting considerations is the comparison of temperatures on man-made and vegetative roofs and wall finishes. Work by Wood identified the ability of some plants to remove n-hexane and benzene from the indoor air. However, plants can also harbour insects, pests and insecticides, and fertilisers, if used, can also be a health risk. Hydroponic conditions highlighted a close relationship between

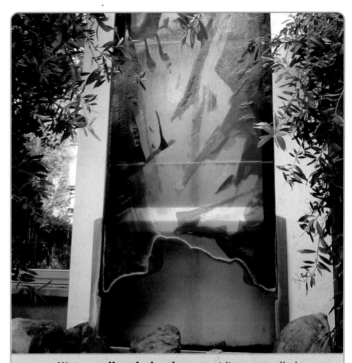

Water wall and planting, providing controlled
humidification at Prisma, Nuremburg
(Architect: Joachim Eble Architects; Photo: the author)

VOC-metabolising bacteria and root systems. More information can be found at www.plants-for-people.org.

Modelling and simulation

There is less potential to observe and record characteristics of ventilation in existing buildings than, for example, lighting. So to judge the effectiveness of a ventilation design strategy it is often necessary to perform some form of modelling exercise. This can range from simple calculations to wind tunnel testing to computational fluid dynamics (CFD) images from simulation programs such as FLOVENT.

Methods such as salt baths have been used in recent years to assess strategies at an early stage. The more complex methods are not necessarily the most effective for all situations,as modelling tools have limitations. They may be tedious or difficult to use, require additional expense, specialist skills or lengthy training outside the scope of many design offices. The techniques are still being developed.

Ventilation and cooling rules of thumb

- Work as a design team.
- Aim to achieve as much as possible passively, and ensure all mechanical plant is efficient, cleanable and properly controlled.
- Reduce summer heat gains by appropriate orientation and fabric design.
- Using low-energy lighting is a major step in reducing heat gains.
- Buildings must be airtight so that, whatever the system, it can operate as efficiently as possible.
- Openable windows must be well sealed when closed to minimise draughts and infiltration energy loss.
- Avoid locating air intakes and opening windows where pollution and noise are at their highest concentration.
- Reduce source strength by replacing polluting materials with low/no-emission alternatives.
- Extract internally generated pollutants at source.
- If occupants have the facility to change their environment, they are likely to use it to improve comfort.
- Combustion appliances should be room sealed, to avoid the requirement for uncontrollable, open air vents.
- Medium-term average ventilation rates are more important than instantaneous rates.

Consult regulations (CIBSE Guide A, Building Regulations) and guidelines associated with IAQ before undertaking design work.

Natural ventilation

- Controllable natural ventilation requires good structural airtightness.
- Consider and design for all the variables.
- Make optimal use of windows and other external openings to maximise the cooling effect.
- Combine window opening types to control ventilation rates for both summer and winter conditions.
- Make realistic assessments of small power loads. Heat gains greater than 15 W/m^2 are unusual.
- Beware of over-cooling.
- Stack ventilation can be effective up to a depth five times the height from the inlet to the exhaust.
- Night ventilation applied to a high thermal capacity structure can reduce the maximum daytime temperature by 2–3°C.

- Driving pressures under natural ventilation are low (10 Pa), so design for low-duct pressure drop.
- Filtration of air under natural flow is virtually impossible; some form of supply or extract fan is necessary to overcome the resistance of the filter.
- Offices should not exceed 27°C more often than a few hours in the afternoon on not more than 10 working days in a typical year.
- The energy efficiency benefits from natural ventilation, and daylight penetration, are most easily obtained up to 6m inwards from the windows. Greater room depth will probably require continuous lighting and mechanical ventilation or air-conditioning.

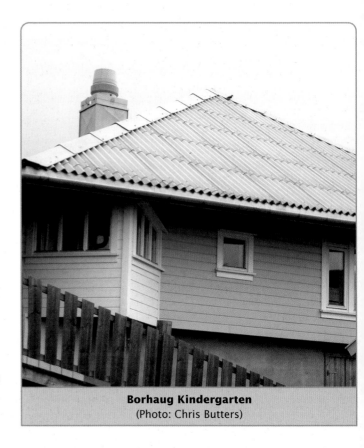

Borhaug Kindergarten
(Photo: Chris Butters)

Case Study 10.7:

Desiccant and solar cooling

Desiccant cooling can be used to condition the internal environment of buildings and operates without the use of traditional refrigerants.

It is an open heat-driven cycle which utilises a desiccant wheel and thermal wheel in tandem to achieve cooling and dehumidification. Because it is a heat-driven cycle, there is the potential to use any low-temperature source: gas, hot water, waste heat, including solar thermal energy.

A research project involved analysing the energy performance and control strategies of two systems (in Lincoln and Edinburgh) over a period of one year, assessing the potential energy savings and reduction in greenhouse gas emissions compared to other cooling options. In addition, an assessment was made of what could be achieved if solar or gas/solar hybrid energy was used to drive the cycle based on real meteorological data and the actual performance of the two case study systems.

A desiccant cooling model was developed and validated with data from the two systems. A solar heating coil was modelled prior to the regeneration coil, and it was possible to show a 76% reduction in primary energy consumed and CO_2 produced, demonstrating that there is potential in the UK for using solar energy to drive the desiccant cooling cycle.

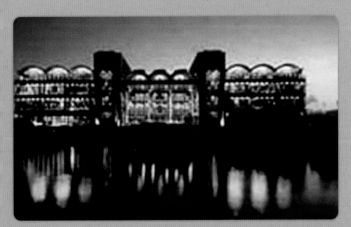

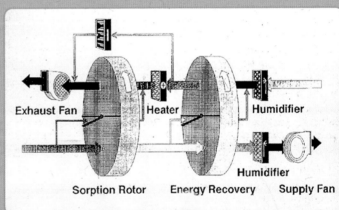

Photo Permission: University of Lincoln

Mechanical ventilation

- The specific fan power should be included in the specification and checked at commissioning.
- Ensure the system is not making things worse – badly placed intakes, poor maintenance.
- AHUs should be as close as possible to the ventilated space, to minimise the length of ductwork.
- Good duct design should achieve airflow which is as laminar as possible to reduce the pressure drop, and hence fan power and noise.
- Ductwork should have a large cross-sectional area to produce energy-efficient, low velocity systems with lower pressure drops.
- Ensure sufficient space is provided for horizontal/vertical ducting, to integrate it with the building structure and avoid complex routing.
- Ensure that main and peripheral plants are switched off when not required – that is,
  - toilet extractor fans
  - kitchen fans
  - warm air curtains
- Check that windows are not being opened to avoid overheating during winter.
- Ensure door closers operate effectively and are not jammed open.

Cooling

- Maximise passive cooling.
- Be prepared to challenge whether air-conditioning is absolutely necessary.
- Undertake an option appraisal to identify the most appropriate, efficient, manageable and occupant-friendly solution.
- Ensure that cooling systems make use of outside air for 'free cooling' whenever possible.
- Set cooling controls to 24°C or higher, unless there are special requirements. Lower settings require more cooling energy and can 'fight' the heating.
- Ensure heating and cooling are not on at the same time! Really, it happens all the time!
- Make sure that any refrigeration plant does not run unnecessarily.
- Ensure that fans and pumps do not run when not required.
- Install variable-speed controls on fans and pumps. These allow motor speeds to be controlled according to the demand instead of running at full power continuously.
- Consider 'coolth' recovery to reduce loading on, and energy consumption of, plant, but also consider the pump and fan power implications of installing such devices. 'Coolth' recovery can increase pressure drop and fan power by 50%.
- Avoid excessive humidification.

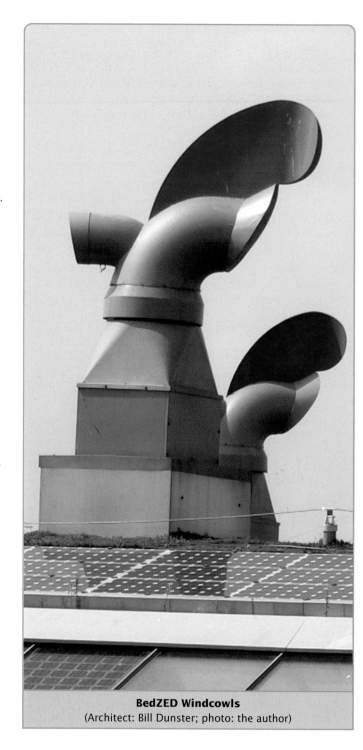

BedZED Windcowls
(Architect: Bill Dunster; photo: the author)

Bibliography

Also see bibliography in Chapter 7.

Search the following:

- BRECSU publications list for good practice case studies, guides and general information leaflets – many of which are free – covering airtightness, energy efficiency, cooling and strategic issues (www.bre.co.uk).
- *Building Services Journal* for PROBE Studies www.usablebuildings.co.uk.
- Carbon Trust at www.energy-efficiency.gov.uk for ventilation, cooling and energy efficiency in buildings of a similar type.
- CIBSE publications list at www.cibse.org.
- International Energy Agency site (www.ecbcs.org) for Low Energy Cooling under Annex 28 and Hybrid Ventilation Annex 35.
- Usable Buildings Trust www.usablebuildings.co.uk.

Ventilation and cooling control strategies are regularly published in Building Services Journal Case Studies.

Useful free publications from BRECSU

GIR 31 (1995) *Avoiding or Minimising the Use of Air-conditioning.* BRECSU.

GIR 56 (1999) *Mixed Mode Buildings and Systems – An Overview.* BRECSU.

GPG 290: (2001) *Ventilation and Cooling Option Appraisal – A Client's Guide.*

GPG 291: (2001) *A Designer's Guide to the Options for Ventilation Cooling.*

Other publications on specific issues

Fanger P.O. et al. (1990) *A simple method to determine the olf load in a building,* Fifth International Conference on Indoor Quality and Climate (Indoor Air '90), Vol. 1, pp. 537–42.

BRE I/P 13/94 (1994) *Passive Stack Ventilation Systems: Design and Installation.* BRE.

GP Case Study 308 (1997) *Naturally Comfortable Offices – A Refurbishment Project.*

GPG 224 (1997) *Improving Airtightness in Existing Homes.* BRE

Fjeld, T et al. (1998) *The Effect of Indoor Foliage Plants on Health and Discomfort Symptoms among Office Workers* Indoor and Built Environment Vol. 7, No. 4, pp. 204–9.

GPG 257 (1998) *Energy-efficient Mechanical Ventilation Systems.* BRE

Berge, B. (1999) *Ecology of Building Materials.* Architectural Press.

ECON 19 (2000) *Energy Use in Offices.* BRE

Simonson, C. J., Salonvaara, M. and Ojanen, T. (2001) *Improving indoor climate and Comfort with wooden structures.* VTT Building Technology, Espoo.

Digest 464 (2002) *VOC Emissions from Building Products.* BRE

DTU *Moisture Buffering of Building Materials* (2005) Department of Civil Engineering Technical University of Denmark Report BYG·DTU R-126.

Gaia Group (2005) *Design and Construction of Sustainable Schools*, Vols 1 and 2. Scottish Executive. Free from Gaia.

Design guides

BRE Digest 399 (1994) *Natural Ventilation in Non-domestic Buildings.* BRE.

CIBSE AM10 (1997) *Natural Ventilation in Non-Domestic Buildings,* March. Members. CIBSE.

Roalkvam, D. (1997) *Naturlig Ventilasjon.* NABU/NFR (in Norwegian).

Allard, F. (1998) *Natural Ventilation in Buildings: A Design Handbook.* James & James.

CIBSE AM13 (2000) *Mixed Mode Ventilation.* CIBSE.

Chapter 11
Renewable technology

In which we investigate current attempts to harness the ever-present renewable energy resources in the wind, water, earth, sun and biomass, and how, when applied alongside better conventional design, these can contribute to achieving sustainability objectives.

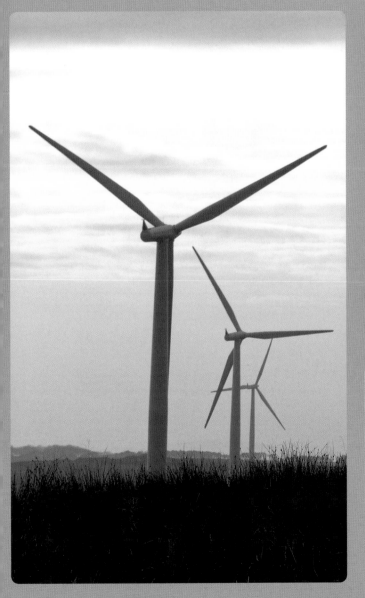

'In technology reality must take precedence over public relations, because nature won't be fooled.'

Richard Feynman

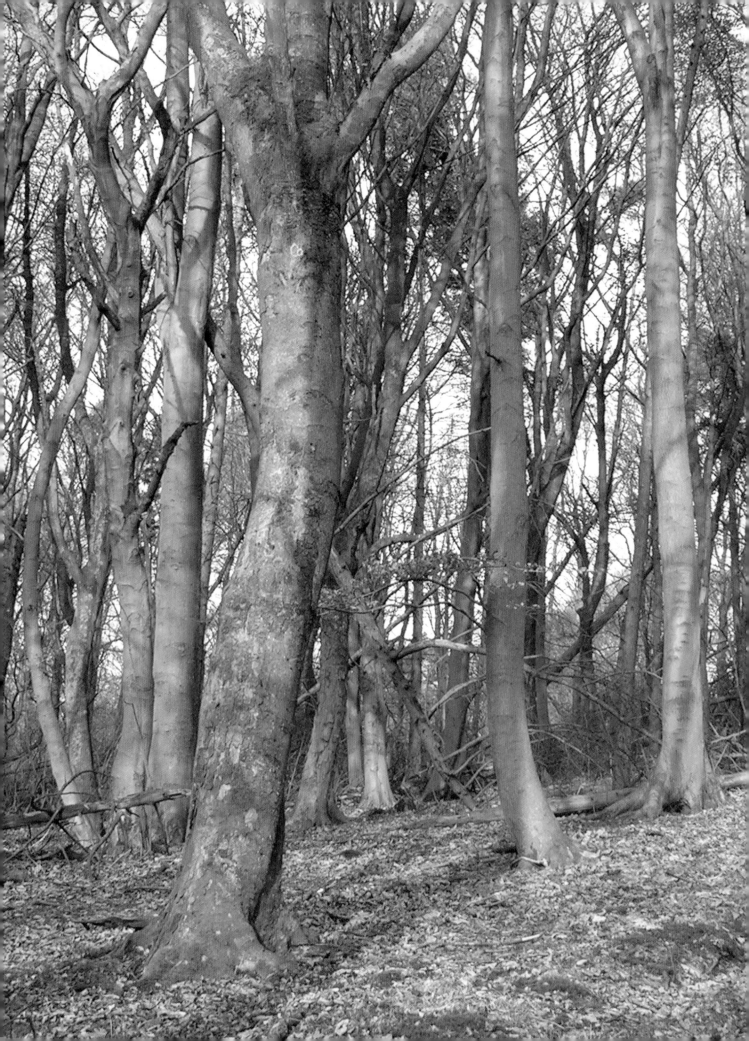

Contents

(Facing page)
Carbon sink
Photo: the author

(Previous page)
Wind Turbines, Shotts
Photo credit: Michael Wolshover

Renewable technology

Introduction

We are in an era of excitement again about renewable energy. This is welcome but caution is required to ensure that decision-making is sensible, and generates the most appropriate responses. Renewable energy technologies need to support good practice rather than substitute for it.

Simply adding technology to buildings does not demonstrate sustainable design. It is important to achieve the right balance of cost, functionality and lifetime benefits. Issues such as build quality and maintenance are crucial, and the basis for any renewable solution is better conventional design.

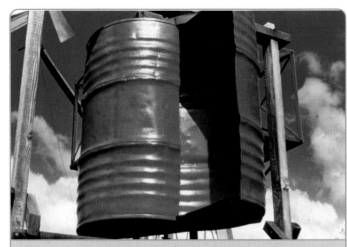

Savonius Rotor 1970s
(Photo permission: Centre for Alternative Technology)

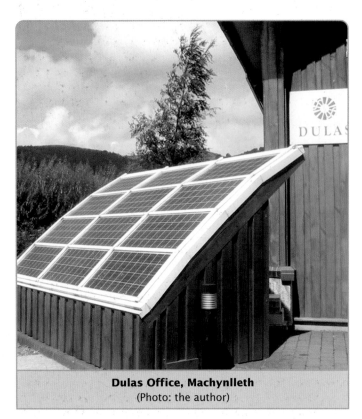

Dulas Office, Machynlleth
(Photo: the author)

The need to develop renewable resources is undeniable. The benefits include:

- the opportunity to reduce pollution due to fossil fuels
- improved security of energy supply
- more predictable costs
- improved efficiency of generation and transmission compared to the grid
- development of a renewables industry
- real cost benefits in an environment of polluter pays.

Extreme sensitivity is required to ensure that development is appropriate. Renewable technologies cannot and should not be the first choice in design. Some technologies are expensive and impractical, and are themselves the source of waste and pollution that can put pressure on ecosystems. Energy generated from renewables has to be used wisely to justify the investment. The term eco-minimalism has been coined to promote an approach that – in counterbalance to the contemporary excitement – looks at passive solutions first and foremost. It has much to recommend it.

Development

Sustainable development requires that we cultivate energy from natural processes in such a way as not to deplete them and not to result in social harm, environmental pollution, waste or short life. Environmental pollution, specifically climate change, is currently the principal motivation for interest in energy conservation and in renewable energy technologies as alternatives to fossil fuels.

Interest in renewable energies has waxed and waned for over 30 years. In the 1970s, the principal pollutants of concern associated with energy were oxides of nitrogen and sulphur (NOx and SOx) emitted from power stations. Predominant south-westerly winds in the UK gave rise to acid rain in Scandinavia and led to international interest in cleaner energy generation. International pressure during the 1970s' oil crisis was also a significant driving force. This led to concerns for the future availability and cost of oil. It coincided with some of the early experimentation in alternative 'green' lifestyles, as well as development of commercial opportunities for renewable energy. Sadly, some early research into economic viability was shamefully misleading.

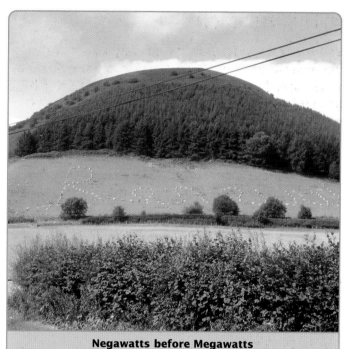

Negawatts before Megawatts
In rural environments people hold very different views about renewable energy versus the alternatives. The only sensible solution is to make radical reductions in energy consumption so that the optimal use is made of whatever is generated
(Photo: the author)

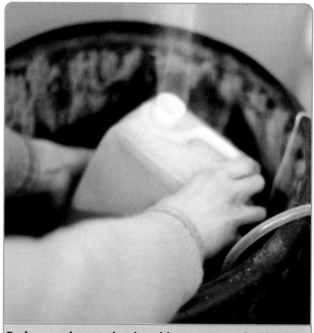

Early experimentation into biogas generation (1970s)
University of Hull (Photo: Howard Liddell)

More recently, international concerns about global warming and security of supply have led to real commitment to increasing the contribution of renewables to our energy needs, which are increasing. The inherent dangers, unresolved waste management issues and sheer cost of nuclear power make its adoption unfeasible if common sense prevails.

The early experimental period led to the founding of institutions such as the Centre for Alternative Technology, where study of clean technologies has combined with experimentation in farming and alternative lifestyles.

For a long time, renewable technologies in the UK were probably stigmatised by this linkage and unfounded assumptions about the lifestyle implications. These suggested that they were only relevant to those who wished to 'give up' on quality of life. In practice, some technical choices (low-tech solar panels or composting toilets) might impose lifestyle changes whilst others (grid connected wind) probably do not.

There remains a need to discuss the social, financial and environmental implications of different technologies within the framework of a wider understanding of sustainable development. It is important that technical responses are sensible and robust, manageable and affordable, and in particular that they are compatible with the user and management skills, needs and aspirations. Experience from exporting technologies to developing countries highlights many cases of waste and short life due to lack of basic skills and spares.

Highly intermittent attention to renewable energy means that it has been difficult to maintain any consistency in approach. It has taken a combined cognisance of environmental hazards, commercial opportunities of technology development and concerns about security of energy supply for serious attention to renewables to become an international issue. The present commercial climate, however, still gives largely unbridled support to the ongoing availability of cheap fossil fuels. Renewable technologies can rarely compete economically, especially as expectations of financial payback are generally very short. Dependence on subsidy, when it is unlinked to any issue of longevity, is notoriously unreliable.

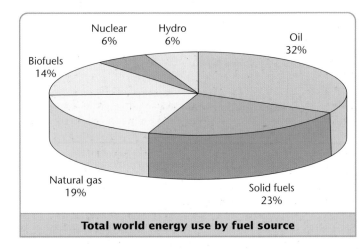

Total world energy use by fuel source

However, fossil fuels are increasingly recognised as generating costly and perhaps irreparable environmental damage. As a result, there is increasing attention to developing long-term fiscal policies which assist clean technology development. International agreements now oblige participating countries to make commitments to energy efficiencies. The Kyoto Agreement commits the UK to reduce greenhouse gases by 12.5% by 2012 from 1990 levels. At the time of going to press there is no agreement beyond Kyoto.

In Europe, there are now increasing efforts to stimulate renewable energy provision through tax incentives and political pressures to meet set targets. The UK strategy involves energy efficiency and fuel switching to less carbon-intensive fuels such as gas, renewables and 'sensible' CHP. Measures such as the Carbon Tax Levy – linked to environmental impact – dovetail with the Non-Fossil Fuel Obligation in encouraging expanding markets, widely seen as significant to reducing costs.

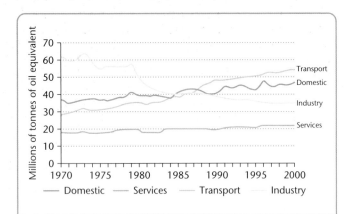

Change in energy consumption by sector
Between 1970 and 2000 energy consumption by sector changed substantially, with rises of 96% in transport, 27% in the domestic and 17% in the service sectors. Industry use fell by 42%. Recently the rate of increase in transport has slowed and industrial use has increased. Overall energy use increased by 1% between 1999 and 2000

'Polluter pays' principle

Asserts that the full cost of controlling pollution should be carried by the polluter without subsidy or tax concessions. The cost of pollution is internalised and reflected in production costs.

Case Study 11.1:

Centre for Alternative Technology, Machynlleth

Founded in 1975, on the site of an old slate quarry, by Gerard Morgan-Grenville, the Centre for Alternative Technology (CAT) is Europe's leading environmental visitor attraction. The seven-acre visitor complex has a wide range of buildings which explore different building techniques, and a number of interactive exhibits to demonstrate a wide range of energy, small-scale farming, and water and waste management techniques.

A significant part of the ongoing exploration at CAT is the implementation of renewable energy technologies on the site.

Data collected from 2000 has been collated by the CAT and shows that 64% of their total consumption of 75.5 MWh of electricity was produced by renewables.

The centre has a 13.5 kW solar roof, two 3.5 kW hydro turbines, various wind turbines of up to 75 kW that were not monitored at this time, and a 600 kW wind turbine exporting directly to the grid. The remainder is supplied from a back-up diesel generator and the grid.

Consumption of non-renewable power was higher than normal due to the construction of a large building.

A water-powered cliff railway can take up to 14 adults at a time up or down the 60 m incline. It operates on the principle of 'water balancing'. The two carriages are connected by cable via a winding drum at the top. Water is run into a tank beneath the upper carriage until it is just heavier than the lower carriage and its passengers. The parking brakes are released and gravity does the rest.

It is one of the steepest cliff-railways in Britain, with a 35° slope and set at a velocity of about 1 m/s. The speed is controlled by a hydraulic pump combined with a regenerative braking system, allowing the surplus energy from the hydraulics to pump some of the water back to the top. This water can be seen from time to time spouting into the pool next to the Upper Station.

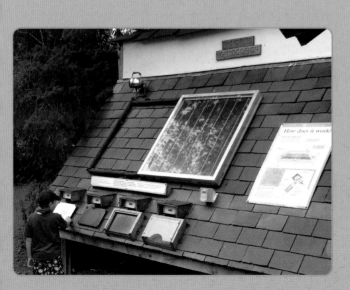
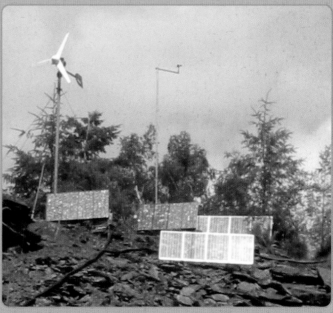

Photo credits: the author

Eco-minimalism

There is growing concern that the potential benefits from some renewable technologies are being oversold. Expensive technologies with short life, suspect manufacturing processes (often themselves energy and chemically intensive) and hence high embodied pollution are not evidently more sustainable than quality, conventional design based on a good understanding of buildability and scientific principles. Even basic calculations highlight that real priority areas for attention are design fundamentals, not technical add-ons. Certainly, the use of renewable energy technologies should never be considered in isolation from demand-side reduction. Both peak loads and run time of equipment should be considered.

Technical illiteracy is rife, leading to situations where buildings of so-called specialist organisations and even those boasting a demonstration of photovoltaic (PV) technology have toilets bearing handwritten notes: 'Beware very hot water'. It happens disturbingly often.

A thermostat plus spray taps would have been cheaper than the PV panel and a genuine contribution to energy efficiency. It will always be more cost-effective to use low-energy bulbs, good control, draught-proofing or more insulation than to install PVs or a wind turbine to an existing inefficient building. For new builds, the very best possible standards of energy efficiency and control should be prioritised before add-on technology.

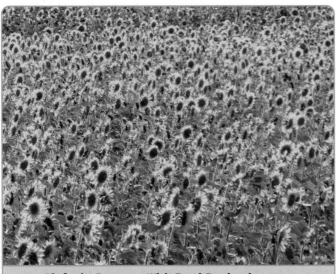

Biofuels Compete With Food Production most biofuels in the UK would be imported
(Photo: Howard Liddell)

Renewable technologies

Biomass

Energy is contained in plant matter and animal waste, and can be burnt to provide electricity, heat or steam. If the original product is free of chemical treatments, then the waste products can be returned to the land, as fertiliser. Plant matter can also be converted to a liquid or gaseous supply to produce alcohol fuel, biogas and plant-oil-derived diesel.

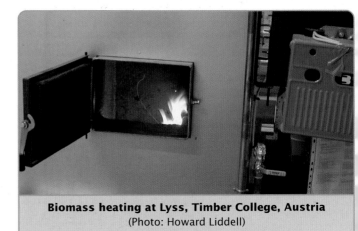

Biomass heating at Lyss, Timber College, Austria
(Photo: Howard Liddell)

Use of organic waste for energy can be integrated into waste management strategies. Emissions from the combustion of biomass are cleaner than emissions from fossil fuels. Biomass is used extensively in developing countries, and in the developed countries large- and small-scale applications are becoming popular. The main sources in the UK are residues from pulp and paper operation, forests, agriculture, urban woodlands and animal waste. Some crops are grown specifically for energy. However, biomass energy is truly renewable (carbon neutral) only when the rate of planting equals or exceeds the rate of use. Landfill gas is a special case of biomass energy in that it is latent rather than renewable. It is formed from the natural breakdown of waste materials over time that generates methane, a particularly intense greenhouse gas.

Biofuels account for 82% of world renewable energy sources. Most of the hydro accounts for 15% and wind power 2.5%. Of the 3.0 Million Tonnes (MT) of oil equivalent of primary energy use accounted for by renewables, 2.2 MT was used to generate electricity and 0.8 MT to generate heat. Global renewable energy use grew by 8% in 2000 and has doubled in the last seven years. It accounted for 2.8% of electricity generated in the UK in 2000.

Case Study 11.2:

Ely Power Station

2002

Constructed by FLS Miljo, and located in Sutton near Ely, this £60 M, 36 MWe facility consumed around 200 000 tonnes of straw collected from farms within a 50-mile radius, and generated 270 GWh of electricity every year, which is sufficient to satisfy the needs of 80 000 dwellings.

The power was sold to NFPA under a NFFO3 contract. The plant was also capable of burning a range of other biofuels and up to 10% natural gas. It is claimed that this is the UK's first and the world's largest and most efficient straw-fired power station. The facility was opened in January 2002 by Brian Wilson, Minister for Energy.

In June 2004 ELY PCR took over the operation and maintenance of the plant allowing them to burn a wider range of fuels. This opened up the potential for reducing fuel costs and increasing security of supply.

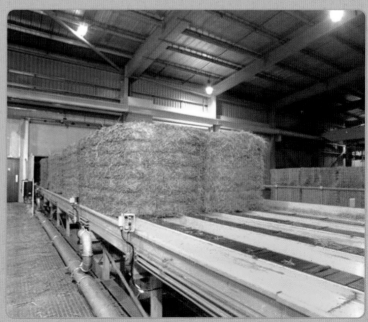

Photo: Energy Power Resources

Case Study 11.3:

Kinlochleven Community and Sports Centre, Argyll

Architects: Gaia Architects, 2001

The 964 m^2 single-storey building has a slate roof over a combination of masonry and timber-clad, timber-frame walls. It is highly insulated with dynamic insulation to the main hall and natural finishes throughout. A woodchip boiler was selected to provide a carbon-neutral development.

The space-heating requirement is met via underfloor heating, cast into the floor slab. The woodchips, sourced from a nearby sustainably managed forest, are stored in a 10 m^3 hopper and feed a 120 kW boiler. The woodchips are supplied dried to 15–18% moisture content, and bought as measured heat and/or hot water at a competitive unit rate of 2.8 p per kWh.

The fuel is automatically fed to the biomass plant, where it is burnt at a temperature of 1350°C. A control panel modulates the fuel-to-air ratio by monitoring the flue gases, to achieve maximum combustion efficiency. Once the heating has been satisfied, a 'slumber mode' kicks in, which maintains an ember bed on the burner, until more heat is called for. Temperature control works in the same way as that of a conventional boiler and supplies 82°C flow, 71°C return. The overall system efficiency is 85–90%, dependent upon the moisture content of the fuel. A 100kW standby LPG burner is in place in case of boiler shut-down during severe weather. Modem monitoring from the supplier's office enables flow and return temperatures to be checked, fault indication, and fuel monitoring to ensure accurate and timely fuel reordering.

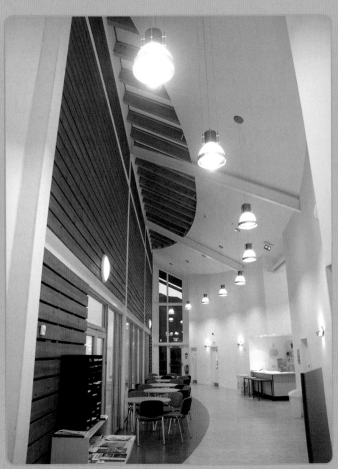

Photo: Gaia Architects

Photovoltaic (PV)

PV cells convert solar radiation into DC electricity. It is adequate for 12/24-volt DC supply, but must be converted using an inverter to AC for most purposes, including export to the grid in the case of excess generation. Storage is required for use outside daylight hours. Systems are built up in arrays from modules to the required size. Principal applications until relatively recently were in remote locations, marine navigation, transmitters, water pumping or battery charging, where the alternatives of grid connection or local generation were unfeasible or expensive. They are now being heavily promoted to the building industry.

Costs have fallen rapidly, as take-up of photovoltaic technologies has increased, but they are difficult to justify unless there has been serious attention to reducing energy and power requirement by every possible means.

The cost of PV cells is presently £300–800/m^2 depending on efficiency. A high-efficiency array of 10 m^2 in southern England has a power output of about 1.5 kW and would generate around 4 kWh/day in midsummer and about one-third of that in midwinter. These seasonal variations generally necessitate that a back-up power supply is provided. It is rarely sensible to try to meet a peak load, and instead designs should seek to meet a base load that reduces the need for new or upgraded infrastructure. They can be utilised in conjunction with another energy source, usually wind.

The main advantages of PV systems are that they are silent, have no moving parts and require minimal maintenance. They produce no emissions in use. Cost has fallen and efficiency risen, but they are very expensive and cannot pay for themselves during their useful life. Most research and development is aimed at increasing the efficiency and reducing the cost, although there is also attention to cleaning up the manufacturing process, which controversially is reliant on solvents and heavy metals. Technical advances have significantly reduced the embodied energy.

Energy used to manufacture a crystalline silicon PV cell now equals four to five years of power generation from it. The expected lifetime is, on average, 20–30 years. Hence, each 1 kW panel is estimated to save 0.5–1 tonne of CO_2/year, or a net 5–25 tonnes in its lifetime.

Typically, PVs are roof mounted, in a domestic situation. More recently, in commercial buildings it has become popular to incorporate the PV cells into the building envelope. The argument is that by serving a dual purpose the net cost of photovoltaics or active solar collectors can be substantially reduced by replacing roof light-shelves, curtain walling or cladding systems that would otherwise need to be introduced. This depends on them having a comparable functional design life.

Doxford Solar Office, Sunderland
– the first speculative office building to incorporate building-integrated photovoltaics and, at the time, the largest ever constructed in Europe
(Architects: Studio E Architects, 1995, photo: Studio E Architects)

System	Approximate Installed Cost £/m
PV curtain walling, glass/glass crystalline	780
PV curtain walling, thin-film amorphous	280
Double glazing	350
Stone cladding	300
Polished stone	850–1500
PV rain-screen cladding	600
Steel rain-screen over-cladding	190
PV roofing tiles (housing)	500
PV modules on a pitched roof	650
Roofing tiles – clay or concrete	32
Timber roofing (larch)	34
Slate	less than 50

Table 11.1 Approximate costs of building cladding materials from Ralph Ogg & Co, Perth and BIPV projects, 2000, ETSU report S/P2/003 28/REP

Case Study 11.4:

The Eco House, Nottingham

Architect: David Wilson Homes, 2000

Located on the University campus, this four bedroom house was built to demonstrate the integration of existing renewable energy technologies such as evacuated tube solar water heaters, PV roof, lightpipes, solar chimney and rainwater collection.

Since then, ground source heating/cooling, PV extractor fan, PV trackers and wind turbines have been added.

Monocrystaline photovoltaic roof tiles cover 15.9 m^2 of the south-facing roof space, inclined at 52°. They are designed to produce 1250 kWh of electricity per year and supply a peak power output of 1580 W – 30% of the demand.

Two self-operated, sun-tracking PV arrays installed alongside the house operate with the roof array. Together, these systems result in approximately 75% of the building's electricity demand being satisfied by PV.

Mounted on the south-facing portion of the frame, a 3 m x 1 m solar collector provides adequate hot water during the summer months and pre-heats water during the winter.

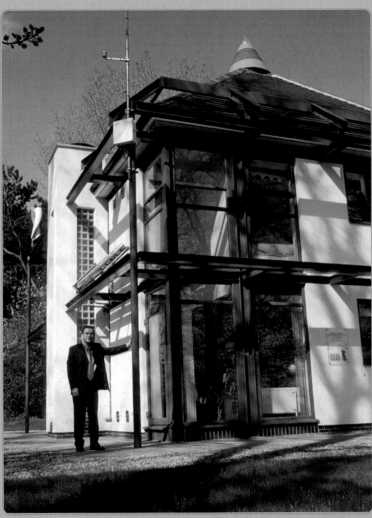

Photo: University of Nottingham

Case Study 11.5:

Sainsbury's petrol station, Greenwich

Architects: Chetwood Associates, 1999

The 57 m² roof of the petrol station at Sainsbury's Millennium store, Greenwich, London, contains 90 PV modules each rated at 75 W and wired together in 10 parallel rows.

The DC electrical output is converted through inverters providing the petrol station with its electricity needs, and any excess is exported to the grid via Sainsbury's on-site CHP generation unit.

The installation also has two wind turbines that provided power for a free plug-in port for charging electric cars, to encourage the use of cleaner transport options. These plug-in ports have now been removed.

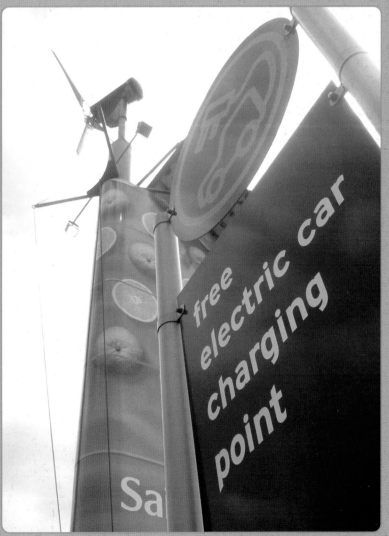

Photo: the author

Case Study 11.6:

University of Northumbria

Refurbishment, 1994

The Northumberland building was used as a demonstration project for building integrated photovoltaic (BIPV) rain-screen cladding in 1994.

It has been extensively monitored to identify energy output and how it compares with durability of standard cladding systems.

Benefits of BIPV are the ability to offset some costs, but they are required to perform at least as well in traditional terms.

465 PV modules were used in a south-facing 286 m² array, tilted at 25° to vertical. Each has an 85 W output, giving maximum DC output of 39.5 kW. A peak monthly energy output, in August 1995, gave 3106 kWh DC converted into 2940 kWh AC.

The monitored figures predicted an annual output of 30 MWh. Assuming a system lifetime of 25 years, the electricity cost is 42 p/kWh.

The building façade is shaded by surrounding buildings of similar size and by a chimney in front of the façade.

Shading occurs mainly in the morning and during the winter season, reducing the annual output, and increasing cost, by 25%.

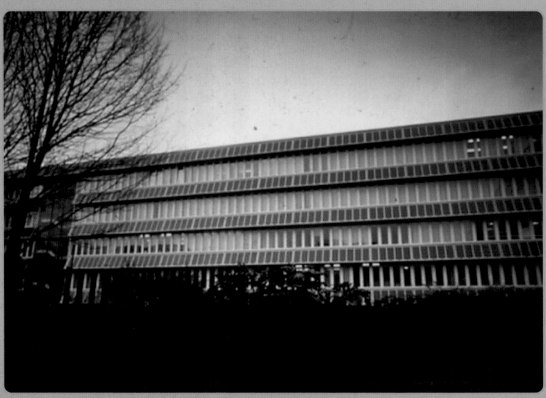

Photo: University of Northumbria

Solar thermal

Solar energy can be used for heating air or water. The solar energy available in the UK is around 900–1300 kWh/m^2/year. Climate data suggests that this is increasing in the south and decreasing in the north.

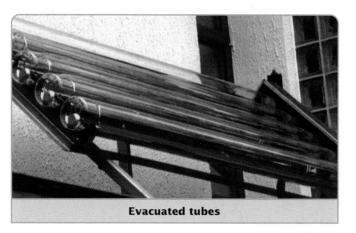

Evacuated tubes

Flat-plate collectors (FPC) consist of water-carrying pipes in contact with an absorber surface. Back and side insulation prevents heat losses, and a transparent cover has the effect of retaining the solar radiation, creating a greenhouse effect. Efficiency is influenced by the amount of insulation, outdoor temperature, fluid temperature and construction. Typical efficiencies are 40–50%, but 70% is possible; increasing levels of sophistication increase cost.

Domestic hot water is required to be delivered at a temperature of around 60°C, to eliminate legionella, and some boost will be required at certain times of year. During winter antifreeze is required, or systems should be drained. The most advanced FPCs heat a little water at a time and store it. More sophisticated collectors absorb energy onto selectively coated black fins placed within evacuated tubes. These have higher operating temperatures.

All types collect direct and diffuse radiation, so operate under cloudy conditions. It is generally assumed that the more expensive the collector, the more efficiently it will perform.

However, controversial research to compare different collectors indicated that the cheaper FPCs outperform the more expensive evacuated tubes. The arguments appeared well founded but the results have not been confirmed.

In the UK, collectors should face south, inclined to the horizontal at an angle equal to the latitude to capture maximum solar energy. Typical installation costs are £300–750/m^2, providing 300 kWh/m^2.

A typical domestic installation is about 4 m^2, meets 20% of the demand and saves about one tonne of CO_2/year. Solar-warmed water can also be used in combination with the desiccant open-driven cycle to provide cool and dehumidified air in an environmentally benign alternative to traditional air-conditioning systems. The system requires heat to regenerate a desiccant material at temperatures readily achievable by solar energy.

As well as warming water, collectors can exploit the ability of any surface that is warmed by the sun to be a source of energy. Air moving passively or assisted mechanically across such surfaces and within designed channels can deliver pre-heated air directly or indirectly to top up heating systems. The low-tech, low-cost approach is being increasingly exploited for a range of applications, as it offers designers a variety of opportunities to provide a cost-effective alternative to commercial systems.

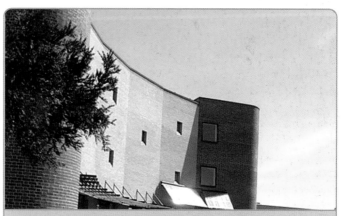

Solar thermal
The extension to Plymouth College of Further Education has domestic hot water provided by evacuated solar tube collectors that serve as both a canopy over the entrance area and absorb the solar energy to heat the building's domestic water requirements

The designers claim that the solar collectors supply hot water for the sanitary needs and approximately 60–80% of the catering domestic hot water needs. The pump is of a small domestic size and the system gives an overall good reliable performance

Hydro power

Hydroelectric plant enables potential energy present in water to be converted into kinetic energy with the use of turbines that drive generators. The amount of energy available is dependent on the flow of water and the head, which can be anything from 1 to 300 m. The technology is simple. Large-scale hydro power is a well-established form of renewable technology.

Small-scale hydro is occasionally worth considering for buildings close to rivers and streams. Technology improvements mean that previously unfeasible projects with low head and flow might be worth considering. As with all other renewable applications, the electricity produced is DC. In the UK, most of the hydroelectric potential is in Scotland.

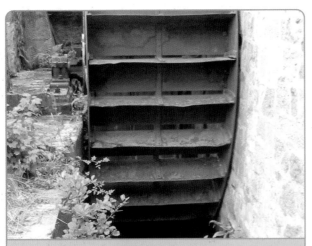

Small-scale hydro
..is occasionally worth considering for buildings close to rivers and streams
(Photo: the author)

Wave and tidal energy

The main advantages of wave and tidal power are the large energy fluxes available and predictability of conditions. As a consequence, many devices have been designed to extract power from waves (kinetic energy) and tides (potential energy) and convert it into electricity. Two wave energy devices are described here.

The Salter Duck is designed such that a wave approaches the 'beak' of the device, making it oscillate. The rounded base prevents waves impinging from the side. A high conversion efficiency of the incident wave power is achieved by extracting the energy at the point where there is minimum reflected energy.

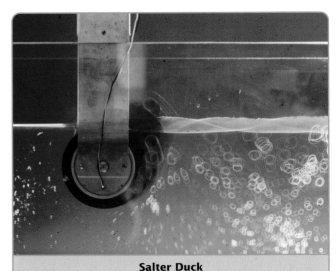

Salter Duck
A time exposure of a duck absorbing power from the waves. Around 90% of the energy was being captured
(Photo: Jamie Taylor, Edinburgh University)

The Oscillating Water Column exploits the amplitude of wave. These force the water level to rise and fall in a vertical cylinder, compressing and decompressing enclosed air. The oscillating stream of high-velocity air is fed to a special turbine, with unidirectional blades, that rotates regardless of the direction of the air. A 75 kW prototype operates on Islay, which feeds into the grid. The technique is being researched for use shallow waters.

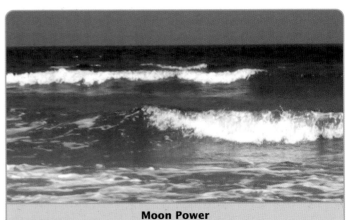

Moon Power
Tidal energy exploits height to take the potential energy from water (Photo: the author)

Geothermal

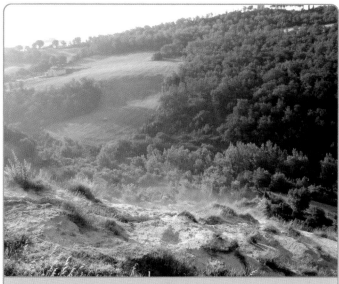

Hot Rocks
The UK only has a few areas of mainly low-grade heat
(Photo: the author)

Geothermal energy is derived from heat deep within the earth. It can be used for heat or electricity generation. Geothermal energy has huge potential for a reliable power generator, with resources identified in over 80 countries and utilisation currently in 58. Of those countries, 21 are producing electricity from water at temperatures as high as 400°C, which is brought from underground reservoirs to the surface and flashed into steam. The best sites are those that correspond with fault lines in the earth, geysers and volcanic regions, but in many places it is possible to drill deep within the earth to reach high-temperature locations.

Throughout the UK, the ground maintains a constant year-round temperature of 11–13°C, with a few hotspots of largely low-grade heat. Ground source or geothermal heat pump systems have been developed to make use of this energy for heating of buildings (www.earthenergy.co.uk provides information on systems and a geothermal map). It is a viable option for single houses, especially new build with high insulation levels, where the capital costs are reduced. Systems are sized in the same way as any other performing the same function, heat losses, floor area and occupancy pattern.

A typical three-bedroom house will require an 8 kW system, comprising 250 m², 300-mm-diameter boreholes at £5900.

The payback period could be in the region of five years. A typical smaller housing association development system might be closer to 4 kW at £4200. Larger commercial systems are more cost-effective (£1000/kW), as the same infrastructure can be used to meet heating and cooling loads. It becomes viable to use central plant with district heating when a group of houses is being built at the same time. (Trench systems in which the pipes are laid close to the surface cost less, as drilling equipment is not required. Problems of freezing ground have been experienced with this technique.) This will provide all of the space heating and provide DHW at 45°C. An immersion is required to boost water temperature to the required temperature and eliminate the risk of legionella.

Use of a heat pump means that an 8kW system uses only 2kW of electricity. However, as the price and environmental impact of electricity is three to four times that of gas, the benefits may be marginal. The heat pump is maintenance free and has a long lifespan. The pump warranty is supplier dependent, but usually around two years. However, parts are abundant and cheap. The systems are low maintenance and parts have standard warranty – there are no hidden maintenance costs. A ground loop has a 25-year guarantee and life expectancy is 50–75 years. Local skills can be employed to undertake installation. The local authority will need to be contacted, but no planning permission is required, because the pipe is installed underground, in a borehole or covered trench.

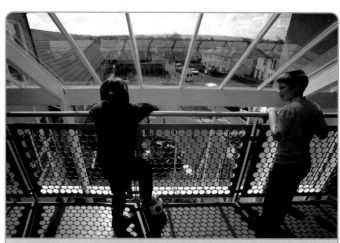

Shettleston Housing Association
Hot water is provided from combined geothermal/solar panel heating and cooled mine-water discharged from the heat pumps is used to feed the WCs
(Photo: John Gilbert Architects)

Wind

Wind turbines are now predominantly used for electrical generation. Offshore and onshore wind farms provide electricity for grid distribution and individual machines find good application in isolated places where they can offset infrastructure costs. Connection to the grid removes the requirement for battery storage, but it is often the prohibitively expensive cost of grid connection in rural locations that is the driver behind investigating wind or other options. Wind power tends to be available when required – at night and in cooler seasons – giving it significant advantages over solar energy in the UK.

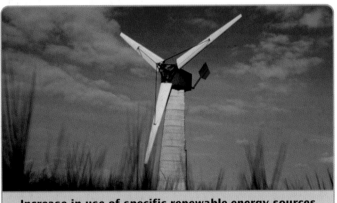

Increase in use of specific renewable energy sources
(Photo: Howard Liddell)

Recent advances have lowered costs dramatically and increased performance, particularly of large turbines. Wind power is now a viable major contributor, and the fastest growing source of renewable energy. Power output of a wind turbine is dependent on the area swept by the blades. The UK is the windiest country in Europe, and for a while Scotland led the world in wind power technology and had some of the first developed wave turbines.

Although wind power can be utilised almost anywhere, the setting is critical due to the changes in wind speed with topography. Doubling wind speed results in eight times the power output, so optimum siting is important. Sites are selected on the mean velocity, which requires historical wind data related to height.

There are also restrictions based on birds' migratory paths. It is also important to consider the implications of space, visual intrusion and noise. Modern turbines also shut down in very high winds to reduce hazards. The efficiency with which energy can be extracted is about 30% and cost is £500–750/installed kW peak output. Professional maintenance is required and this should be considered in costings.

A source of some contention was the low rate paid out to small producers wishing to sell to the grid compared to the purchase price. This has changed dramatically with the increase in ethical suppliers of electricity and the availability of Renewable Obligation Credits.

Fuel cells

Fuel cells run on hydrogen – a colourless, odourless, tasteless gas that can be generated from water, natural gas, propane, methanol, ethanol or landfill gas. The fuel cell consists of two electrodes sandwiched around an electrolyte. Oxygen passes over one electrode and hydrogen over the other, generating electricity, water and heat. The fuel cell transfers chemical energy to DC by separating the proton and electron present in the hydrogen or in a hydrocarbon fuel. In the latter case, a 'fuel reformer' is used to extract the hydrogen.

Fuel cells can be combined as required and small demands can be catered for, whilst maintaining high efficiency. They have no moving parts, produce no noise and require minimal maintenance. As with all energy there is a cost of extraction, and in this case the production of hydrogen gas is energy intensive and therefore net gains are reduced, potentially with significant associated pollution, unless the hydrogen can be produced using clean energy.

A truly 'zero emissions' system is possible only if renewable energy is used to release the hydrogen molecule from hydrogen. In this case the output of the fuel cell operation is electricity, heat and water, with the water able to undergo electrolysis to repeat the hydrogen cycle.

Any other system has associated emissions. The major drawbacks are that fuel cells are heavy and very expensive. Technological advances or cost re-assessments are required if the fuel cell is to become a useful source of renewable energy.

Case Study 11.7:

Lerwick district heating scheme

Shetland Islands Council Charitable Trust, 1999

The Shetland Islands Council Charitable Trust decided, in 1977, to construct a district heating scheme in Lerwick to use the heat from the Council's proposed Waste to Energy Plant at Greenhead. It was not until 1999 that the scheme became operational and the first 10 km of mains were laid. The plant currently supplies about 280 houses and 70 non-domestic properties, including a hospital, two schools, a fish factory and two care centres, plus dairy, retail and commercial properties.

The incinerator burns domestic rubbish from Shetland and Orkney, which amounts to 26 000 tonnes of waste per year and gives an output of 6.8MW. The district heating uses a centralised boiler and distributes the heat via insulated underground pipes. Heat contained in the pipes is transferred to the buildings' internal wet heating system via a heat exchanger; no water is transferred to the buildings. Some of the advantages of the scheme to its customers are lower heating costs and reduced maintenance costs against a boiler system.

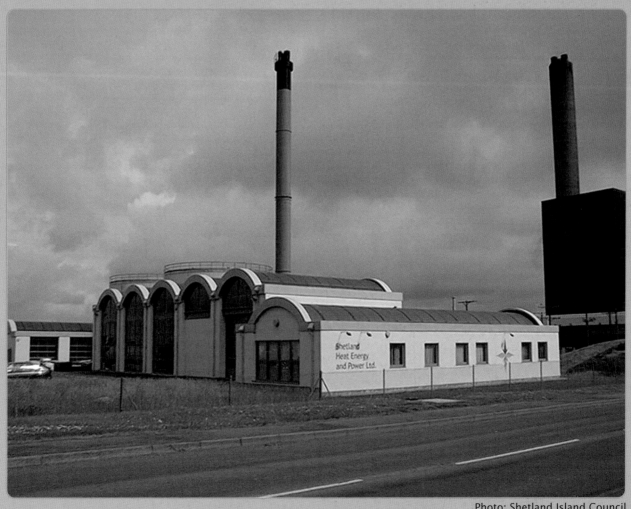

Photo: Shetland Island Council

Autonomy

Sustainable development requires that systems operate with minimal reliance on external inputs of energy or other resources. Indeed, the limits to growth are not the amount of people, cars or things, but the unrecyclable resources that they consume in manufacture and use, and the unmanageable waste or toxicity produced.

To this end there have been a number of studies of individual houses and also developments at a larger scale to investigate the resource throughputs and the potential to develop such autonomous systems with independence from grid-based systems. They extend beyond energy use to other forms of resource management. This implies the need to develop feedback loops in which resources form cyclic systems, rather than the linear ones which characterise our present unsustainable systems.

Future potential

Shell UK predict growth in all the major technologies, with the fastest growth anticipated in solar, PV and wind. The UK government is committed to achieving 10% of the UK's electricity from renewables by 2010. Presently, the figure stands at 2.5%. New and Renewable Energy – Prospects for the 21st Century summarises much current strategy. To assist the uptake of renewables, the UK government has undertaken research into funding needs, and its Performance and Innovation Unit's 2002 report recommended:

- £25 m for offshore wind
- £15 m to help farmers and foresters establish energy crops
- £10 m dedicated to innovative PV schemes
- £10 m for PV and other technologies utilised directly on homes, business and community buildings
- £10 m for fundamental research on the next generation of renewable energy technologies
- £5 m for demonstration and testing of wave and tidal technologies (UK research leads the world)
- £4 m for advanced metering and control technology so electricity grids can best harvest PV and other small-scale technologies
- £18 m for development and demonstration of advanced energy crop technologies for clean and efficient production of heat and electricity.

A study commissioned by the Scottish Executive reported a total renewable energy resource in Scotland equal to 59 GW,

three-quarters of the UK's current installed generation capacity. All of it, including relatively expensive offshore capacity, could be produced at less than 7 p per unit by 2010 (excluding grid strengthening costs). Wind accounts for more than half of the renewable energy potential, followed by wave and then tidal power. The Executive's current target for renewables is 18% by 2010.

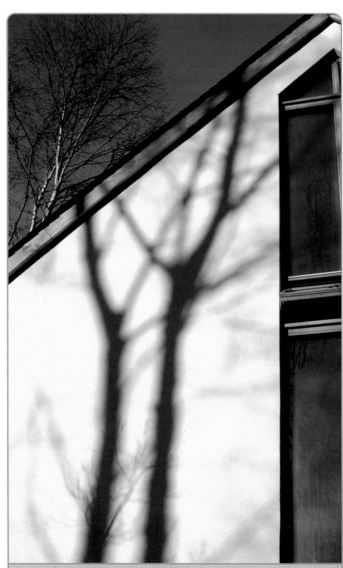

Glencoe Visitor Centre
Built from and heated by local trees
(Architects: Gaia Architects Photo: Michael Wolshover)

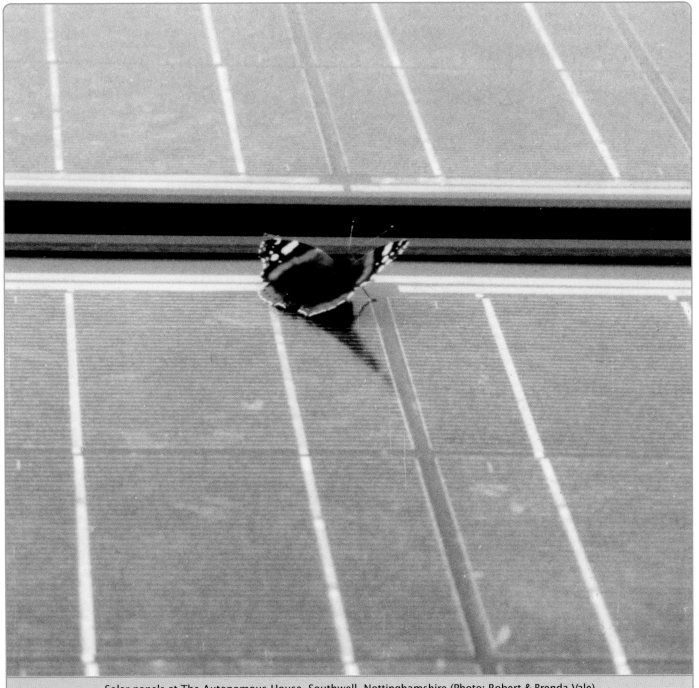

Solar panels at The Autonomous House, Southwell, Nottinghamshire (Photo: Robert & Brenda Vale)

Bibliography

Historic and general

There is an extensive range of guidance on renewable energies going back over three decades. Some of the early materials on specific technologies remains very relevant to the non-specialist and there are a number of good general text books.

Frequent policy shifts mean that technical and commercial advances have been haphazard. This is reflected in the lack of coherence in the information and it is easy for designers to get out of touch. Funding regimes are volatile.

There is an abundance of case study publications from government agencies and the technical press has contemporary project literature that is often ahead of books. A number of publishers now specialise in renewables.

Historic and general

Dickson, D. (1974) *Alternative Technology and the Politics of Technical Change*. Fontana.

Boyle, G. (1975) *Living on the Sun – Harnessing Renewable Energy for an Equitable Society*. Calder & Boyars.

Chapman, P. (1975) *Fuel's Paradise – Energy Options for Britain*. Penguin.

Lucas, T. (1975) *How to Build a Solar Heater*. Mentor.

Vale B. and R. (1975) *The Autonomous House* Thames and Hudson

Boyle, G. (1996) *Renewable Energy – Power for a Sustainable Future*. Open University.

BSRIA (1996) *Sustainable Housing*. BSRIA. A study of energy/water supply and drainage/sewerage technologies and their application at scales from a single house to a cluster, village or town.

BSRIA (1997) *Sustainable Housing - options for independent energy, water supply and Sewerage* BSRIA

Twidell, J. and Weir, T. (1998) *Renewable Energy Resources*. E. & F. N. Spon. Undergraduate study, including fluid mechanics and heat transfer, but also detailed applications.

EUREC Agency (2002) *The Future for Renewable Energy 2 – Prospects and Directions*. A useful summary of the available technologies, with refreshing honesty about issues like costs and the secondary effects of manufacture and disposal, such as pollution. An in-depth review of why renewables are not yet truly sustainable technologies and the life-cycle issues that need to be tackled in order to get there.

Web Sites

Department of Trade & Industry – The DTI New and Renewables programme is a source of policy guidance. The website is the source of information on contemporary policy. www.dti.gov.uk/energy/sources/renewables/index.html

Centre for Alternative Technology (CAT) – extensive experience and a large range of publications are available at www.cat.org. including comprehensive guidance with good references to journals and suppliers.

Energy Saving Trust. www.energysavingtrust.org.uk/

The European Renewable Energy Research Centres Agency. www.eurec.be/

Future Energy Solutions (was ETSU) Extensive publications lists are readily available on all the different technologies, including a vast record of commissioned reports, fact sheets, demonstration projects and case studies, categorised under energy from waste, biomass, wind, tidal, solar, fuel cells, small-scale hydro. There are hundreds of titles. www.aea-energy-andenvironment.co.uk/

Wind energy

McGuigan, D. (1978) *Small Scale Wind Power*. Prism Press.

Piggott, H. (1978) *It's a Breeze: A guide to choosing wind power*. CAT.

Winddirections, Journal of the European Wind Energy Association.

Hydro, wave, tidal

McGuigan, D. (1978) *Small Scale Water Power*. Prism Press.

DoE (1990) *Taking Power from Water*. HMSO. Review of tide, hydro and wave power technologies, programmes and UK potential.

Solar thermal

Halliday, S. P. (1998) *Solar Air Conditioning – Technical Assessment & Demonstration*. Gaia Research

Duffie, J. A. and Beckman, W. A. (2001) *Solar Engineering of Thermal Processes*. John Wiley.

Gordon, J. (2001) *Solar Energy – The State of the Art*. ISES.

Halliday, S. P. (2002) *Solar Desiccant Cooling*. Applied Thermal Engineering.

Andren, L (2003) *Solar Installations*. James & James.

Santamouris M. (ed.) (2003) *Solar Thermal Technologies for Buildings*. James & James.

Weiss, W (2003) *Solar Heating Systems for Houses*. James & James.

Solar PVs

Thomas, R. (ed.) (2001) *Photovoltaics and Architecture*. E. & F. N. Spon. An overview of how PVs work, and a useful guide for architects and engineers to assess feasibility.

Geothermal

Armstead, H. C. V. (1983) *Geothermal Energy – Its past, present and future contribution*. E. & F. N. Spon.

Fuel cells

Bockris, J. O'M. (1991) *Solar Hydrogen Energy*. Optima.

Biofuels

Kovarik, B. (1981) *Fuel Alcohol*. IIED.

Horne, B. (1996) *Power Plants*. CAT. Comprehensive guide and a useful contacts list.

El Bassam, N. (1998) *Energy Plant Species*. James & James. Explains how biomass works, harvesting and storage, conversion and economics.

Sims R. E. H. (2002) *The Brilliance of Bioenergy*. James & James.

Royal Commission on Environmental Pollution (2004) *Biomass as a Renewable Energy Source* RCEP

Biomass and BioEnergy Monthly. Pergamon Press.

District heating

Renewable energy in district heating. DBDH Journal 4/2000 (www.dbdh.dk).

Heat Pumps

McGuigan, D. (1981) *Heat Pumps*. Garden Way.

Renewables design tools

Design of PV systems – CD from Construction Resources (info@ecoconstruct.com).

EUREC Agency – *Photovoltaic Information Strategy to Architects (PISA)*. A useful, free, CD.

Chapter 12
Water and sewage management

(with special thanks to Nick Grant, www.elementalsolutions.co.uk)

In which we consider the flow of water and wastewater through buildings and rain falling on and around buildings. We look at its efficient and, sometimes, creative use, appropriate treatment of discharged wastewater and the potential for reuse.

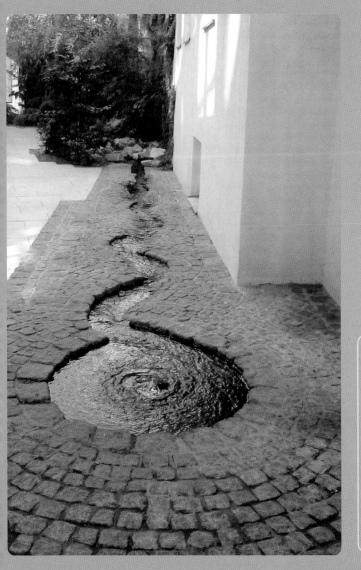

'The society which scorns excellence in plumbing because it is a humble activity, and tolerates shoddiness in philosophy because it is an exalted activity, will have neither good plumbing nor good philosophy. Neither its pipes nor its theories will hold water.'

John W. Gardner

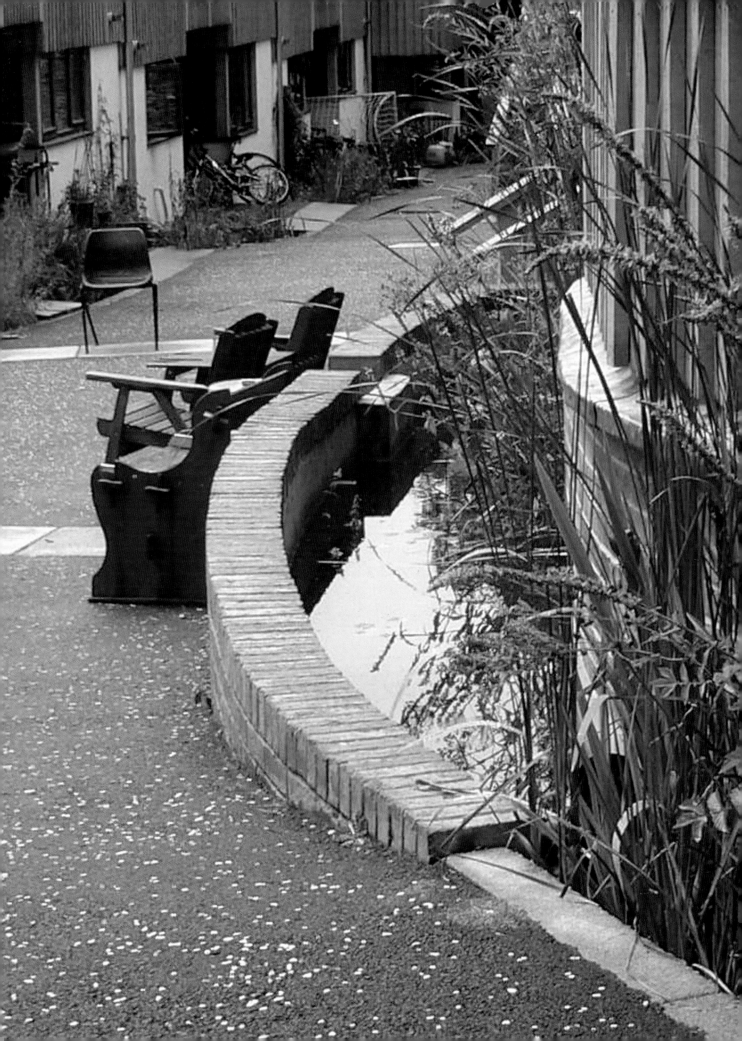

Contents

(Facing page)
Springhill Co-housing, Stroud
(Photo: the author)

(Previous page)
Water Feature at Prisma in Nuremberg
(Photo: the author)

Water and sewage management

Introduction

The aim of sustainable water management is to ensure that use is efficient and pollution is minimised, so that water returns to the environment in a benign form. Sustainable water management is relatively easy to achieve. However, whilst there are notable exceptions, many designs either ignore it or seek to produce a 'statement' that does not stand up to detailed environmental scrutiny.

Most water enters our buildings as purified drinking quality and leaves as sewage. The extent of our water use affects the infrastructure, storage requirements and energy required for delivery and purification. Yet, in general, we use it very inefficiently. For example, we mix and dilute wastes that our bodily systems have spent the whole of evolution separating and concentrating.

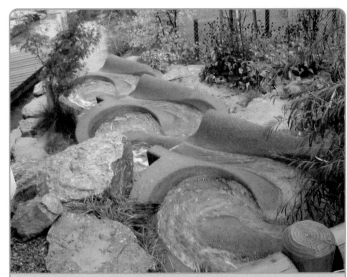

Street scene with open flowing water
An award-winning ecological housing project at Arkadien Asperg, Germany by Joachim Eble Architects, with landscape and water design by Herbert Dreiseitl
(Photo: the author)

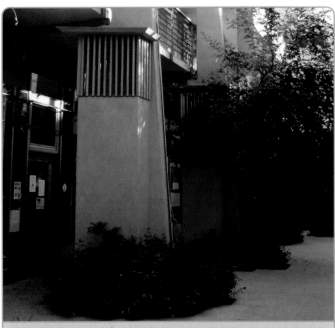

Half open drain pipes at Prisma serve their purpose using half the material of traditional systems
(Photo: the author)

The extent to which we pollute water adversely affects ecological systems, our health and ultimately our quality of life, yet we are less than conscientious with respect to chemical and bacterial pollution.

Wastewater can be a resource if purified for non-potable uses such as toilet flushing. If properly managed, some valuable nutrients can be returned to the land. Rainwater can be used as a substitute for treated water for some household uses, but rarely is. Impervious surfaces that dominate the built environment make rainwater a nuisance rather than an asset, and with increasing propensity to flooding, water management has become a serious issue.

There are many opportunities for water conservation and benign disposal, but the wide availability of mains water, sewerage and storm water drainage connections means that water issues are rarely considered in building projects. However, there are benefits to such considerations at the earliest stage in design and refurbishment, and these are increasingly a requirement on the part of planners.

The UK is still very reserved in its approach to using and expressing water in the environment – but this is an emerging area of interest because of the benefits to biodiversity and the creative opportunities. This chapter looks at a number of projects where water features have been combined with ecological treatment inside and around buildings.

Context

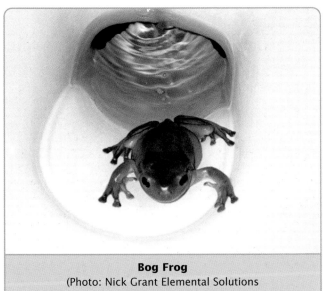

Bog Frog
(Photo: Nick Grant Elemental Solutions
www.elementalsolutions.co.uk)

Good building design responds to the local environment. Sustainable water management is particularly sensitive to context and resistant to standard 'bolt-on' solutions. Good practice water efficiency measures should be considered for all projects, but will always have to be balanced alongside other design issues.

There is a tendency to assume that solutions such as reed beds, compost toilets, greywater recycling and rainwater systems are inherently sustainable regardless of the context. This is not the case. Analysis is always required to determine an appropriate design solution.

For most sites with a reliable water supply, and a suitable 'sink' for wastewater, conventional solutions are probably more practical than innovative 'demonstrations' and statements.

Conservation of water is the major issue in buildings which are already connected to mains services. Solutions such as dry toilets may not only be a sustainable option, but the only practical one for the most constrained sites: public toilets in SSSIs, developments in remote locations and buildings on rock or heavy clay. Indeed, these can be the easiest to assess as the limited options determine the solutions.

In many situations the designer is presented with complex choices; motivation, impact, management and cost will all influence the most sustainable solution.

Main considerations

- *Conservation*. Use water more efficiently to reduce waste.
- *Delight*. Use water to create a dynamic energy in and around buildings – supporting biodiversity and play.
- *Pollution*. Minimise organic waste to landfill. Consider the impact of sewage treatment and discharge, and consider the treatment options.
- *Rainwater drainage*. Minimise the impact of the built environment on the flow of rainwater back into the natural environment.
- *Environmental impacts*. The benefits of water saving or wastewater treatment measures should not be cancelled out by, for example, increased energy or chemical use.
- *Education*. Environmental benefits can be multiplied if the context is inspiring and the technique is replicable.
- *Closing the circle*. Consider using the waste from one process as the input to another.
- *Economics*. Sustainable economics takes into account a wide range of costs and benefits over the installation's lifetime, but many 'sustainable' approaches are cheaper even in crude capital cost terms.

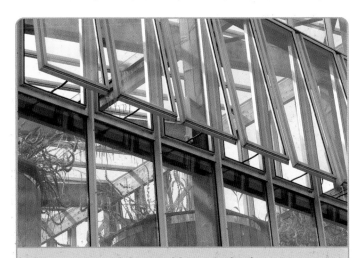

Living Machine at BedZed
There is a tendency to assume that solutions such as reed beds, compost toilets, greywater recycling and rainwater systems are inherently sustainable regardless of the context. This is not the case. Living Machines might sound like the holy grail but in many situations they can be very energy intensive
(Photo: the author)

Case Study 12.1:

Gibson Mill, Autonomous Visitor Centre, Hebden Bridge

Architects: Ecoarc Architects, 2005

Owned by the National Trust, Gibson Mill is a nineteenth-century cotton mill that sits at the heart of Hardcastle Crags near Hebden Bridge. It has been brought back into use as a facility for visitors and for the local community. The brief required the renovated mill to be a model of sustainable development, being run with minimum adverse impact on its environment. The lack of any mains services inspired a totally autonomous design.

A private water supply and wastewater treatment was the only practical option for this remote site, but the autonomy brief also called for sewage solids to be treated rather than tankered away. Dry compost toilets were considered for the public but rejected by the client in favour of conventional-looking but efficient WCs. As well as the 'no tanker' brief, access to the public toilets is by a narrow bridge, so a sludge-free system made sense.

The solution chosen was based around the Swedish Aquatron separator. This simple passive device uses surface tension to separate the solids from the flush water for composting in one of two prefabricated bio-chambers located in the room under the toilets. The separated liquid effluent from the Aquatron flows to an unpowered dosing device, which delivers pulses of effluent along an infiltration trench. The sandy soil provides filtration and biological treatment without odour, pollution or energy use and not a reed in sight.

Located across the river from the Aquatron system, the staff and cottage loos are served by compact compost toilets. The historic buildings precluded the use of larger vault-type toilets, which are more robust but would have required excavation of the building floor.

Fortunately, a reliable and pure spring was found that was just high enough to supply all the buildings by gravity without the need for pumps or treatment. Finding a free source of water pouring out of the hill might seem to make water efficiency measures redundant; however, dramatically reducing the water use simplifies wastewater treatment and disposal, demonstrates best practice, and has performance and reliability advantages.

The visitor toilet block is served by robust but super-efficient four-litre WCs with traditional leak-free siphons and Ifö Cero waterless urinals. When temperatures dropped to minus 13°C during winter everything froze solid, but the urinals continued to work without risk of bursts or flooding. Once the WCs had thawed they worked fine, with no leaks or damage to the tough mechanism. With limited power, hot water was not considered feasible for the remote toilet block, but the use of spray taps minimises the discomfort from washing hands in unheated water whilst also further reducing effluent volumes.

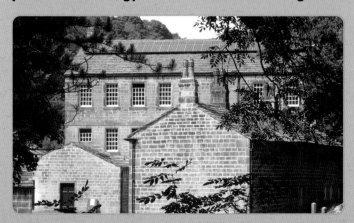
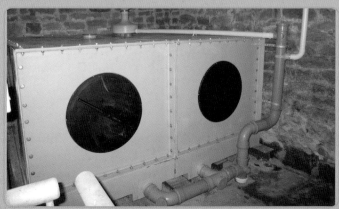

Photos: Elemental Solutions

Conservation

Water economy is beneficial even where there is not an obvious water shortage:

- Conservation through specification of efficient water systems, such as WCs, can significantly reduce infrastructure requirements and costs, and deliver savings in metered water use.
- Contrary to most expectations, water and energy efficient solutions can have significant performance benefits that justify their inclusion regardless of water saving. Examples include odourless flood-proof urinals, WCs that flush first time and are quick to refill, taps that run hot without a long wait, improved hygiene from auto-shut-off taps, etc.
- Reuse of 'greywater' or collection of rain locally for non-potable uses such as gardening and toilet flushing can also save metered water. However, it will often increase infrastructure costs except for sites with no other source of water.
- Where sewage is to be treated on site or wastewater is to be infiltrated into soil, reducing the volume has compound benefits.
- Over-abstraction depletes groundwater supplies and reduces surface water flows in summer. Even parts of the UK that might be perceived as wet can suffer severe shortages in summer. This directly reduces the flow of streams and rivers downstream.

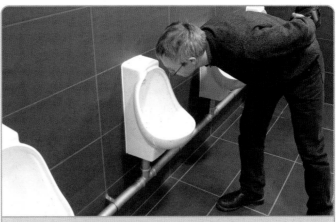

Airflush waterless urinals
An olfactory inspection of at the National Trust's headquarters in Swindon. The complete absence of odour means no urinal blocks or airborne chemicals
(Photo: the Green Building Store)

- Water conservation also has associated energy savings. Treating and pumping mains drinking water and treating the resulting sewage typically requires about 1 kWh/m^3. This equates to about 220 kWh (200 kg of CO_2) per year for a four-person household. Where hot water is conserved, much greater energy savings can be achieved.

Financial savings are generally modest – except for industrial processes or major leakage. Emphasis therefore needs to be on design and performance rather than just cost savings.

Many water-economising features, such as four-litre WCs, waterless urinals and spray taps, can be routinely specified as standard, with 80% water savings readily achievable.

For sites with limitations on water supply or effluent disposal, specialist solutions such as vacuum and dry toilets, rainwater collection and wastewater recycling may be justified.

Personal preference and better functionality may also be a driver. Compost toilets may be chosen because they lack odour and splash, and are silent in use. Alternatively, prejudice or bad experience can prevent use of dry or low-water-use toilets or waterless urinals.

A growing range of efficient products such as WCs, taps and showers are available at prices comparable with less efficient products. However, labels may be meaningless, and evidence of performance should be sought and compared with benchmarks. Indicative benchmarks may be found for some showers and spray taps in the *EA fact cards* and BRE IP/2/00.

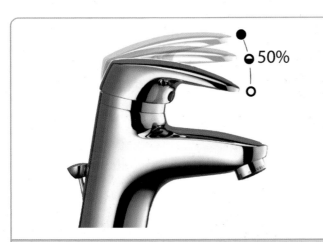

Water brake taps
Centre-cold and regulated aerators provide small but worthwhile water and energy savings, with no loss of function
(Photo: the Green Building Store)

Case Study 12.2:

Gallions Housing Association, Thamesmead

Architects: PRP Architects, 2002

Gallions Ecopark is an affordable housing scheme of 39 houses at Thamesmead. It was developed by Gallions Housing Association. The homes contain a combination of cost-effective and practical water- and energy-efficient design solutions that are easy to use.

The water-saving features include low-volume baths, water-efficient showers, spray taps, flow regulators, mixer taps (in the kitchens), Swedish low dual-flush toilets (4/2.5 litre) and water butts. Gallions have monitored the use of water in a number of houses using residents' water bills, and initial indications show that the average resident uses 109 litres per day. This is 27% less than the national average of 150 litres per day, although this data has yet to be verified.

Throughout the development, the landscaping is sensitive to the needs of the environment. Paved areas are limited and the use of half-open pavement areas allows rainwater to penetrate the ground and reduces run-off. Rainwater is biologically treated before entering the local canal system and street water passes through oil separators before reaching the biological treatment area.

The financial benefits of the Ecopark approach will be quantifiable once the monitoring has been completed. This uses a variety of methods, including telemetric monitoring systems and utility bills. An additional four properties offsite are used as a 'control' against the Ecopark homes. These control dwellings are of a similar size and age to the Ecopark homes, and are built to standard Building Regulation requirements.

A visitor centre has been developed on site with an accompanying 'naked house' exhibition home. This showcases the sustainable elements of the design and construction, and includes 'hands-on' interactive exhibits. Gallions Housing Association runs n educational programme with local schools to promote an understanding and acceptance of the principles of sustainability. Tenants are encouraged to understand and perpetuate the sustainable principles and features.

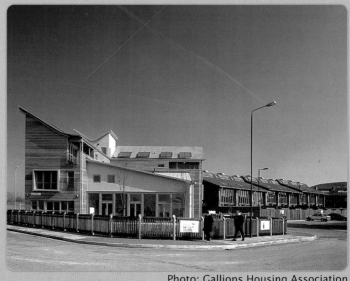

Photo: Gallions Housing Association

Delight

The few examples of real creativity provide inspiration as to the real possibilities in how we use and manage our water resources.

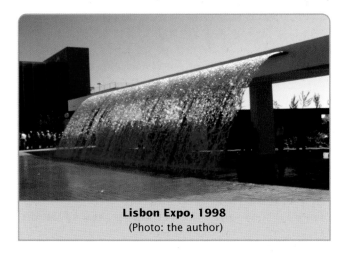

Lisbon Expo, 1998
(Photo: the author)

Water features are increasingly seen as an intrinsic part of the approach to the built environment. Projects such as Schafbrühl (Tübingen) incorporate elements that facilitate play and also enhance biodiversity. At both Prisma (Nuremberg) and Okohaus (Stuttgart), water is incorporated as a functioning aspect of the indoor environment, and street features are also commonly incorporated as a significant aspect of approaches to public space and even school design. In the UK, we remain very reserved on this issue.

Pollution

In the UK, lead, nitrates, aluminium and pesticides are among those pollutants found above safe limits in water. Few of the chemical compounds found in water are monitored regularly and EC directives cover only a fraction of them. Many remain unidentified. Whilst much originates in industrial discharge and agricultural practice, there is also a great deal over which the building designer and user can have a positive influence, including reducing pollution from rainwater runoff, leachate from buildings and landscape elements, landfill and water-borne waste.

The UK still lags behind much of Western Europe in recycling domestic solid organic waste, such as food, paper and card. Most of this ends up in landfill, and contributes to the generation of polluting leachate and to greenhouse gases such

as methane and carbon dioxide. Recently, targets have been introduced requiring significant increases in recycling.

Reduction, reuse and recycling should be a first consideration. Provision for composting and recycling (e.g. space for separate bins) can be incorporated at any scale. Rainwater run-off and treatment options for greywater and sewage are dealt with later in this chapter.

Innovation

All 'green' technologies face a potential perception problem. Shortcomings will inevitably be blamed on the innovative 'environmental' aspects. When conventional urinals smell or WCs don't flush, it is not considered exceptional. If, however, waterless urinals or efficient WCs under-perform for any reason, then the lack of water will be blamed. Therefore, 'green' technologies need to out-perform the standard specification if they are to gain acceptance.

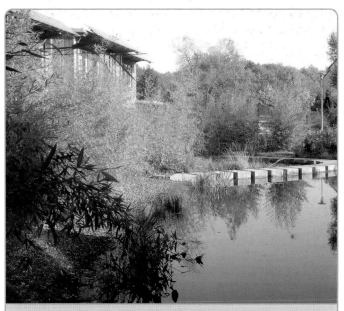

Multi-faith Ecological School at Gelsenkirchen, Germany with integrated gardens and ponds
(Waterscape: Atelier Dreiseitl; photo: Ian Cameron)

Case Study 12.3:

Hopwood Park Motorway Services, M42

Bob Bray Associates, 2000

The site is almost impermeable, and so surface water has to be collected and treated prior to discharge direct to local watercourses.

The HGV park comprises a self-contained drainage system with water flowing across a grass filter strip to a stone 'treatment trench' sized to intercept and clean the 'first-flush' run-off from the tarmac surface. There are no gullies, pipes or oil separators.

Run-off then flows to a spillage basin designed to contain tanker spillages and finally to an attenuation pond. Flows in excess of the 'first-flush' volume overtop the trench and are collected in a swale that leads to the attenuation pond. Day-to-day run-off therefore experiences four 'treatment stages' before release at 'greenfield rate' to the adjacent wildlife reserve, helping to maintain the baseflow in a tributary to the Hopwood stream.

The remainder of the site subdivides again into three: the fuel filling area, coach park and access roads; the car parking area; and the amenity building. Each area collects and treats run-off in different ways, but always ensuring that water flows through a series of SuDS features before controlled release to the Hopwood stream.

Hopwood Park Motorway Service Area is the first site in the UK to demonstrate a clear 'management train' with 'treatment stages' reflecting the pollution risks likely in each sub-catchment. It demonstrates how pollution, particularly oil-based contamination of run-off, can be managed using the SuDS approach to drainage.

The development has been intensively monitored since 2000 and has demonstrated the effectiveness of the 'management train' in dealing with pollution, the importance of treating pollution 'at source' to protect wetland amenity features and the cost-effectiveness of SuDS maintenance both on a regular basis and when occasional silt removal is required in small linked wetland features.

Water leaves the site at 'greenfield rate' of five litres per second per hectare and meets the storage requirements for the 1-in-25 'storm return period'.

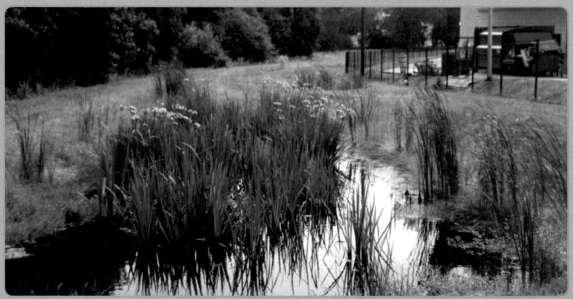

Photo courtesy of Robert Bray Associates Ltd, www.sustainabledrainage.co.uk

Case Study 12.4:

Matchborough First School, Redditch

Worcestershire County Council, 2001

Rainwater is collected from $725\,m^2$ of roof, filtered and stored in a $15\,m^3$ concrete tank. To ensure security of supply should the pump fail, the rainwater is pumped to header tanks, which also allow mains water back-up.

The capital cost was around £4200 plus installation and the estimated annual rain utilisation is $350\,m^3$.

Matchborough was also retrofitted with a SuDS solution after the proposed pumped scheme to the sewer was found to be both costly and unable to deal with the whole site.

The run-off is collected in open basins that link together with a shallow swale round the playground, leading to a final wetland. There are two controls within the site and a final controlled outfall at the end of the wetland. An interceptor swale collects run-off entering the site from adjacent housing.

All SuDS features are open to provide maximum interest for the site, ease of management and wildlife interest. The Head Teacher has supported the scheme and involved children in the system with a dipping platform and algae removal in the early stages of establishment.

All overflows from the rainwater harvesting system enter the SuDS system into the conveyance and storage swale.

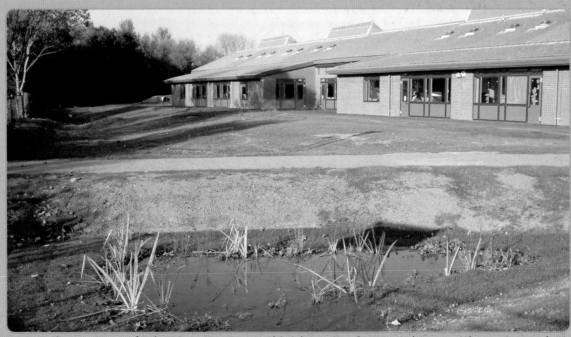

Photo courtesy of Robert Bray Associates and Rainharvesting Systems Ltd, www.rainharvesting.co.uk and www.sustainabledrainage.co.uk. Permission: Nick Grant

Rainwater drainage

Storm water can be more problematic than sewage because of high peak flows. Storm water connections are now discouraged. Some water companies offer reduced fees if it can be shown that no roof or surface water discharges go to the mains sewer.

The increasing attention to rainwater drainage in recent years is in part because relatively easy solutions have been identified to mitigate the downstream problems of flash floods and overloading of treatment plants receiving combined sewer flows. A contributory factor has been concerns over the potential for climate change to exacerbate problems. The problems are caused by the use of impervious surfaces for roofs, paths, roads and parking, and the tendency to move water rapidly away from these areas through piped systems. This prevents rainwater naturally filtering into the ground and instead creates rapid run-off polluted with animal faeces, tars, vehicle fuel and oil. The contemporary solution to dealing with water that falls as rain is known as Sustainable Drainage Systems (SuDS). It aims to:

- Control flooding
- Prevent pollution
- Provide amenity
- Recharge groundwater
- Reduce the load on sewage treatment plants.

SuDS is an approach rather than a specific technology. It aims to return water to the natural environment at an appropriate rate and quality. Typical systems use permeable surfaces, swales and filter strips to capture and convey run-off, simultaneously removing pollutants and buffering peak flows. If the site is suitable, infiltration is encouraged. Some systems include storage for irrigation or WC flushing. Usually, interceptors, pipes and gullies are avoided but some systems, combine hard and soft technologies. The use of petrol interceptors has pros (can catch a tanker load of fuel and hold it for recovery) and cons (if they do not get emptied). Systems need to be designed to cope with the construction process and not just the building in use.

Environmental impacts

The environmental benefits due to water saving or cleaner effluents could be cancelled by, for example, increased energy or chemical use. There should be an assessment of the relative environmental impacts that are being traded. Although difficult in absolute terms, a comparison between competing technologies is usually possible as the quantifiable differences are often significant. Examples of trade-offs include:

- Water wasted in dead legs vs. energy loss from trace heating or pumped loops
- Effluent quality vs. energy input or treatment system size
- Extensive system with zero energy use vs. intensive system with small footprint but ongoing energy use
- Water saving from vacuum or drying toilets vs. energy use
- Water saving from domestic greywater system vs. energy and chemical use.

Sustainable sewage treatment requires attention to the capacity of the receiving environment. Where sewage is collected in a cesspool and removed by tanker, vacuum toilets may have a lower net energy use than conventional ones. Ideally, buildings should not be placed in sensitive locations, but where this has already happened creative solutions are needed. Where a freshwater lake, loch or SSSI is at risk from sewage effluent, then energy or chemical use may be justified. At the other end of the scale, it rarely makes environmental sense to expend resources treating sewage to a very high standard before discharging it to soil, unless this overlies an aquifer.

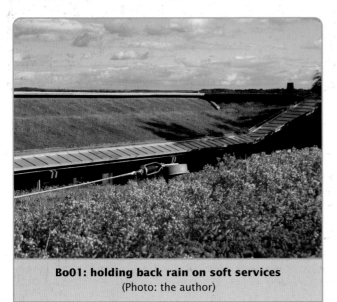

Bo01: holding back rain on soft services
(Photo: the author)

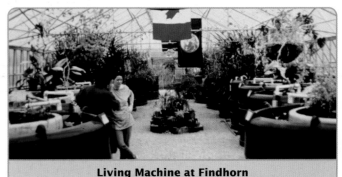

Living Machine at Findhorn
(Photo: Howard Liddell)

Education

A replicable design will generally be affordable and acceptable to builder, owner and user. Achieving this will require that a range of design issues are addressed, including management in use. Recently, increasing interest in water management issues has resulted in a number of experimental projects, some with artificially imposed restrictions such as water autonomy or complete on-site sewage treatment. In a high percentage of 'eco demo projects', an inappropriate solution for the site or one which is too expensive or energy inefficient may have resulted – a reed bed in a city context or a powered treatment plant in a rural one. Whilst these can serve as valuable test beds and have useful spin-offs, such as creating wider interest, they may not merit replication. As only about 4% of the UK population is off the mains sewer, such systems are likely to have minimum uptake and distract from issues with far greater potential to make a difference.

Water management requires better understanding of the closed circles inherent in natural systems. Good design and management education should concentrate on developing an appreciation and understanding of where water comes from and where what you put down the drain goes, why to turn off the tap when brushing teeth, and when and what to bag and bin. Recently, there has been a tendency to assume that it is

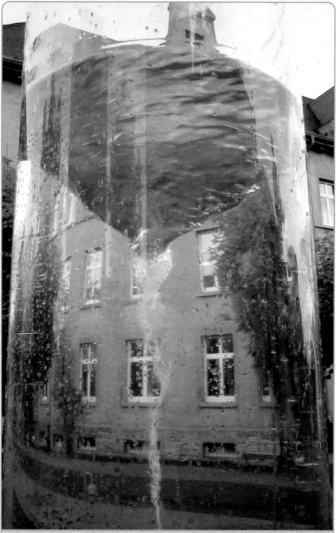

Street toy in Loretto, Tübingen
Water provides for plants and play in the urban environment
(Photo: the author)

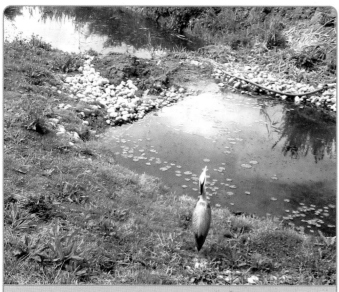

Brenzett Primary School sewage treatment system
(Photo: the author)

educational, for example, to install inappropriate green icons such as reed beds in urban schools. This is rarely so.

The real challenge is to educate through the interpretation of genuinely more sustainable solutions, which might otherwise go unnoticed. Much more could be learnt from a visit to the local sewage or water treatment works than from implicitly promoting the idea that a reed bed would be a good thing to have in a town garden.

Case Study 12.5:

Autonomous Environmental Information Centre

Centre for Alternative Technology, Wales. Architect: Pat Borer, 2001

Increasing visitor numbers put a strain on the site's reed-bed sewage system and sewage from a new building needed to be treated separately. The site was ideally suited to the use of a Swedish separating system that collects and composts solids. The liquid effluent is treated biologically by using the slate tip, on which the building sits, as a biological filter. Unlikely to be widely replicated, it illustrates the principle of using what is available. If the site had been on impermeable clay, then ponds may have been considered. The WCs are four-litre and the urinals are waterless.

A rainwater system was installed for demonstration and research, but has suffered from coloration due to gutters holding stagnant water and leaves, a lesson in the importance of checking details. A new type of high-quality, twin-vault, urine-separating compost toilet is installed as an additional working demonstration. Electronic sensor taps with regulated sprays (1.8 l/min) were chosen to counter CAT's low-tech image, but mechanical taps would have given the same savings at lower cost. The hot water is conveyed at 'mains' pressure through small (10mm PEX) pipes, thus minimising the dead leg and addressing legionella concerns without the need for high flows or trace heating.

This project is a mixture of reproducible best practice and very site-specific solutions. The overall style is modern and efficient. The electrically insulating nature of the slate waste site caused some problems with the electronic taps, which need an earth connection. The avoidance of sludge generation is an important principle at CAT, where everything is composted and soil is in short supply.

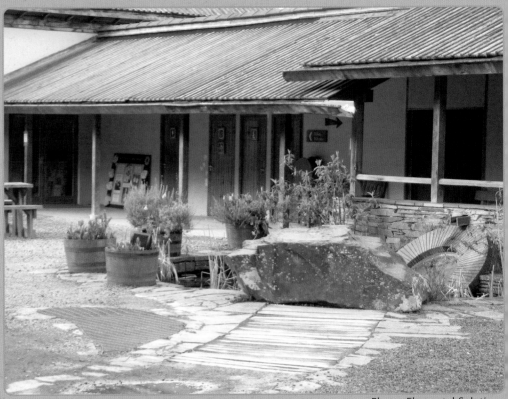

Photo: Elemental Solutions

Closing the circle

The best systems consider the local hydrology, soils and hydro-geology rather than bolting on a context-insensitive technical fix.

Rainwater

The local treatment and reuse of wastewater (including rainwater) for toilet flushing and other non-potable uses such as irrigation is increasingly popular. Generally, it is more effective to implement water efficiency measures such as low-volume WCs before considering reuse, although there are situations where reuse has compound benefits, such as the attenuation of storm water flows.

An obvious case for recycling or reuse, for example, would be one in which a large roof area suitable for rainwater collection is matched to a large demand for non-potable water (e.g. for vehicle washing or toilet flushing). Similarly, many industrial or agricultural processes use clean water for cooling or rinsing, which can then be reused without treatment for cleaning.

Local reuse benefits from economies of scale and is rarely cost-effective at the single household level. In some countries, subsidies are available that reflect the wider benefit of reducing storm water flows and demand on aquifers and watercourses.

Where a high water table is present, then consider a shallow well for non-potable water abstraction with rainwater infiltrated nearby. This uses the immediate environment for filtration and storage, and avoids the problem of preventing rainwater tanks floating. Solutions need not always be re-invented.

Nutrients

Plant foods in wastewater can be returned to the soil. The main sustainability driver for nutrient recycling is usually the protection of watercourses that can suffer from excess nutrients. In Sweden and Germany, separating toilets have been used which collect nitrogen- and phosphorus-rich urine in large tanks for agriculture. Whilst increasingly common in Scandinavia, such systems are unlikely to become mainstream in the UK in the foreseeable future.

Effluent

If there is a requirement for sewage effluent to be treated to a very high standard, then the cost of a reuse scheme may be partly covered by necessary upgrade costs. Technologies such as membrane bio-reactors (MBRs) and sequencing batch reactors

(SBRs) are commercially available and produce high-quality effluents suitable for non-potable reuse after disinfection.

However, before labelling such schemes as sustainable, it is necessary to perform some life-cycle analysis to compare with other water supply and efficiency options.

Indirect reuse outside the property boundary should not be ignored. Examples include high quality effluent returned to rivers, and sewage and rainwater infiltrated into the ground to replenish aquifers.

Where the public sewer is available, connection is usually required and it rarely makes sense to use on-site treatment. Possible exceptions include where the available treatment works is close to its capacity or where effluent is to be reused or recycled on site.

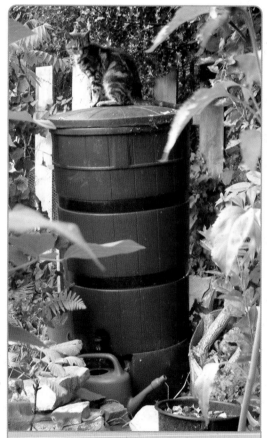

Water butts can be transformed with sympathetic planting
(Photo: Ian Franklin)

Case Study 12.6:

Boatemah Walk, Lambeth, London

Architects: Anne Thorne Architects Partnership, 2003

Boatemah Walk is a three-storey block of 18 flats and is part of Lambeth Council's regeneration of Angell Town estate. The original design brief was for a greywater recycling system to a green roof and standard WC and taps specification. ech$_2$o consultants were asked to design a rainwater harvesting system for the flats after the decision was made to abandon the greywater recycling scheme.

As the most important part of any sustainable water strategy is to reduce demand at point of use before sourcing water from elsewhere, they changed the WC specification from six-litre single flush to the IDO 4/2.5-litre dual flush), and specified flow regulators at 4 litres/minute to all basins and at 10 litres/minute for the showers. Incorporating rainwater harvesting into the design at such a late stage could have been problematic, but due to strong support from Mendick Waring (main engineers) and Sandwell (design and build consultants), it was achieved with little difficulty. Rainwater from the roof is filtered and stored in a 15 000-litre capacity underground tank, sized to make optimum use of rainfall on the site. The stored rainwater is pumped on demand to a header cistern which feeds the WCs in the flats. No UV disinfection has been specified as the rainwater is used for WC flushing only; thus, the environmental load of using rainwater is reduced. The system is metered so that the exact amount of WC flushing demand offset by rainwater can be quantified. It is estimated that 220 m^3 of water will be saved a year from the WC specification and a further 176 m^3 from using rainwater on the site.

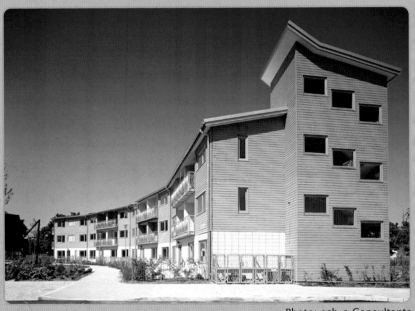

Photo: ech$_2$o Consultants

Sewage treatment options

Where a mains sewer connection is not feasible, the appropriate sewage treatment technology will require assessment of many factors:

- The physical aspects of the site
- A destination for treated effluent and storm water
- The volume and nature of wastewater that is to be generated
- The regulator's decisions about disposal routes and effluent quality.

The environmentally and economically preferred route is usually to 'soakaway', unless wastewater volumes are too great for the available land area or the site is otherwise unsuitable (e.g. high water table, groundwater protection zones, impermeable soil, steep slopes, bedrock, nearby private water supplies).

A well-designed system in suitable soil will provide excellent treatment with no energy consumption and maximum use of natural processes and on-site materials (soil). In marginal cases a 'soakaway' system may become feasible with improved design and water efficiency measures. If a 'soakaway' is not possible, then a suitable drain or watercourse must be identified and an appropriate effluent quality determined.

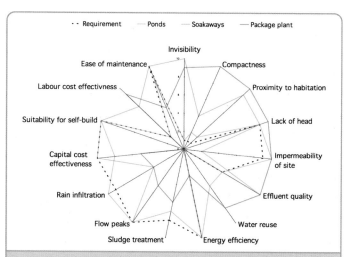

Example of context analysis for a range of system choices
(Diagram: Elemental Solutions)

Radical solutions

Technologies that avoid the problem rather than end-of-pipe solutions are sometimes difficult to retrofit and must be considered at the design stage:

- Dry toilets – avoid the generation of wastewater and the need for a water supply.
- Greywater irrigation or reuse – reduces or eliminates the generation of wastewater to be treated and saves drinking water.
- Storm water source control and rainwater reuse – reduces the load on combined sewers, eliminates point-source pollution, and can eliminate the need for storm sewers or flow-balancing tanks.

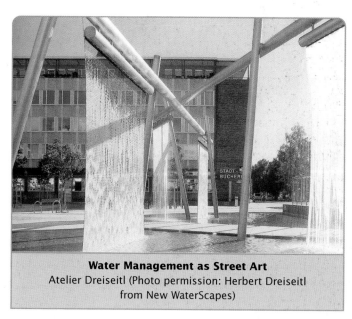

Water Management as Street Art
Atelier Dreiseitl (Photo permission: Herbert Dreiseitl
from New WaterScapes)

Extensive systems

These are large and robust, zero or low energy consumption. Choice of system depends on soil type, available falls and area, etc. Loading rates are limited by oxygen transfer between atmosphere and wastewater and/or retention time:

- Passive ponds and lagoons – large, ideal in heavy clay, may incorporate aquaculture.
- Leachfields – hidden, good solution in suitable soil (arguably 'passive intensive').
- Land treatment – low cost, possible 'planning' issues.
- Wetlands, horizontal-flow reed beds – performance and clogging issues to address.
- Sea or river – in all systems the wider environment continues the treatment process.

Case Study 12.7:

Hollow Ash, Herefordshire

Self-build conversion, 1996

The combination of a difficult site for drainage and an environmentally aware client led the installation of a compost toilet. This made particular sense in view of a number of factors, including a very heavy clay soil and no watercourse for effluent discharge. An efficient WC was also added (discharging into the compost chamber) on the assumption that grandparents would be nervous of the dry toilet. In practice, the dry toilet is preferred by all but the smallest visiting children, as there is no smell, splash or sound. There is no septic tank and the warm greywater passes through the compost toilet to aid the process of decomposition.

A potable rainwater system with a small UV filter, backed up by mains water, results in very low water bills and the occupants prefer the taste. The rainwater system has worked well but is experimental, requiring some adjustment and maintenance that would be beyond the scope of most householders. Normally, potable use is not recommended, but with the compost toilet there would have been little other use for the water. The system has achieved ultra-low water use, but the energy use by UV is substantial and there is an issue about manufacture and disposal of UV tubes containing mercury. Total water use is 37 l/person/day (about 75% less than average) of which 5 litres is mains (about 3% of average), but energy use for rainwater pumping is 0.21 kWh/m^3 and for UV treatment 3.75 kWh/m^3. The energy consumption is four to eight times greater than for mains water, but could be reduced by improved control.

The minor problems encountered in this particular system include using a submersible pump rather than gravity to discharge wastewater from the chamber and reliance on mains electricity to run the extraction fan, resulting in smell during power cuts (overcome to some extent by using a battery backup), difficulty in maintaining an airtight external seal to the chamber, which occasionally resulted in a smell and sewage fly problem, and plastic rubbish being thrown down into the chamber by children.

Whilst managing with the water that falls on your roof is a nice idea and an interesting experiment, this project has been a good lesson in the benefits of keeping things simple.

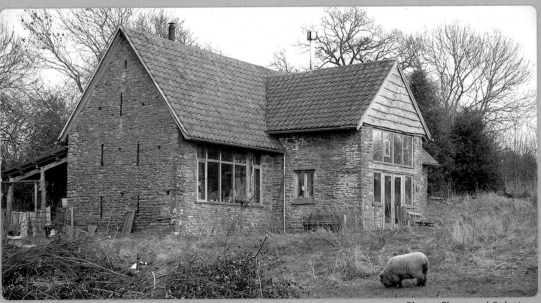

Photo: Elemental Solutions

Case Study 12.8:

Withy Cottage, Herefordshire

Nick Grant's self-build home and office, 2002

Another rural self-build in Herefordshire which provided the opportunity to try a range of largely simple measures. As with Hollow Ash, a septic tank gives way to a compost toilet chamber, over which the super-insulated house was built. The compost toilet was an aesthetic as well as environmental consideration, and provides a very elegant solution for a rural self-build. Lessons learnt from Hollow Ash have resulted in an odour- and fly-free system. A four-litre, leak-free siphon WC provides an extra toilet and discharges directly into the compost toilet. All hot water pipes except to the bath are 10mm micro-bore, which means that taps and shower run hot quickly with minimal waste.

Taps are single-lever ceramic mixers with eco-brake cartridges and aerators or sprays as appropriate. These have a click-stop to provide a gentle reminder not to use full flow unless required and also only provide cold water in the central default position, thus saving energy as well. All outlets are fitted with dynamic flow regulators to stabilise flow and pressure throughout the house, whilst offering modest savings when taps are run at full flow. An A-rated washing machine was chosen for low water use and there is no dishwasher, despite claims that they save water.

Hot water is mains pressure from a thermal store and a number of water-saving shower technologies have been tried. However, the current set-up is a fairly standard shower-head with a 6 l/min flow regulator. The house is heated with a single small wood stove, which also provides winter hot water. As the days lengthen and the stove is left unlit, solar water heating takes over, with minimal requirement for immersion heater back-up (less electricity than the standby for a gas boiler).

A household rainwater system was a conscious mission, but large recycled fruit juice barrels collect rainwater for garden use. Extensive use of mulch and organic matter reduces water requirements for the large vegetable garden.

All these measures result in a household water use that averages only 52.5 litres per day, per full-time occupant.

As there is no septic tank, greywater is dispersed in a blockage-resistant 'Trench Arch' infiltration system. More information at www.elementalsolutions.co.uk.

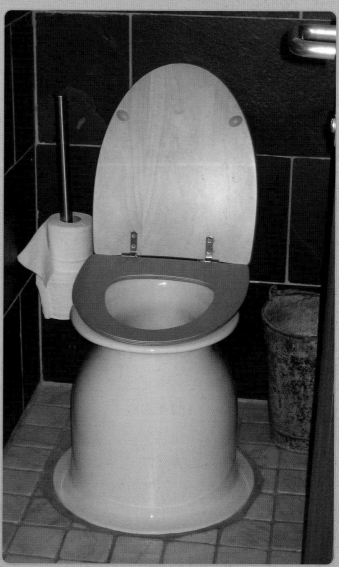

Photo: Howard Liddell

'Passive intensive'

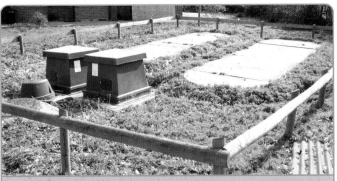

Intensive systems
A package treatment plant with the capacity to treat the wastewater from 200 people
(Photo: Elemental Solutions)

This evolved from extensive systems but offers a smaller footprint at the cost of engineering complications. These systems use a vertical-flow regime, making use of gravity to improve the availability of oxygen:

- Trickling filters (bio-filters).
- Sand filters – little used in the UK but can produce very good effluent, various types.
- Vertical-flow reed beds – sand filters with plants.

Extensive with energy input

These are large systems typically with aeration to reduce odour or improve effluent quality. They are usually inefficient in energy and space terms, but may have a green image:

- Aerated ponds and lagoons – aeration is sometimes added to cope with seasonal variations and occasional odours. Some 'green' domestic systems use an order of magnitude more electricity than some package plants.
- Living machines.

Intensive systems

These typically reduce the system size by using mechanical aeration. Some use chemicals to achieve oxidation, precipitation or nutrient removal, and some systems combine biological and chemical processes. Treatment stops when power fails:

- Activated sludge – conventional municipal-scale technology, many variations.

- Membrane bio-reactors (MBR) – a new technology which combines membrane filters and biological treatment to produce high-quality effluents suitable for reuse.
- Sequencing batch reactors (SBR) – an activated sludge process ideally suited to small-scale plants. High-quality effluents may be suitable for reuse and solids may also be treated.
- Package plants – compact pre-built and easily installed systems for small- to medium-scale applications. Many process technologies available. Energy use, cost and effluent quality vary considerably between designs.

Hybrids

Combinations of any of the above, typically an intensive first stage followed by an extensive polishing and buffering stage, such as a pond or wetland:

- Rotating biological contactor (RBC) followed by a horizontal-flow reed bed.
- Trickling filter followed by grass plot or soakaway.

Detailed guidance on the choice of appropriate systems is beyond the scope of this chapter, but the case studies touch on a few of the many options and associated issues. Generally, the more energy-intensive systems can be tailored to any situation if power is available, whilst natural systems are more site sensitive.

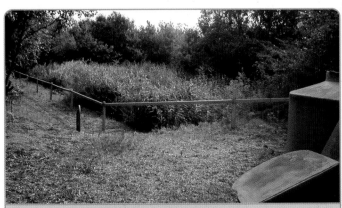

Hybrid System
Package plant followed by horizontal-flow reed bed. The reed bed provides buffering and tertiary treatment, reducing BOD and suspended solids to low levels
(Photo: Elemental Solutions)

Case Study 12.9:

Burwarton Village, Shropshire

Drainage replacement, 1995

Burwarton is a small village in rural Shropshire with a popular pub and a resident population of about 150. Half the village was connected to a failing treatment system, with the rest on failing septic tank systems. The local soil is heavy clay and the antiquated drainage system receives surface water infiltration and storm water run-off from about 2000 m². Plenty of low-cost farmland ideally located between the village and a brook was available. These factors, combined with a commitment to a 'green' solution, made a pond system the clear choice.

Heavy clay eliminated the need for liners and the large ponds buffer the unavoidable storm water input. The ponds are followed by a wetland area. There is no discharge to the small brook in the summer months when its flow, and available dilution, is low. With little opportunity to address wider aspects of water management, this 'end-of-pipe' solution was the practical option.

Comparison of CAT and Burwarton case studies. Burwarton has impermeable soil and plenty of space but little fall. The treatment is in effect 'powered' by wind and sun. CAT has highly permeable slate, little area but plenty of vertical fall, with the treatment 'powered' by gravity and natural convection. A site with little space, no fall and impermeable soil would probably require energy input for treatment, or a radical solution such as dry toilets or the less sustainable pumping or tankering off site.

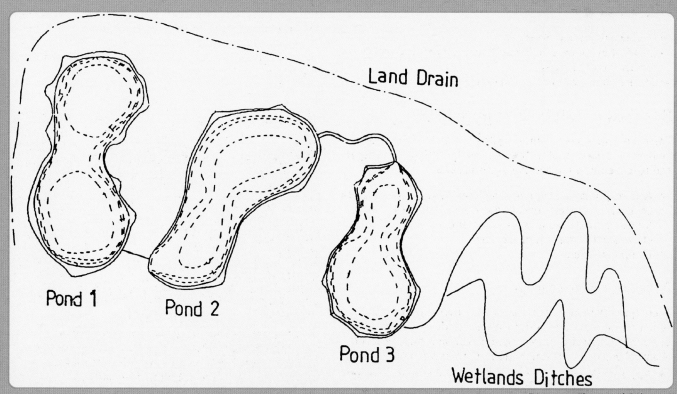

Diagram: Elemental Solutions

Case Study 12.10:

Glencoe Visitor Centre, Glencoe, Argyll

Architects: Gaia Architects; Water Consultant: Elemental Solutions, 2002

The assumed sewage treatment solution for this green flagship project was a wetland. However, this would have required a large land take on a site with little flat ground and significant quantities of quarried aggregate. In addition, such a system would have been at odds with the very sensitive treatment of landscape and ecology that was an important part of this development. The more radical solution adopted was to rebuild and upgrade the existing trickling filter using long-life stainless steel mechanical components and reused high-performance plastic media from a local sewage treatment works.

As with Gibson Mill, the water supply was from a spring, so water efficiency would seem to be unnecessary other than as an educational demonstration. However, radical but replicable

water efficiency measures, including waterless urinals, four-litre, leak-free WCs and spray taps, meant that the existing settlement tank could be retained.

Unfortunately, the urinals were of a type requiring very regular and specific cleaning, and this has led to maintenance problems. Additional treatment stages could have been added to further clean the effluent, but the final watercourse provides high levels of dilution and ongoing treatment, so to do so would have added to the overall ecological (and financial) impact of the system.

A rebuilt and upgraded bio-filter (trickling filter) was chosen as a greener alternative to an extensive wetland system for this particular site.

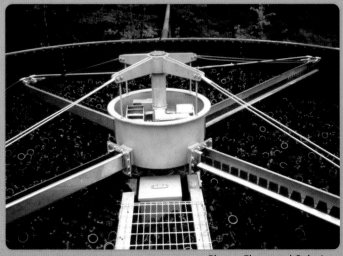

Photo: Elemental Solutions

Design checklist

Legal

- EA/SEPA, consents and concerns.
- Planning.
- Building Regulations.
- Environmental Health.
- Water Regulations.
- Wayleaves, land ownership, shared systems.
- Maintenance contracts.
- Performance guarantees.

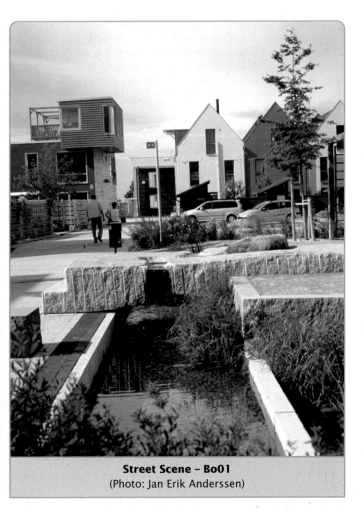

Street Scene – Bo01
(Photo: Jan Erik Anderssen)

Site features

- Soil type and permeability.
- Sensitivity of receiving body: are nutrients a concern (lakes and lochs) or bonus (biomass irrigation)?
- Can the wider environment be considered as part of the treatment system?
- Available area.
- Proximity to habitation.
- Public access: safety, vandalism.
- Available fall. Flat sites suit ponds, horizontal-flow reed beds and leachfields, sloping sites suit trickling filter, sand filters and vertical-flow reed beds.
- Availability of local materials: filter sand, gravel, slag, stone, topsoil, clay.
- Availability of electricity on site.
- Access for machinery and materials.
- Access for sludge removal.
- Visual and aesthetic considerations: invisible or feature?

Client/user details

- Can the problem be eliminated at source? (e.g. cheese factory whey fed to pigs; dry toilets; swales rather than storm drains.)
- Budget.
- Available maintenance skills.
- Number of people served.
- Per capita water consumption: can this be reduced?
- Need or potential uses for water or nutrients on site (e.g. dry climate gardens, biomass coppice).
- User acceptability and expectations: mountain bothy vs. hotel.
- Cultural issues.
- Unusual inputs: for example, photographic chemicals, sterilising fluids.
- Image: system may have to be 'distinctive' to obtain funding.
- Risk.

Economics

'Sustainable solutions' need not be more expensive than good-quality 'non-sustainable' ones. More efficient versions of toilets, taps, showers and washing machines can be added to any project and will be competitive with good-quality, but not poor-quality, alternatives. It is rare, but informative, to compare options on a life-cycle basis considering energy, water charges and materials.

The cost benefits are self-evident in:

- waterless urinals and smaller boilers
- when using smaller pipes and pumps for lower flows
- some natural treatment systems – soakaways and passive ponds
- sustainable urban drainage schemes.

Significant expense can be accumulated through:

- poor design
- overly complicated and inefficient systems
- low-volume production, expensive prototypes – prices should fall with increased uptake
- high-quality products that include environmental features as part of a general high specification – the mistake is to attribute the over-cost to the efficiency measures and to expect a payback which would not be required if the item was simply expensive.

Much of the benefit of implementing efficiency measures accrues to society (through delayed investment in new infrastructure such as reservoirs and treatment works) and to the environment by reducing the need for expensive future clean-up.

Notes and assumptions relating to the graph shown are as follows:

1 Investment in a simple cistern displacement device costing £5 (fitted) and saving 1 l per flush. Four people each using the toilet five times per day and paying £1/m^3 for water and £1/m^3 sewage charges.
2 Replacement of a 9 l WC (10 l actual flush) with a 4.5 l (actual) at a cost of £350 installed. Other assumptions as before.
3 £350 invested at 6% tax free, interest re-invested annually.
4 £30 invested in fitting a dual-flush siphon retrofit saving three litres (30%) per flush.
5 £1500 invested in installing a rainwater recovery system that utilises 75% of all the rain falling on a 60 m^2 roof in an area with 800 mm of rainfall per year. Annual running costs and repairs assumed to average £15. Savings of sewerage charges not included as effluent volume remains the same.

The payback period is where the line crosses the x-axis. The £5 Sava-flush has the shortest payback period but investment is limited to £5 per WC. Assumptions can be altered to get different results.

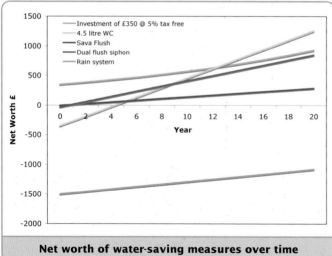

Net worth of water-saving measures over time
(Graph: Elemental Solutions)

Case Study 12.11:

Woolfardisworthy Sports and Community Hall, Devon

Architects: Gale and Snowden Architects, 1999

Woolfardisworthy community commissioned a sustainable multi-use hall to be an asset for future generations. A super-insulated timber frame uses minimal thermal bridging and airtight construction to reduce heat loss. Passive solar heating, triple-glazed windows and optimised daylighting are included. The WCs are two- and four-litre dual flush, fed by rainwater pumped directly from the storage cistern. This rainwater system is a standard German system, but the WC function is dependent on the pumps functioning.

Waterless urinals are installed, of the oil trap type. The services engineers optimised hot water pipe sizes and pipe runs so as to minimise the dead legs without resorting to pumped loops, which add complexity and increase energy consumption.

The times for showers and basin taps to run hot are reported to be acceptable. The wash basin taps receive pre-mixed warm water through 10mm pipes, which avoids issues of scalding and minimises legionella risk whilst saving water and energy. The showers are standard commercial models with 6 l/min dynamic flow regulators.

The building and services are reported to be working well. Water and energy use is being monitored.

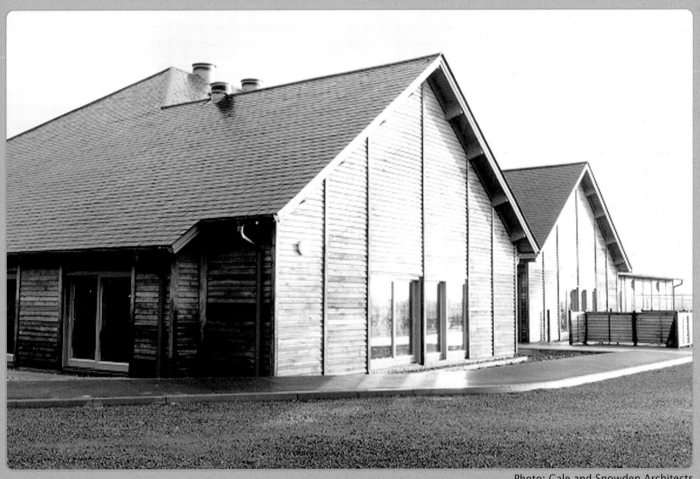

Photo: Gale and Snowden Architects

Water – rules of thumb

- Autonomy does not equal green – connect to mains drainage if available.
- Where possible, infiltrate rainwater into the ground rather than into sewers.
- Avoid single-issue solutions. Consider as wide a picture as is practical and appropriate, including function, maintenance, water use, effluent quality, chemical use, energy consumption, materials, land use, aesthetics.
- Check commissioning, maintenance and product reliability.
- Make prioritised lists of site-specific issues and opportunities.
- Pay attention to efficiency measures, as they are almost always cheaper and more environmentally benign than recycling or harvesting.
- Check manufacturers' and designers' green claims.
- Do not be fooled by iconic green features such as plant and animal life, but apply standard criteria such as energy use, embodied energy, materials content, land take, etc.

- Remember that terms such as 'natural' and 'water efficient' are often meaningless in a product sales context.
- Use low-cost sub-metering, as it allows performance to be measured and problems spotted.
- Realise that, for most sites, reproducibility and public acceptability may be more important than absolute environmental performance if good practice is to spread.
- For very sensitive sites, radical solutions and change of personal habits may be acceptable or necessary.
- Do not underestimate the importance of detail and quality in design and installation.
- Balance absolute greenness and performance without considering it a compromise, e.g. if a WC will meet a specification at 3.8 l but using 4 l means it outperforms technologies using 6 l, then the compromise will be worthwhile.
- Balance risk and benefit. 'No-risk solutions' may simply move the risk off site.
- Never compromise health. Improvements in water and sanitation have saved more lives than modern medicine.

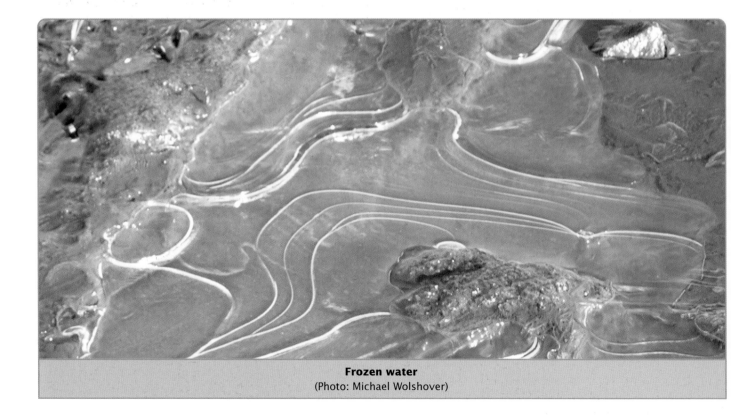

Frozen water
(Photo: Michael Wolshover)

Bibliography

SEPA: (undated) *Designs that Hold Water – Sustainable Urban Drainage Systems explained*. Video. www.sepa.org.uk

Harper, P. and Halestrap, L. (1999) *Lifting the Lid*. Centre for Alternative Technology, Machynlleth. The definitive UK dry-toilet book, also covers household nutrient recovery and composting.

WRAS, Water Supply (Water Fittings) Regulations (1999) SI Nos. 1148, 1506. Water Industry, England and Wales. www.wras.co.uk/directory.

WRAS IGN No 9–02–05 (1999) *Marking and Identification of Pipework for Reclaimed (Greywater) Systems*. www.wras.co.uk/directory

Grant, N. and Griggs, J. (2000) *BRE Good Building Guide* GBG42, Part 1, *Reed beds: application and specification* and Part 2, *Reed beds: design, construction and maintenance*. CRC Ltd.

Martin, P. et al. (2000) *Sustainable Urban Drainage Systems – Design Manual for Scotland and Northern Ireland*. CIRIA, Publication Code C521.

Water Regulation Advisory Scheme (2000) *Water Regulations Guide*. CIRIA.

BRE Water Centre (2000) *Water Conservation: IP 2/00, Low Flow Showers and Flow Restrictors*. Available from CRC Ltd.

CIRIA C539 (2001) *Rainwater and Greywater Use in Buildings: Best Practice Guidance*. CIRIA.

Environment Agency (2001) *Water Resources for the Future: A Strategy for England and Wales*, March. This document and the associated regional ones give an excellent analysis of the problems of water supply in the UK. Free, as above.

SEPA (2003) *Ponds, pools and lochans – guidance on good practice in the management and creation of small waterbodies in Scotland*. SEPA.

Dreiseitl, H., Grau, D. and Ludwig, K. H. C. (2005) *New Waterscapes Planning, Building and Designing with Water*. Birkhauser.

Grant, N., Moodie, M. and Weedon, C. (2005) *Sewage Solutions; Answering the Call of Nature*, 3rd edition. Centre for Alternative Technology, Machynlleth. Introduction to sewage treatment, conventional and alternative.

Environment Agency (pending) *Conserving Water in Buildings Fact Cards*. Practical information, publication list, posters on water efficiency and updated contact list of equipment suppliers.

Guidance on water management, pollution and SUDs is available from: Scottish Environmental Protection Agency (www.sepa.org.uk) and Environment Agency (www.environment-agency.gov.uk)

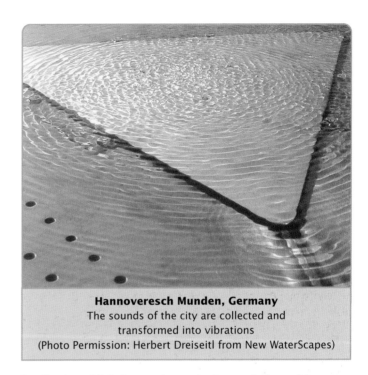

Hannoveresch Munden, Germany
The sounds of the city are collected and transformed into vibrations
(Photo Permission: Herbert Dreiseitl from New WaterScapes)

My thanks to Nick Grant, who worked extensively on this chapter. Nick runs the water and wastewater consultancy Elemental Solutions (www.elementalsolutions.co.uk), and is a director of Solution Elements Ltd and NatSol Ltd. His experience ranges from practical product development to theoretical research into water efficiency and wastewater treatment and reuse. In 2000 he wrote the guidance document for reed beds and sand filters, which supports the UK Building Regulations. In 2001 he produced the *Conserving Water in Buildings* best practice fact cards for the Environment Agency. Nick shares Gaia's 'eco-minimalist' approach to sustainable construction based on good design and sound science, rather than bolt-on solutions and green icons. Nick is a keen theorist, but also extremely practical, having designed and developed commercial products, constructed sewage treatment systems, and designed and built his own water- and energy-efficient house and office.

Chapter 13
Construction processes

(with special thanks to Adrian Leaman for the section on post-occupancy evaluation, www.useablebuildings.co.uk)

In which we investigate construction as a process, not an act and building as a process, not a product. We highlight a broad range of the pitfalls that can undermine sustainability criteria, how to overcome them and how to learn from engaging in constructive feedback.

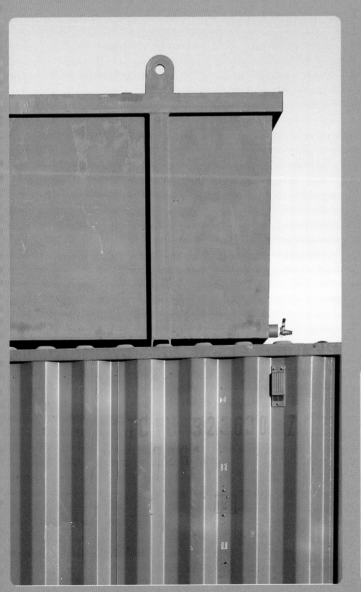

"If we are to move forward... towards mainstreaming ecological design as an integral part of building for the 21st century, then it is crucial that it is accessible, economic, genuinely environmentally-sound, gimmick-free and not stigmatised as a style"

Howard Liddell, from *Eco-minimalism – less is more* (2006)

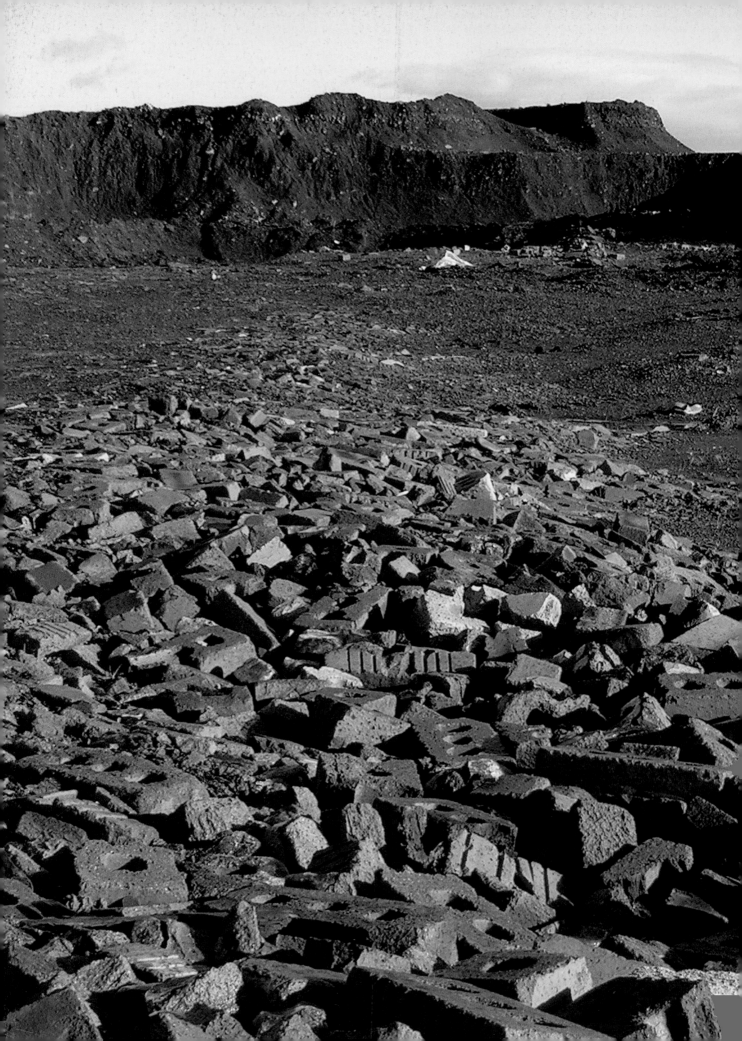

Contents

(Facing page)
Discarded bricks
Photo: Michael Wolshover

(Previous page)
Photo: Michael Wolshover

Construction processes

Introduction

There are two principal strands of concern with regard to sustainable construction and process. One relates to the activity involved on site, to ensure that this is undertaken in an environmentally sound manner. Most available guidance has been focused here. Initiatives such as 'considerate constructors' and 'CEEQUAL' are helpful in promoting and monitoring the attitude and methods for delivering buildings attentive to the environment and to neighbours' rights and needs. They provide good guidance on site management. They are increasing used as contractual requirements. It is not unusual now to see construction sites adorned with flower boxes, although the presence of these, or 'green' hoardings, doesn't guarantee good practice.

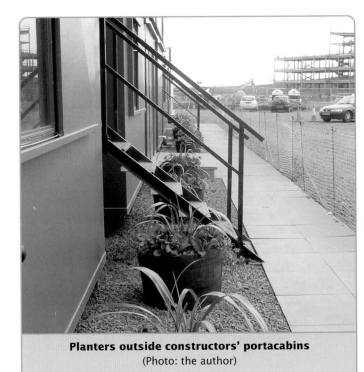
Planters outside constructors' portacabins
(Photo: the author)

Planters outside portacabins and 'green' hoardings are increasingly common. The image of the construction industry has changed dramatically. Health and safety and job security were early targets and this has been followed by voluntary schemes which include environment targets. These are now used routinely by most major builders.

Significantly less attention is generally given to the second strand: ensuring that projects themselves are delivered in accordance with the aspirations for sustainable development. There is generic guidance available on only a limited range of aspects.

Appropriate and aware strategies throughout the process of procurement, design, tender, cost review and handover, for instance, have the potential to underpin aspirations, whilst lack of attention to future management can undermine. Problems can arise from the outset with lack of attention to those most affected, or because members of the design team fail to take seriously a client's aspirations, have different priorities or inadequate knowledge. Lessons can be learned through a coordinated approach to feedback and this can be fed forward into future projects. It is attention to these elements that comprises a significant amount of this chapter.

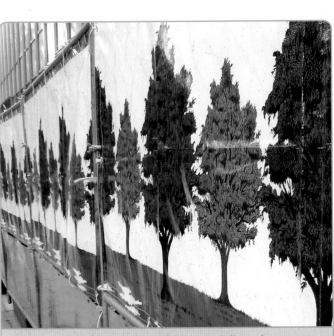
Hoardings on a Japanese building site
(Photo: the author)

Scope

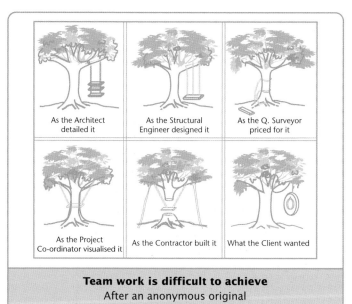

As the Architect detailed it	As the Structural Engineer designed it	As the Q. Surveyor priced for it
As the Project Co-ordinator visualised it	As the Contractor built it	What the Client wanted

Team work is difficult to achieve
After an anonymous original

Documents such as the *Green Guide to the Architects' Job Book* have since developed to address the process issues in depth. It is an environmental *aide-mémoire* to enable built environment professionals to include environmental considerations as part of their remit and formalise the management of environmentally sound practice. It is intended to provide information, at each stage of the Plan of Work, which will assist delivery of buildings that are functional, efficient, joyous and healthy, both internally and in their impact on the wider world. The *Green Guide* and the *Environmental Code of Practice* should be referred to for more in-depth guidance than provided here. The BREEAM series has increasingly responded to pressure to look at process and incorporate these aspects, although it does not form part of the appraisal.

Often, the sustainability aspirations are the most vulnerable throughout the design and tender phase, with trepidation on the part of designers, great pressure on cost targets, often with inadequate information, and pressures on time often threatening aspects of environmental quality. This is especially true when teams are inexperienced in dealing with the issues. Matters arising before, throughout and after operations on site are all relevant.

The key issues that require attention in relation to the process of sustainable construction are:

- The delivery of the aspirations for a building from inception to handover and beyond, such that it can meet the increasingly common social expectation that it is an appropriate development.
- The process of construction itself, to ensure that the methods of building and the impact of construction on the community and the environment – both local and global – is as benign as possible.
- The process of feedback so that experiences can be shared and contribute to continual improvement.

The dearth of information on the delivery of sustainability objectives of projects is surprising, given the far-reaching and long-term impact. It probably stems from the fact that project managers have not yet embraced the sustainability agenda constructively. The *Environmental Code of Practice for Buildings and Their Services* was perhaps the first document to deal with sustainable construction as a process and not a product. It led to a study of the issues arising during the design, construction and demolition of a wide range of projects, including the Centre for Understanding the Environment, Bishopswood Environmental Education Centre and Linacre College, and an in-depth advocacy study during the construction of the BRE Office of the Future.

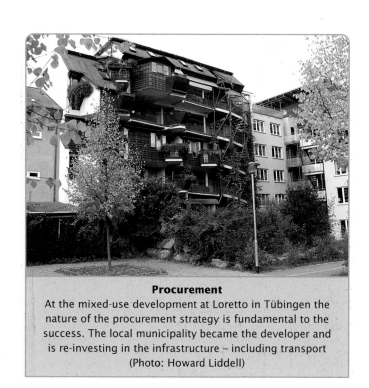

Procurement
At the mixed-use development at Loretto in Tübingen the nature of the procurement strategy is fundamental to the success. The local municipality became the developer and is re-investing in the infrastructure – including transport
(Photo: Howard Liddell)

The sustainability baton

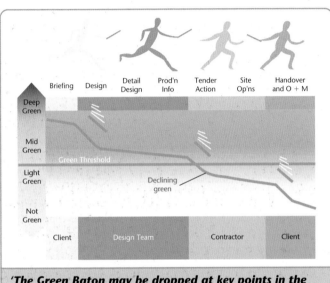

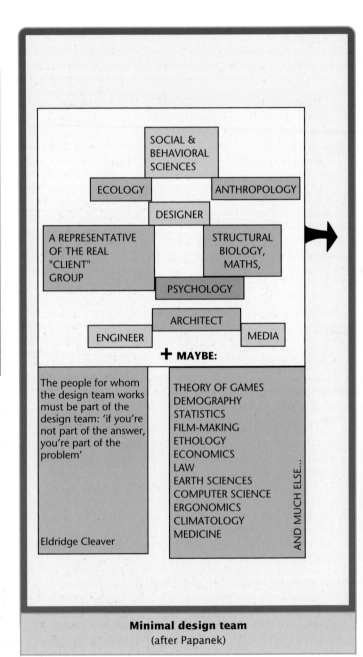

'The Green Baton may be dropped at key points in the process ... Once dropped it is difficult to pick up again and regain lost ground.' Howard Liddell

The construction period is described here in set periods – with dominant levels of responsibility transferring as the project progresses. Howard Liddell's concept of the 'green baton' illustrates that at each stage in the procurement process the sustainability agenda is vulnerable. There is a high risk of the 'sustainability baton' being dropped throughout the process and particularly as responsibilities are transferred from the client to the design team to the contractor and back to the client.

The effect of any compromises will inevitably depend on the aspirations at the start-out. It is vitally important, and necessary, to start with high aspirations and to involve the widest range of interests in the design process.

A project with low expectations and little support will find it difficult to withstand the wide range of pressures and be unlikely to have green credentials at all by the time it is delivered. These pressures cannot be underestimated. For an inexperienced client or design team it will be helpful to employ a specialist to set the aspirations and to oversee their progress throughout the construction period. For clients it is necessary to seek real evidence of delivering sustainable projects, as many more people now claim this experience than can factually support it.

Minimal design team
(after Papanek)

Case Study 13.1:

Woodhouse Medical Centre, Sheffield

Architects: Robert and Brenda Vale, 1989

Woodhouse Medical Centre (WMC, 640m² gross) is the smallest building studied in PROBE. The single-storey medical centre on the outskirts of Sheffield is domestic in scale and construction. It was commissioned from Robert and Brenda Vale by two medical and one dental practices and is divided into three individual units. Opened in 1989, it was built to very high standards of insulation (wall U-value 0.2 W/m²K, roof U-value 0.1 W/m²K) and includes several other low-energy features, such as mechanical ventilation and heat recovery, gas condensing boilers and low-energy lighting. It was also completed within the strict financial and spatial constraints of the local Health Commission, with no additional funding for the low-energy features.

WMC has the lowest CO_2 emissions per square metre of any of the PROBE buildings. It is well liked by occupants despite several gaps in their understanding of the design intent – which appeared to stem from little contact between the designers and the building's end-users during and after handover. For example, the heat recovery room ventilation units were

generally assumed by users to provide a form of year-round airconditioning, and hence to provide improved summer comfort. In fact, they had no bypass, so would actually tend to increase air temperatures. Similarly, the natural ventilation strategy relied on openable windows to promote the stack effect through the corridor and if necessary to cross-ventilate with outlets through openable roof windows near the ridge in corridors and public areas. However, the roof windows were not used because they are high up and impossible to reach. In addition, the intended cross-ventilation of doctors' surgeries via high-level windows to the corridors proved impossible owing to the need for acoustic privacy. One practice decided to retrofit split DX air-conditioning room units in a number of spaces.

Daylighting levels within the building are poor, resulting in a high use of electric lighting in the building with the exception of the central corridor, where the lighting levels were high. Yet, despite this, the Woodhouse Medical Centre achieves an outstandingly low heating and electrical lighting use.

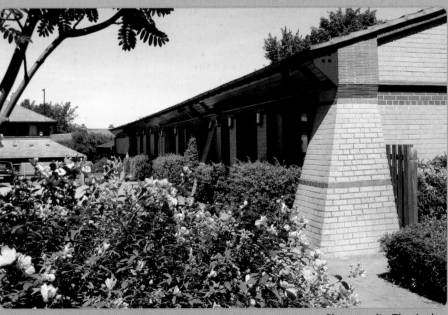

Photo credit: The Author

Key issues

The following six attributes are vital considerations in any project:

1 Stewardship of projects is a vital and overarching aspect in delivering, both in the first instance but also in ensuring their performance over time. Too many aspirations for sustainable projects are undermined by failure to identify appropriate targets, tools and benchmarks, or to look to long-term manageability.

2 Support communities – identify and meet the real needs, requirements and aspirations of communities and stakeholders, and involve them in key decisions.

3 Enhance biodiversity – do not use materials from threatened species or environments, and improve natural habitats where possible through appropriate planting and water use.

4 Create healthy environments – enhance living, leisure and work environments; do not endanger the health of the builders or users, or others, through exposure to pollutants, toxic materials or harmful organisms.

5 Use resources effectively – do not consume a disproportionate amount of resources, including money, energy, water, materials and land, during construction, use or disposal; do not cause unnecessary waste due to short life, poor design, inefficiency or less than ideal construction and manufacturing procedures; and be affordable, manageable and maintainable in use.

6 Minimise pollution – create minimum dependence on polluting materials, management practices, energy and transport.

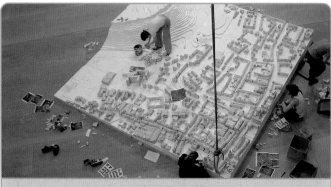

Community consultation
Communities enjoy workshops where they can discuss and define their individual and common needs and aspirations.
(Photo: Howard Liddell)

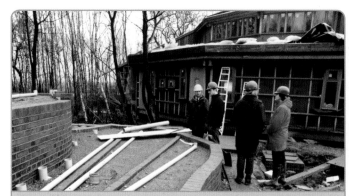

Site visit: Bishopswood Environmental Centre, Hereford
(Photo Permission: The Author)

Procurement

In the wake of the Latham and the Egan Reports, significant effort is presently directed to innovative procurement. Many contractors remain cautious and conservative. In respect of sustainability issues, there is no evidence to indicate that delivering the green baton intact need be hindered by any form of procurement – PFI, design and build, traditional design team-led procurement or hybrids of these – although continuity is likely to be a key to success under any system. Goodwill, good dialogue and agreed targets are fundamental.

Scepticism or lack of ambition or commitment by key players can always undermine any procurement system. Any form of innovation runs a risk of losing elements of importance to the final building, and its ongoing management, if their significance is not understood or contractual in the chain of delivery.

Experience to date indicates that the expectation that long-term thinking would accompany long-term responsibility incurred under PFI proved to be misguided, at least in many of the early projects. Close involvement in decision-making of users and others with a commitment to long-term project success, however that involvement is managed, is more likely to be a recipe for success.

A recent visit to Norway to investigate school design identified that a consistent factor in the most successful schools was the extent of community and parental involvement. Those projects with the greatest pre- and post-design and construction stage involvement were generally judged to be the best performing. The reasons for this are unclear. It may be that the consultation process enabled the designers to better understand how the project would be used and hence to design for this. On the other hand, it may be that the involvement encouraged users to understand the complexities or to be more forgiving about performance.

Case Study 13.2:

Donald Dewar Leisure Centre, Drumchapel, Glasgow

Architects: Glasgow City Council, 1999

The Drumchapel project was the first proposed for dynamic insulation in the UK. The McLaren project, however, was the first to be built and the Drumchapel project was able to benefit immensely from the experience gained. The design team, building control officers and contractors all made visits to McLaren in order to learn about the do's and don'ts of detailing, constructing and commissioning airtight roof voids, etc. Operation and maintenance training for Drumchapel staff is to be undertaken jointly by the architects of the two buildings. The intention of the training is to familiarise staff with the basic principles of the approach, but also the operational regimes. The aim is to move the staff away from the misguided belief that buildings are self-regulating, and to show that their attention and intervention can have an important positive or negative influence on comfort levels and energy efficiency.

Interestingly, during a hot spell in 2005 complaints were received that the fitness suite, which was designed with culvert ventilation to avoid the need for air-conditioning, was too hot. The client phoned a number of other fitness suites with air-conditioning and found that all of them were also overheating – a reminder not to blame the innovative technology.

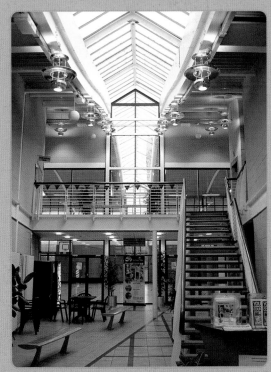

Photo: Howard Liddell

Case Study 13.3:

Range of procurement methods

Three different methods of procurement were in evidence in the schools visited on the tours, and although the procedures employed in Norway and Germany do not correspond exactly to equivalent circumstances in the UK, they were close enough to be recognisable under familiar UK terminology. These are as follows (see Table 13.1):

- **Traditional – design team led with traditional tender**
- **Design competition – mostly with traditional tender**
- **Contractor led by:**
  - **PPP/PFI equivalent**
  - **Design and build (novated design team at tender stage).**

Half the schools visited were procured by traditional means, a quarter by competition (with traditional tender), a quarter by contractor-led means and one, Kvadraturen, following a design competition.

In terms of the perception of the schools by the study group:

- **All of the traditionally procured schools were well received**
- **Half of the schools procured by competition were reviewed well and half reviewed poorly**
- **Only one of the contractor-led schools (Oserød) was well received – the rest were reviewed poorly.**

I	Kirchheim	Traditional
2	Borhaug Nursery	Traditional
3	Pfennigäcker	Traditional
4	Farsund	Design Competition
5	Gelsenkirchen	Design Competition
6	Kjeldås	Traditional
7	Vanse I	Traditional
8	Oserud	Design/Build (Novtd)
9	Borhaug Snr	Traditional
10	Schäfersfeld	Traditional
11	Loretto	Traditional
12	Pliezhausen	Design Competition
13	Oddemarka	PPP
14	Herne	Design Competition
15	Vanse 2	PPP
16	Hechinger Eck	Design/Build (Novtd)
17	Kvadraturten	PPP

Table 13.1 School procurement and rating
(Table by Howard Liddell)

A/B: Setting the aspirations

The outset of the project is likely to be the time of greatest aspiration in respect of environmental quality and sustainability objectives for client, architect or, occasionally, both. The level of understanding of, and commitment to, the sustainability agenda will vary. It is useful to identify the level of commitment on the part of the client (this may, for example, take the form of a model brief or a design quality framework) and then ensure that this is fully translated into the design.

All projects will tend to find aspirations above the legislative minimum are at risk and it is likely that important aspects will be undermined as it progresses from first thoughts to completed building. However, much can be achieved with appropriate guidance.

Outset

It will be useful at this stage to agree to:

- design in an interdisciplinary manner
- make the landscape and biodiversity fundamental to the design
- optimise passive use of building form and fabric
- minimise expenditure on building services through passive design
- a sustainable development policy statement
- seek the best possible guidance on sustainability issues to ensure a contemporary and holistic approach
- consult with stakeholders, including future user groups
- think long term
- adopt life-cycle costing
- use healthy and benign materials
- set targets – for energy and water consumption, percentage of local and reused/recycled materials
- be prepared to innovate with the right advice
- avoid gimmicks and oversizing
- think through building control and management
- develop, early on, a handover strategy with the eventual user
- a feedback strategy (including post-occupancy appraisal) and terms of engagement
- meet regularly during the defects liability period.

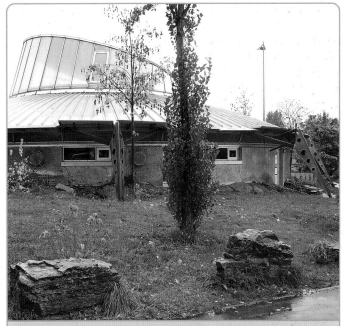

Self-build
At this project in Germany the local children designed and built their own community centre with the help of their parents. They all developed a range of new technical and social skills in the process and the result is well cared for
(Photo: the author)

A commitment to, and planning for, community consultation will assist in making a project run more smoothly and potentially contribute to long-term quality and security. This is important, as concern for security of a project after handover can sometimes be a principal determining factor of many aspects. Community consultation can enhance a project but also enhance the community by:

- providing the opportunity for a community to broaden its horizons and providing hands-on experience
- bringing people together from otherwise diverse experiences and walks of life and enhancing a sense of community – for example, Eco City in Belfast, where children lived physically close together separated by peace walls
- providing a community with a sense of ownership which will potentially be passed on from generation to generation.

C/E: Protecting the aspiration

At this stage every aspect of the design team job has to be viewed through a sustainability filter: money, materials, lighting, controls, landscape, fabric, form, orientation, energy, fire protection, heating, waste, IT, ventilation, cooling, transport, water provision, coordination, changing legislation, policy, building management.

This is the point at which to achieve a truly sustainable project. All of the design team will be required to negotiate and agree to resolve cross-cutting issues. The client, quantity surveyor, environmental engineer, services engineer and project manager have to take on board issues of design for manageability and life-cycle costing; the indoor environmental impact of materials needs to be discussed; the design quality and energy aspects of lighting strategies need to be agreed; a biodiversity strategy and a transport plan may need to be placed firmly on the agenda; and the importance of construction details and build quality, such as airtightness detailing, and eventual deconstruction need to be considered. Failure to make these a core aspect of the detailed design will have already undermined the aspirations. It is not possible to overestimate how difficult it is; this is why I wrote this book! However, the industry has already moved a very long way and this trend is not reversible. This is the time at which benchmarks of performance, labelling of materials, products, building and process need to be agreed and, for many, some potentially new knowledge acquired.

All construction activity affects wildlife and plant species. In building terms, most protection is given to greenfield sites and yet there is no evidence that these are by their nature most interesting or diverse, or that our current knowledge is adequate to protect the biodiversity increasingly apparent in the urban/brownfield environment. Biodiversity action plans are increasingly used as a guide to positive measures that may include rehabilitation of degraded habitats or the creation of new habitats. This is an area where there has been significant development of guidance in the last decade.

F/G: Production information and tender

Failure to make the fundamental sustainability aspects contractual is likely to further undermine the project. The tendency at this stage is to take aspects core to the design and label them sustainability options, thereby highlighting them to the bidders and making them the clear target for cost-cutting.

The point at which the folly of this becomes apparent is when the sustainability option is a designed offset of another cost – for example, where hygroscopic materials are used to offset a humidification/dehumidification load.

At this stage it is vitally important to:

- set performance targets, which relate to the project aspirations
- ensure the contractor understands the issues and potential benefits, if necessary by pre-tender seminars on sustainability aspects
- provide adequate information in prelims to avoid substitution without approval
- provide supply chain guidance for unique elements that may be new to the bidding contractors
- encourage contractors to join the 'Considerate Constructors Scheme' and to set clear targets and record achievements, and if appropriate set a target under CEEQUAL or a BREEAM assessment for the construction phase
- look for real verifiable experience of important aspects such as airtightness and materials specification.
- in order to ensure proper handover, the client or their representative of the future facilities' management staff should be part of the process and maintain a log book.

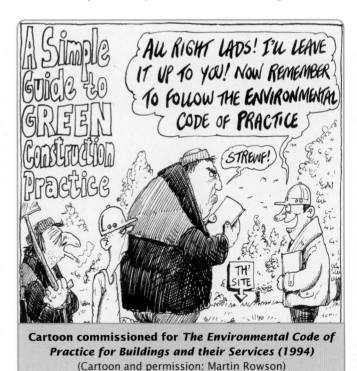

Cartoon commissioned for *The Environmental Code of Practice for Buildings and their Services* (1994)
(Cartoon and permission: Martin Rowson)

Case Study 13.4:

Glencoe Visitor Centre, Glencoe, Argyll

Architects: Gaia Architects, 2002

The site agent was the key to the delivery of a high standard of green design and specification. Gaia Architects undertook a pre-tender seminar and also asked contractors for their environmental buildings experience at interview. But the winning contractor R. J. McLeod of Dingwall did not have experience of a building of this nature. This turned out not to be a hindrance to the effectiveness and quality of the end product.

There was a large amount of dialogue between the architects and the site staff – especially the joiners. The contractor became interested in the sourcing of material from unconventional supply-chain routes and genuine sense of partnership grew throughout the contract period. The project cost was not significantly higher than for a conventional building and was delivered within budget.

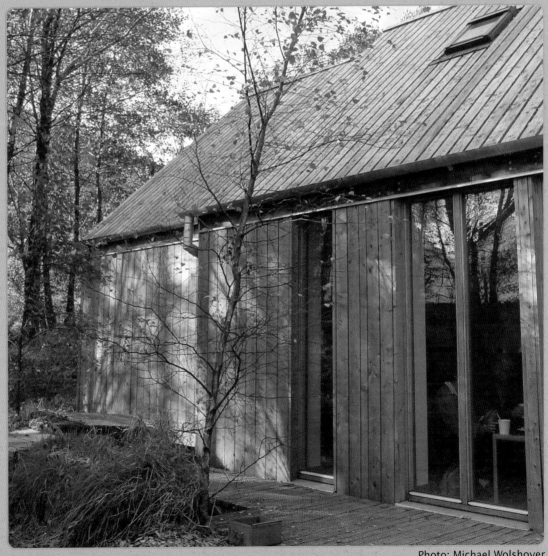

Photo: Michael Wolshover

> ### Contractor benefits of sustainable construction
>
> * Reducing waste saves money
> * Less time in repairing environmental damage
> * Reduced risk of legal costs (fines)
> * Better company profile
> * Improved tender opportunities
> * Reduced neighbour disputes
> * Reduced demand for resources.

H: Tender action

This is likely to be a very sensitive period in the cycle of procurement. There are various ways in which the sustainability agenda can be at risk:

* The bills and specification are not clear enough
* The pricing contractor (subcontractor) does not pick up novel specifications
* The pricing contractor ignores the price implications of a novel specification
* A 'fear factor' creeps into the pricing due to unfamiliar elements
* Failure to identify important suppliers except through conventional supply chains
* Tenders too high and a re-tender or ruthless cost reduction exercise takes place.

In order to overcome or mitigate these risks, it has been found to be useful to have a period for information exchange prior to the tendering process. Bidding contractors may be given the opportunity to respond to a presentation of the key sustainability aspects of the building.

This can take away the 'unknowns'. It also underlines the fact that when special items are specified they are crucial and should not be overlooked, substituted or compromised.

J: Mobilisation

The pre-site start stage is the principal point where environmental and health issues are subsumed to demands for cost reductions in pursuit of short-term budgetary aims, regardless of evidence or pleading that cost-in-use savings can be made.

Once a tender has been accepted and the contract let (or close enough to benefit from an early meeting), then certain items should be put in place at the very beginning to underline that sustainability involves the process as well as the product:

* An environmental statement for the finished building should be established
* Method statements, targets and information on environmental matters and procedures should be established with subcontractors
* Key performance targets should be underlined and monitored
* Any specialist materials should be highlighted and supply-chain issues identified
* Any specialist commissioning over and above normal practice should be clarified and method statements evolved at an early stage (e.g. pressure testing)
* Handover, training, and operation and maintenance procedures should be addressed at an early stage
* Any additional resource implications should also be agreed.

The attention given to site safety is vitally important, but it is notable that making health and safety simply a site issue is a disconcerting example of misunderstanding the process aspects of construction.

> 'Of the 75 000 synthetic chemicals which are now in common commercial use, less than 3% have been tested for carcinogenicity. In 1994, 2.26 billion pounds of toxic chemical were released into the environment, of which 177 million pounds were known or suspected carcinogens. Most testing of chemical toxicity is undertaken on the basis of exposure at work by adults. We are ignorant of the effects on children and other species which might be vital to the ecological make-up of the planet. No one knows the cocktail effect. It is permitted only because the victims are anonymous.'
> – Steingraber in Living Downstream

Case Study 13.5:

Toll House Gardens, Fairfield, Perth

Architects: Gaia Architects, 2004

The construction of low-allergy housing required some amendments to the normal procurement process. The Architect offered to arrange a pre-tender seminar in order to reduce the number of unknowns that the tenderers would be dealing with. This was declined. The first tenders returned very high, and the contractors admitted that a 'fear factor' had been operating because of the innovative aspects. A seminar with the three lowest bidders was arranged. It involved explanations of the innovative aspects and a schedule of reductions. A subsequent re-tendering exercise brought the project within budget.

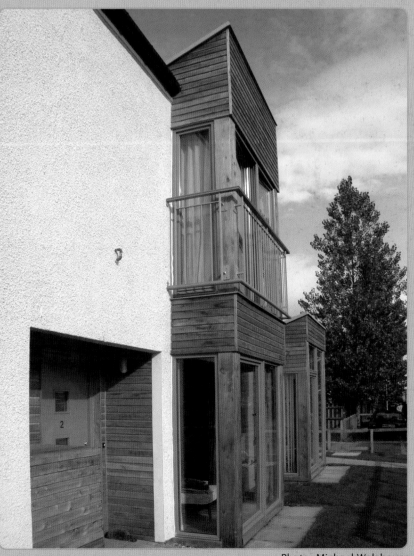

Photo: Michael Wolshover

Polyvinyl chloride (PVC)

Risks
- During manufacture: ingredients such as vinyl chloride monomer emit dioxin and other persistent pollutants that can present both acute and chronic health hazards.
- During use: PVC products can leach toxic additives – for example, flooring can release softeners called phthalates (one of the recognised asthma triggers and also linked to genital deformities, premature births, hormone disruption and cancer).
- In disposal: leaches toxic additives when disposed of in landfill; emits dioxin and heavy metals when incinerated.
- In fire: emits hydrogen chloride gas and dioxin.

Possible PVC alternatives
- Stainless steel conduits.
- Polyethylene (PE), Polypropylene (PP) or rubber sheathing to wiring.
- Copper or PE water pipes.
- Cast iron rainwater goods.
- Linoleum or rubber in lieu of vinyl floor coverings.

Formaldehyde

Formaldehyde is used in hundreds of industrial processes, including the manufacture of paints, plastic products, paper, textiles, carpets, pesticides and fumigants, particle boards, MDF, chipboard and plywood, cosmetics, thermal insulation foams, furniture, biomedical products, leather goods, adhesives, glues and resins.

Risks
- Exposure to high levels or long-term low levels of formaldehyde may cause cancer (emissions still occur after installation).
- Formaldehyde is recognised as an asthma trigger.

Possible formaldehyde alternatives
- Cellulose insulation in lieu of foamed insulation.
- Water-based paint in lieu of wallpaper and associated glues.
- Natural timber in lieu of MDF and chipboard (note: timber naturally contains formaldehyde, but at levels that are acceptable in terms of minimum health risk).

Solvents (chemicals commonly used in paints and adhesives)

Risks
Range from irritation and headaches to dermatitis, colour blindness, brain damage, cancer and even death.

Possible solvent-free alternatives
- Natural water-based emulsion paint.
- Linseed oil-based gloss paint.
- Avoidance of materials containing or requiring glues, e.g. manufactured wood products, wallpaper.
- Where use of glues is unavoidable (e.g. for installation of linoleum or rubber flooring), use solvent- and formaldehyde-free glues.
- Avoidance of timber treatments through detailing.

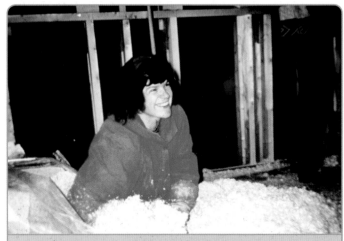

Healthy Materials
Create healthy environments. Increasing pressure for energy-efficient airtight construction puts an onus on specifiers to avoid the use of polluting materials or conditions that give rise to ill-health
(Photo: Dag Roalkvam)

Key site issues

Wildlife

Heavy fines are now applicable for damage to a range of living things: trees, plants, insects, birds, mammals and their habitats. Relevant species can be identified prior to or during works on site. Action must be taken to minimise damage to the site ecology. All site actions are potential threats because of:

- Changes to water quality
- Destruction of habitats
- Vegetation damage
- Interruptions to wildlife movements
- Habitat fragmentation and hedgerow removal
- Dust, noise and lighting pollution
- Damage, removal or burial of rock formations.

Construction activity has become increasingly subject to environmental legislation and biodiversity appraisal is now an expectation. All nesting birds are protected by law and many other species – badgers, voles, reptiles and bats – require constructors to take special care. Guidance is available on appropriate ways to deal with local ecology. See for example the Ecology Year Planner www.carillion.com/sustain-2002/

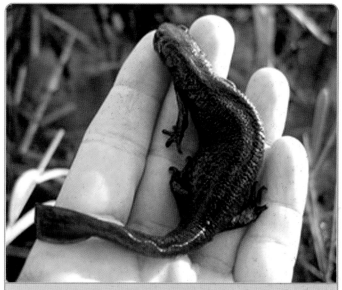

Crested Newt
Construction activity has become increasingly subject to environmental legislation and biodiversity appraisal is now an expectation. All nesting birds are protected by law, and many other species – badgers, voles, reptiles and bats – require constructors to take special care. Guidance is available on appropriate ways to deal with local ecology. See, for example, the Ecology Year Planner, www.carillion.com/sustain-2000
(Photo: Staffordshire County Council)

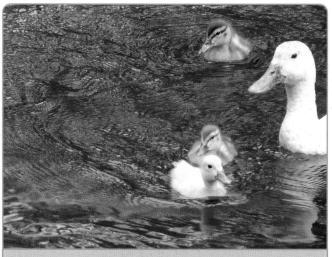

Enhancing Biodiversity
The pond supplying the water balance lift at the Centre for Alternative Technology contributes to the water management strategy and provides a new place for wildlife
(Photo: the author)

Contamination

The contract will refer to specialist guidance on how to deal with specific contamination. Main examples of risks are:

- Contamination encountered during the works
- Handling/excavating contaminated ground and polluting aquifer
- Windblown dust
- Stockpiling contaminated material that leaches
- Spillage of contaminants (e.g. oil)
- De-watering – drawing water from surroundings
- Discharge of contaminated de-watering.

Investigate site history to avoid obvious problems.

Waste

Legally, this is 'any substance or object the holder discards, intends to discard or is required to discard'. The relevant waste strategy issues are: monitoring procedures; raw materials wastage; storage and handling; reduction of landfill tax; potential for reuse and recycling; transport and disposal. It is essential to be aware of:

- Legislation and penalties
- The nature of any potential damage to the environment
- The potential impact on project/budget.

Emissions

Site dust, emissions and odours cause annoyance and health risks. They have legal, site health, ecological and cost implications. The following are essential steps for problem avoidance:

- Check haul routes are suitable
- Use containment methods for demolition
- Keep plant clean, including exhausts
- Keep earthworks damp and revegetate
- Ensure effective materials handling and storage, and watch wind direction
- Clean concrete pour-and-batching regime
- Minimise site cutting, grouting, grinding
- No burning on site.

Water

Relevant issues within the water strategy are: abstraction; disposal; spillage; vehicle washing effluent; solid wastes; surface water run-off; silty water; pumping to grasslands; settlement tanks; lagoons; sewage discharge. The following are essential steps for problem avoidance:

- Evaluate risks
- Identify strategy
- Ensure compliance/monitor
- Emergency procedures.

Noise

'Sound that is unwanted by the listener.' BS5228 (1997) *Noise control on construction and open sites* is key guidance. The following are essential steps:

- Evaluate potential noise/vibration problems and monitor levels before starting
- Inform neighbours

- Minimise and monitor effects during work
- Monitor conditions after works are complete.

Archaeology

Archeological sites are irreplaceable, and early investigation is essential if significant delays and costs are to be avoided. Pre-planning is key. Published guidance and heritage bodies should also be consulted: English Heritage, Historic Scotland, Northern Ireland Environment and Heritage Services, Cadw (Welsh Historic Monuments).

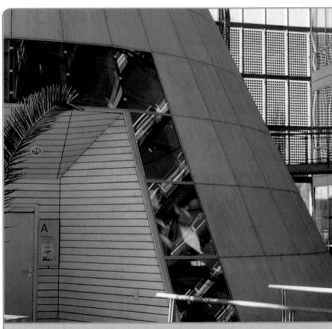

Heritage – The Library at Mont Cernis Academy
Respect for the industrial heritage was a key aspect of the development at Emscher Park
(Photo: the author)

Case Study 13.6:

Brettstapel housing factory and Hotel Post extension

This family-run business in Austria builds 100 houses and a number of much bigger buildings every year.

The houses energy ratings range from standard construction (based on 8.5 litres of oil consumption/year) to Minergie (4.5 litres) and passive houses (1.5 litres). They offer a design service with extensive showroom facilities where clients can specify all the finishes through to site construction.

The construction technique called 'brettstapel' involves bonding of wood strips using wooden dowels to create a massive wood construction for walls, floors and roofs, blowing in insulation and sealing.

Taking in low-quality wood at the factory door, each house is delivered to site on four lorries, constructed to watertight in days and finished within two months.

The technique is gathering momentum in southern Europe and recently factories have opened in Finland and Scandinavia.

This technique enabled the Hotel Post to extend its hotel during a nine-week period from start to finish. The penalty for late delivery was a requirement on the contractor to pay for lost income on unfinished rooms.

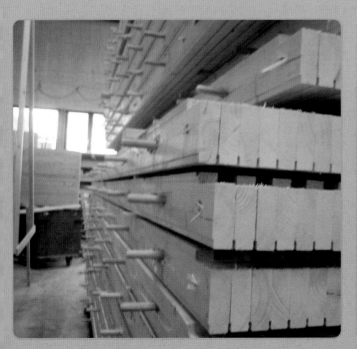
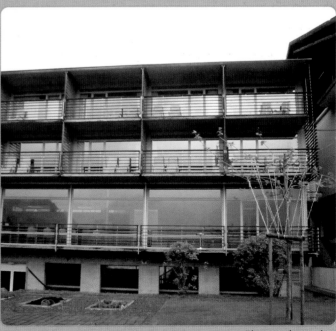

Photos: the author

K: Construction to practical completion

Much is to be gained or lost during the period of delivery of the building itself. The process of construction is often a fairly lengthy one and can be a major pollutant at all levels from local to global. Attention to the sensitivities of local people is important in helping a project run smoothly. Establishing controls within the routine of the site operations will be beneficial:

- Unique or unusual elements, materials, products or services systems should by this stage have been fully explained. However, a site has a large and ever-increasing work-force and key issues should be part of the induction process for new site staff (this is required for health and safety, and could be included with it).
- Environmental issues regarding the building being delivered and the construction related activities on site should be a permanent agenda item.
- Within reason, all relevant sub-contractors should have explanations of key environmental elements and have the important installation aspects highlighted.
- Monitoring, checking and testing routines should be established at the outset.

The design team should ensure that they are informed and present at all key checkpoints.

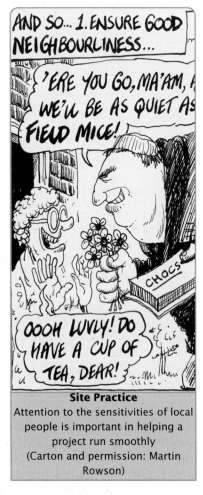

Site Practice
Attention to the sensitivities of local people is important in helping a project run smoothly
(Carton and permission: Martin Rowson)

Commissioning

Particular attention should be paid to the commissioning operations – not just of innovative technology, but also of the routine ones, as they can also undermine a system. Attention is required to commissioning a building for different operational requirements and different seasons.

Checking that products are of the required quality, and that they work as specified and operate according to the manufacturer's recommendations is essential.

Early involvement of the building users and operation/ maintenance staff will be beneficial.

It will become clear at this point how important it was to specify all the testing regimes at the tender period and for these to have been costed out and accounted for.

Handover

At the handover stage the client needs support to be able to use the building appropriately and not misuse or undermine the aspirations through lack of knowledge or understanding of its intent and potential.

The point of formal handover should be very soft, with training and involvement of users and operation/maintenance staff before handover and a 'hand-holding' exercise by the design team and specialist technology/materials installers afterwards.

Essential training is needed for all who can contribute to the smooth and effective annual usage cycles. It should have been written into the original contract. Once the building is under operation there is value in the design team maintaining a direct interest – and this should be properly resourced. Best practice examples show that significant savings, on energy and maintenance costs, can be achieved through effective feedback. In particular, users should be made aware of the difference between snagging and defects (which are design team responsibilities) and operation and maintenance (which are client responsibilities from the moment of handover).

Whilst a health and safety file will contain most of the handbook and operational manuals, it is good practice for these to be indexed and presented in a manner which the client can navigate. The contract will contain clauses relating to appropriate levels of training, but it is not unusual in the last-minute rush to handover for training to be more rudimentary than it should be. It is not adequate for one representative of a specific aspect of a building to talk to one representative of the user. Training should involve as many potential operational staff as possible, and refresher inputs should also be considered.

L: After practical completion

The interface between completion of a project on site, handover, and ongoing operation and maintenance is a key point in the procurement process. If client, design team and contractor have been attentive to the issues and requirements, then the building will be delivered as intended. However, the first period of occupation involves a learning curve as well.

A lack of understanding of controls, regimes or design parameters can reduce their efficiency or undermine them altogether. This is where sustainability as a process and not a product is really demonstrated.

Operation and maintenance

The critical point in the cycle of procurement is when the building becomes the full responsibility of the client and users. No architect or contractor can deliver a sustainable building.

Achievement is a complex interaction of design, designed manageability, client commitment and user understanding. The client needs to understand the various cycles of building management and the difference between routine operation/maintenance and contractual issues relating to snagging and defects. There will be daily, weekly, seasonal and annual routines. These can be identified either in a manufacturer's instructions or in the design team's handbook or advisory documentation. The procedures required will depend on the project size and could extend from identified responsibilities and a good log book to full quality assurance. Identifying the right scale is important to success.

Failure to implement these regimes can negate the warranty for products or services. Buildings, like cars, will also have running problems if they are not well looked after, but ownership of problems is often less clear.

It can be advisable to retain the services of installation companies throughout a handover period in order that problems arising (snagging, defect or maintenance issues) are clearly owned. It is not unknown for companies to walk away from a repair or making good obligation by claiming that it was a maintenance shortcoming rather than a defect. Some design teams now ask to be retained beyond handover to assist in the induction of staff into building-friendly operation and maintenance. This acts as a two-way dialogue, as the design team gain the benefit of feedback as to how the building is performing.

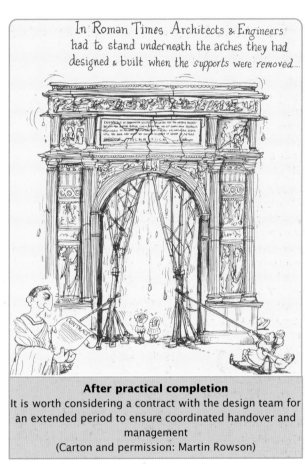

After practical completion
It is worth considering a contract with the design team for an extended period to ensure coordinated handover and management
(Carton and permission: Martin Rowson)

Monitoring

There is significant benefit in monitoring key aspects of a building's resource usage (energy, water, waste materials, etc.). Provided that the techniques are simple and coordinated (as rudimentary as checking monthly invoices and comparing them with projected targets), they need not be expensive or time-consuming. The benefits of identifying problems at an early stage can be substantial. Effective feedback on how a building is operating technically, in terms of human mechanics, spatial organisation, ease of management and communication, has a large potential for resource saving in itself.

As organisations become increasingly subject to analysis with regard to their environmental impact, sustainability and corporate social responsibility, the performance of their buildings, along with their transport strategies, is being brought into sharp focus. There is increasing expectation that companies will understand and seek to mitigate adverse environmental impacts, and to optimise their performance for users, clients, neighbours and other stakeholders. The use of building log books is part of this.

Case Study 13.7:

Eco-cabins, CAT

Architects: Cindy Harris and Pat Borer, 1991

Since the completion of the Eco-cabins in 1991, over 5000 people (mainly schoolchildren), have occupied them for a week-long learning experience. During their stay, they learn about managing renewable energy sources, conservation of energy and water, dealing with sewage effluent, composting techniques and environmentally benign ways of growing food. The Eco-cabins themselves are two self-contained residential units where the electricity supply, the water supply, the waste system and the heating system are all independent stand-alone systems operated and studied by those who stay in them. Each cabin receives an equal share of the generated energy, which is monitored on display boards inside the cabins. The display board gives information of the battery voltage, input and output currents, both instantaneous and cumulative, wind speed, insolation, outside and inside temperatures, and elapsed time. At the beginning of each week the two groups are supplied with a full battery and a full reservoir, with the objective to make these last for the full week. The group quickly learn that they will need to be careful with the given resources if they are to achieve their goal. The result provides a huge learning experience.

Students and schoolchildren staying at the hostel at CAT have large dials in their lobby to remind them how much water and energy they are using. They are allocated a finite amount at the beginning of the week and can see how quickly the water disappears if they constantly use the flush WCs instead of the composters. Likewise, the amount of stored electricity will race away if they leave lights and equipment switched on. They always start profligately and become conservation experts within a very short time.

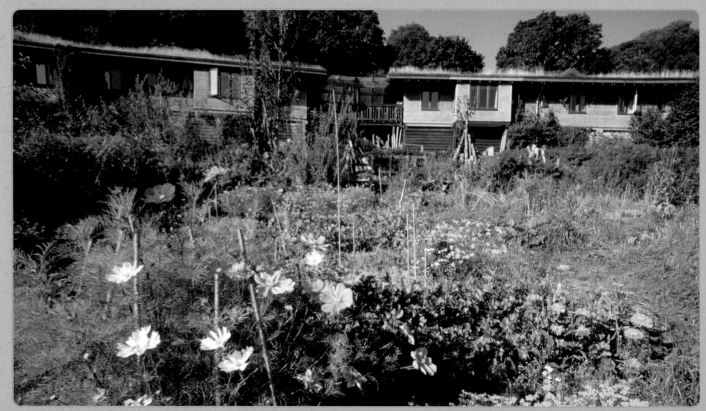

Photo: Centre for Alternative Technology

Feedback

Feedback has recently come to prominence. There are three general types:

1. Review of project performance (perhaps a SWOT analysis by the design team) to learn lessons and identify future opportunities. This is likely to cover issues such as the brief, design, project management, programming and coordination, cost control, build quality, etc.
2. Feedback during the year or so after completion, taking the form of an ongoing relationship with client/users to ensure best operational practice and have pre-emptive rather than reactive maintenance. This can inform, help to fine-tune and ease transition into full, effective operation.
3. Assessing the complete product and its performance in use to highlight both technical and generic issues to do with daily operation and use. This is what is usually understood as POE.

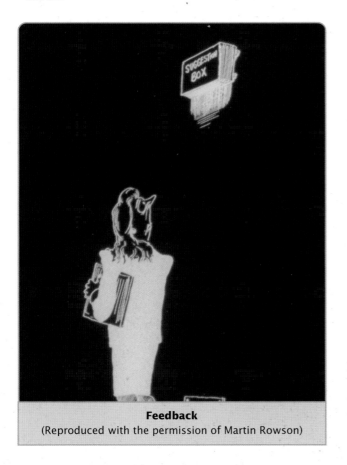

Feedback
(Reproduced with the permission of Martin Rowson)

> **'Feedback in design is a hackneyed yet useful concept.'**
> Building Performance Research Unit (1972)

Post-occupancy evaluation

(This section on post occupancy is adapted and summarised from a paper commissioned by Gaia Research from Adrian Leaman, over which he holds copyright. Adrian also acknowledged the assistance of George Baird and staff at Victoria University, School of Architecture, Wellington, New Zealand. The full paper is available at www.usablebuildings.co.uk)

The notion of deriving feedback from buildings in order to enhance future design is not a new idea. Indeed, some considered it outdated three decades ago. It has been an accepted part of the RIBA Plan of Work for four decades, but even so has never been accepted as a routine part of the design process.

This is changing and the value of post-occupancy evaluation (POE) in the design process is now quite well recognised, although many more are prepared to support it in principle than to actually carry it out.

Practical guidance on POE is not widely available and public domain case studies are relatively few and far between.

Much of what has been written on POE tends to be adversarial or theoretical rather than constructive or based on 'real' buildings. A major exception is the series of studies published in Building Services Journal from 1997 to 2002 under the PROBE acronym (post occupancy evaluation of buildings and their engineering). The PROBE studies are real and in the public domain.

In theory, post-occupancy studies ought to cover all aspects of building performance – space, cost, aesthetics, operations, use, occupant satisfaction, management, environmental performance and so on. They should also take due account of the context in which a building was procured, briefed, designed and occupied. Context usually turns out to have a much more important influence on performance than often envisaged. In practice, POEs are less ambitious, because doing everything on the wish-list is usually too time-consuming, expensive and, sometimes, disruptive. The PROBE studies showed that a good story and meaningful outcomes can be generated by collecting the right fraction of the available data using tried-and-tested methods.

Case Study 13.8:

Queen Margaret's University Campus, East Lothian

Sustainability advocate: Gaia Research, 2004–7

Gaia Research was appointed as Sustainability Advisor for RE-LOCATE, Queen Margaret University Campus, in 2004. The aim was to develop and oversee the sustainability strategy for the relocation of Queen Margaret University from numerous locations in and around Edinburgh to a dedicated new campus in East Lothian. The new campus comprises library, sports, staff and student accommodation and a range of office and teaching spaces. The client body aimed to have the most sustainable campus yet designed and also to be able to show evidence of the achievements.

Gaia Research took the client through a process of defining their sustainability aspirations for the campus. Workshops with the design and management team: project manager, architects, structural and environmental engineers, landscape designers and cost consultants -

stablised the key principles. The design team members themselves then determined what contribution they could each make to delivering the client aspiration. This resulted in a matrix of objectives. Gaia Research then sought to match these with quantitative and clearly defined targets using evidence-based systems. The many qualitative aspects that flowed from the process are also apparent. Gaia Research was then involved throughout the design, tender, construction and handover process to maintain a focus on meeting the targets and to facilitate the highest possible standards. The result is a project with high levels of sustainability at precisely the same budget, thus supporting Gaia's eco-minimalist approach that the most important factors in delivering sustainability are a clear understanding, high aspiration and constant vigilance.

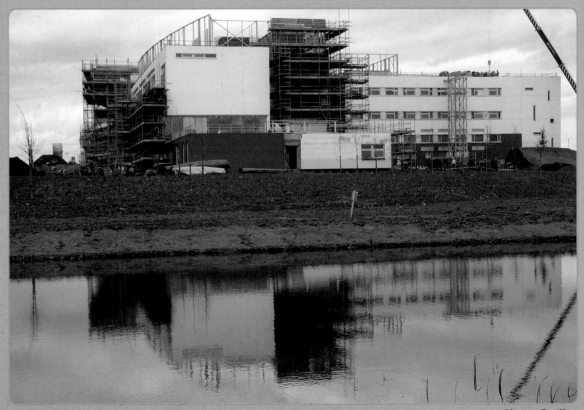

Photo: Carillon

What is POE for?

Post-occupancy evaluation of buildings (POE) tries to answer two broad questions:

1 How is a building working?
2 Is this intended?

POE was coined in the 1970s in the United States to describe the process of assessing buildings in use, initially from the occupants' point of view. The Building Performance Research Unit (BPRU) introduced the phrase 'building performance appraisal' into the UK in the early 1970s. A need was felt to tell more of what POE is about and its implications for early decisions, the design and production processes and the building in use. The performance approach has been defined as:

> *'The practice of thinking and working in terms of ends rather than means ...concerned with what the building (or building product) is required to do, rather than prescribing how it is to be constructed.'*
>
> – Baird and colleagues

Because we live in buildings and use them every day, they can often seem to be simpler than they are. In fact, building designers have the responsibility to understand and resolve great complexity. There are many spatial subsystems to resolve (e.g. site, fabric, shape, services, fit-out, etc.), as well as interacting subsystems (e.g. lighting, temperature and ventilation) and how these relate to the external environment. Buildings are also a mixture of physical ('hard') and behavioural ('soft') systems.

If this were not complex enough, the most problematic and complicating factor is often a building's context. This includes its physical location but also, for example, its procurement, design, operation, management and use patterns. These contextual factors often explain a lot about building performance, such as why the performance of one building may differ substantially from another that is at least superficially similar. Management often turns out to be much more important than designers envisage. To undertake design in a way which meets sustainability criteria is an enormous feat.

Given that buildings in use are 'context dependent' and 'multivariate' in the senses just described, it often is better to

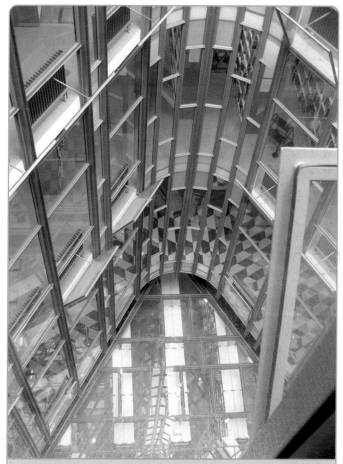

What is POE for?
Post-occupancy evaluation can help to iron out common problems in buildings – such as lights on unnecessarily and windows propped open against the design intent – in the early stages - saving money and increasing comfort and satisfaction (Photo: the author)

approach their evaluation with a 'real-world research' approach. This involves looking at things that are likely to happen in a given situation, rather than at cause and effect. This helps create improvement strategies which involve occupants and management rather than just solely being technically or physically based.

POE techniques

Capturing how an occupied building works can be a mesmerising task. For example, one checklist of techniques has over 150 possible POE analysis methods! A list recently prepared for a UK project has 50 potential methods. With this embarrassment of riches, some of the dangers are that you:

- choose the wrong method(s)
- try to re-invest an approach that has been tried elsewhere
- generate far more data than you can analyse
- subsequently discover that you focused on the wrong area
- use a technique with no robust benchmarks, making it difficult to interpret your findings. (A building may score 2 from 5, but is the average 1.5 or 3?)

POE has taken 30 or more years to stabilise because it has not been obvious which techniques are best. Weakly developed interdisciplinary research and lack of funding continuity are also to blame.

Difficult areas

In order to meet the delivery criteria, PROBE did not attempt to cover directly:

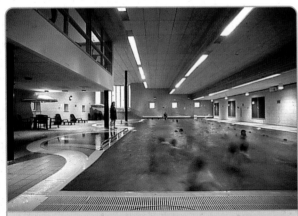

Innovation
The McLaren Centre benefited from a two-year research project to investigate the performance of the innovative dynamically insulated ceiling – but it was the traditional aspects where all of the problems occurred
(Photo: Gaia Architects)

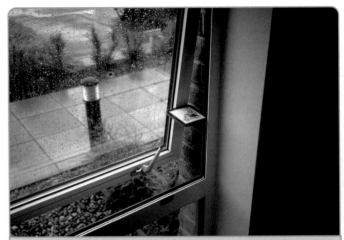

**Personal control of temperature, air and light are important design consideration
(Photo: Bill Bordass)**

1 First costs and costs in use, which are notoriously difficult to pin down:
   - organisations rarely hold cost information on a building-by-building basis
   - they can be extremely reluctant to release what they have
   - it is often inconsistent anyway
   - the results may be vetoed, making it harder to publish the complete study.
2 Aesthetics, which has specialist methodologies not readily applied and compared in all situations.
3 Space efficiency, density or utilisation, which is relatively easy to carry out and can be included, but is rarely asked for.
4 Design and procurement history, which is often quite hard and expensive to study, especially as the design team will usually have dispersed, and can rake up old disputes which may be best left undisturbed.

In the course of their work, the PROBE team developed insights on each of these aspects and concluded that all may find their legitimate place in POEs. The PROBE team also found that most of the salient points about performance can be arrived at either directly or indirectly without needing to cover everything in painstaking detail so long as the results had enough credibility to be taken as an authoritative record. PROBE shows that it is possible to get perhaps 80% of the performance story by collecting less than (say) 20% of available data.

Case Study 13.9:

British Telecom (BT), Brentwood

Architects: Arup Associates, 1999

BT Brentwood has 15 000 m² net of office space on three floors with restaurant and 'winter garden' conservatories. The building has many of the features which earlier POEs have shown to be beneficial to users, such as stable thermal performance and higher provision of occupant controls than are usually found in open-plan workspaces. First results from occupant surveys show that the **approach has probably been vindicated. For example, independently audited perceived productivity gains of 8% are reported.**

A red–green system of lights on interior columns tells occupants which operating mode is current. Red means 'don't open the windows!'. The system seems robust enough for occupants to ignore this if they wish.

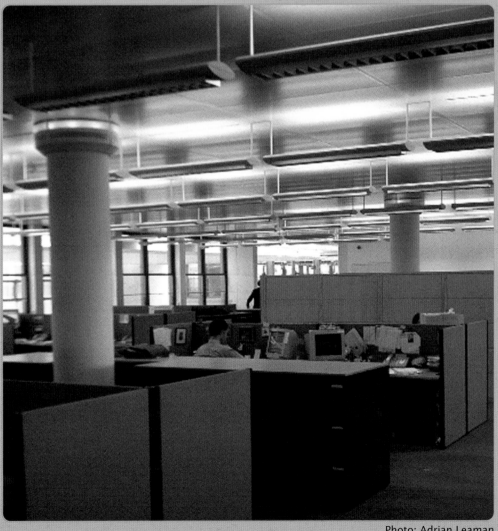

Photo: Adrian Leaman

PROBE benchmarks

PROBE has been relatively successful because it relies on methods perceived to be robust. It does not attempt to include too much, which ensures that the work does not become mired methodologically. This also enables studies to be carried out relatively quickly. It restricted itself to: Energy (with a technical and management emphasis; water assessments were introduced in the third phase); Occupants (using perceived ratings and attitudinal observations from questionnaires followed up by interviews and discussions if necessary); Airtightness (with measured data, introduced in the second phase of the project). It used just three assessment methods, which were known to be practical and robust. All three methods incorporate benchmarks based on performance evaluations of the building in use (not models, simulations or design prescriptions):

1 The energy assessment and reporting methodology (EARM) comprehensively covers building energy performance from both a supply and demand perspective, which helps in a thorough understanding of technical performance, and is helpful with diagnostics. EARM uses 'Typical' and 'Good Practice' energy benchmarks for various building types and may be adapted for uncommon situations.
2 Building Use Studies' (BUS) occupant questionnaire covers occupant issues like comfort, health and productivity in a format which gives useful information across a range of disciplines (e.g. architecture, building services, facilities management), and is also helpful to non-specialists. The BUS occupant survey method has benchmarks for 45 occupant ratings for the UK. It is now used worldwide in comparable formats. Like EARM, this is also applicable across different building types, and may be used for various user permutations. Building Use Studies has a sample of UK buildings which is large enough to include comprehensive occupant benchmarks.
3 An air pressure test to CIBSE TM23 specifications, which examines the airtightness of the fabric. The pressure test has a database and benchmarks for comparison.

In addition, PROBE has:
- A pre-visit questionnaire (PVQ) to collect basic data about hours of use, technical systems, plans and other background information in advance of the actual survey. This provides valuable consistency and is a useful test of the seriousness of the client. If they cannot give you the information, it will usually be best not to attempt the POE.
- A water consumption method, but this is not yet fully benchmarked.
- A supplementary questionnaire on journey to work and transport mode.

A note on scope

Organisational factors like changing staff morale or management quality may affect POE outcomes. People may use criticism of the building as an indirect way of getting at management they dislike. These factors may be detected, but are often hard to study directly.

It may be wiser to avoid subjects like job stress or staff morale in a POE questionnaire, for example, because they give management an excuse for denying you access to the study building. It is best to stick to topics in POEs which are directly building related.

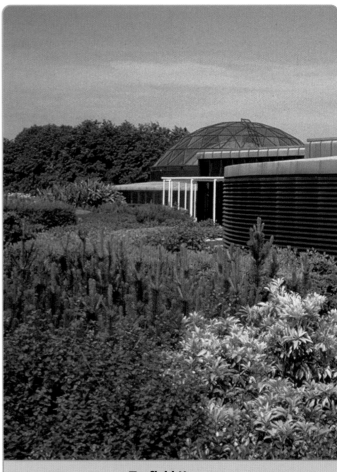

Tanfield House
The highest rated of all the PROBE studied buildings
(Photo: Bill Bordass)

Why isn't feedback better used?

It may be obvious that feedback from buildings in use should be an integral part of the design and construction process – just as it is in most other industries as part of taken-for granted quality control – but this rarely turns out to be so. Despite the growing awareness and presence of POEs and its advocates, the take-up in the UK is still poor, and funding especially difficult. Even the most technically advanced design practices and construction companies struggle to embrace it, even though they may wish to. The reasons are quite complex and embedded historically in how knowledge about buildings is organised and applied. These are some of the reasons:

- Occupied buildings are complex systems that are a challenge to study. There are hundreds of topics which might potentially be embraced. It is hard to distinguish between topics which are 'nice to have' or 'need to know', especially for the inexperienced.
- POEs work best in multiple. One or two may tell you about individual buildings' quirks and features, but they do not tell you about the bigger picture. But, whereas studies of single buildings are relatively easy, it is much harder to maintain them over larger samples of (say) five or more. A sustained programme of POE is harder to carry out, even more so than most realise at the outset. 'Meta-data' (the management and organisation of the full multi-building data set which provides the benchmarks) defeats all but the most stoic. Organisations rarely have the foresight to see this.
- POE projects are often enthusiastically supported at lower levels in organisations, but vetoed higher up. Corporate decision-makers tend to perceive POEs as risky and hostages to fortune, especially when they have never seen or understood what value POEs provide. Those who use POE understand this value and embrace it thereafter. The better managers are prepared to deal with consequences, which in turn helps to improve their skills and awareness. This puts POE at the 'top' of the market because it embraces the very skills that got organisations to the top in the first place! This, in turn, means that POEs tend to report on the better performing buildings.
- Designers and managers from their different perspectives find it hard to extract useful information from POEs. Reports are too verbose.
- POEs by their nature are multi-disciplinary. They have to deal with topics from the supply industry's perspective and from the user side. All these want different things from POEs.
- The industry is not organised to collect POE and feedback information and deal with it. It also sees it as a threat, despite most POEs tending to accentuate the positive in reporting their findings.
- Clients do not see why they should be doing something they hope to take for granted. Nor does government – in spite of the major public interest aspects.
- Academic disciplines do not regard building performance as an area of legitimate interest. It seems both too trivial – even anecdotal – and at the same time too difficult.
- POE does not fit well into career paths and funding stereotypes. As POE has a real-world bias, it also is not very fashionable because it does not theorise overly or draw on models and simulations.
- There is a tendency for those concerned with running buildings (e.g. facilities managers and surveyors) not to talk to those who provide them.
- Professions tend to be territorial, defending their perceived areas of expertise, and are often ill-equipped to include the client's and user's perspectives. Partly, this goes with the job – they know too much about buildings to step back far enough.
- Most designers and builders go straight on to the next job without learning from the one they have just done; this is also related to time/cost pressures.
- Learning curves are quite steep and ill-defined. You need to know a lot in order to do POE. It is basically a real-world not a laboratory problem, and systemic not single issue. Only a handful of schools of architecture (e.g. the Victoria University of Wellington, New Zealand) have courses on building performance.
- The lack of a quality control tradition at the level of the building itself (although products and components within the building do have this tradition). Integration between systems is often the sticking point.
- The 'not invented here' tendency, endemic in the UK, for research organisations not to recognise the work of competitors.

Case Study 13.10:

Elizabeth Fry Building, University of East Anglia

Architects: John Miller + Partners, 1995

The comfort ratings given by the occupants of its offices to the Elizabeth Fry Building are, at the time of writing, the second highest ever recorded by Building Use Studies Ltd in the UK. At the time of the survey it was the highest. On occupant satisfaction, the building has one important physical property on its side – the cellular office. The next task is to achieve the similar excellence in energy and comfort in the open-plan offices that many organisations now require. BT Brentwood shows this may be possible.

These results did not just happen by chance or by the selection of a particular technical system, such as ventilated hollow-core slabs. It came from committed people and attention to detail, which is rare in an industry which puts too much emphasis on time and particularly cost, often to the detriment of quality. Elizabeth Fry's energy performance – although excellent – still leaves room for engineering systems improvement. Services engineers Fulcrum think that with refinements – and specific attention to specific fan power – they might halve the fan energy consumption in a future building. Lighting efficiency and control could also be better. Less is more! Factors for success included:

- A good client. For the past decade at least, the UEA has been seriously trying to obtain better buildings.
- A good brief. UEA takes care in brief preparation, and since the late 1980s has been particularly interested in obtaining buildings with ground-breakingly low energy and maintenance costs.
- A good team. You seldom get the best out of a team on its first job – people are still getting to know each other!
- A good design. The response to the brief led the design team to seek to avoid air-conditioning in the lecture rooms, and they found that Termodeck (with modifications) was appropriate. Initially, the offices were to be naturally ventilated, but Termodeck proved affordable here, provided that the

fabric insulation and airtightness performance was good enough to eliminate the costs of perimeter heating.
- An appropriate specification. The team took advice on aspects of the design with which they were unfamiliar, in particular the Termodeck system, and on obtaining the well-insulated and airtight shell which was so important to achieving their objectives.
- A good contractor. For an innovative solution, a traditional JCT contract worked well, with a main contractor who entered into the spirit of the design, together with that seemingly vanishing species – the client's clerk of works.
- Well built, with attention to detail. Often, the things which cause the most technical difficulties occur at the interfaces, an issue which subcontract packages, coordinated by management, too often ignore.
- Well controlled. Here there was a false start. The client wanted 'fit and forget' stand-alone controls. Although the building is a stable thermal flywheel, its slow response makes it like the proverbial supertanker: difficult to 'steer' until you become familiar with its handling characteristics – and this needs good control and feedback! Fortunately, UEA was able to retrofit a building energy management system and to use it effectively – improving comfort and performance and halving gas consumption.
- Post-handover monitoring and support. PROBE advocated a 'sea trials' period during the first year of occupation (Termodeck UK Ltd now suggest two years). At Elizabeth Fry – as in most other buildings – this did not happen initially. However, following initial problems with controls, and feedback from monitoring, the attention devoted to understanding and fine-tuning has allowed the building to deliver high levels of comfort and energy performance.
- Management vigilance. Universities tend to have limited resources for looking after their buildings. Recognising this, and having some maintenance nightmares from the past, UEA has clear requirements for simplicity and manageability.

Handy hints and tips

Each period between setting out the aspirations and the hand-over of a building is crucial to the success or otherwise of a sustainable project. Make sure that procedures are in place at each stage or the sustainability agenda is at risk. Every participant in the procurement process has a key role to play in the process of delivery of a sustainable product.

- Make sure that the green baton is being passed on to a safe pair of hands.
- And make it contractual.
- Be clear about what you want from the start.
- Establish a project-specific environmental policy for the project delivery before work starts on site and monitor its effective delivery.
- Establish a framework of what is and is not acceptable.
- Use pre-tender seminars to guide all involved.
- Agree key performance targets before the contract is signed.
- Use the tools and guidance available, such as ensuring membership of the Considerate Constructors Scheme and aiming for a CEEQUAL Assessment with clear targets.
- Tie in the client/user prior to handover in order to ensure good-quality operation and maintenance, etc.
- Encourage people to collaborate and learn from experience.
- Consider operation and maintenance issues throughout the construction phase.
- Create an on-site culture of tidiness, waste management, reuse and recycling.
- Monitor key issues once on site, including water, waste, noise, emissions, contamination, wildlife and archaeology.
- Exercise duty of care for waste, including subcontractors' waste, and keep records of waste disposal and transfers for at least two years.
- Be aware that health and safety, or anything else, is not just a site issue.
- Be aware that you are a part of a team with a responsibility to deliver the sustainability baton.
- Resist letting sustainability specification items be the first choice for cost-cutting if savings are to be achieved. Minimise the plant oversizing first.

- Avoid taking anything for granted.
- Generate a good team culture with mutual and shared responsibilities so that people don't start blaming each other.
- If 'it does what it says on the tin' – read the tin!
- Timetable in soft handover.
- Do the feedback.

Remember that a sustainable building is a product that is part of a process.

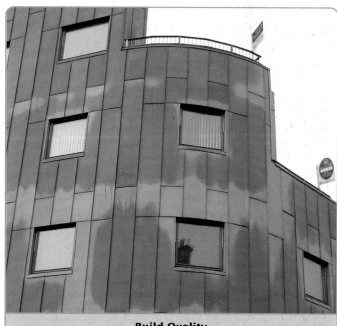

Build Quality
Checks within the construction process, as well as improvements in regulation, should enhance building performance
(Photo: the author)

Bibliography

Robson, C. (1993) *Real World Research*. Blackwell, Oxford.

Brand, S. (1994) *How Buildings Learn*. Viking Penguin.

Halliday, S. P. (1994) *Environmental Code of Practice for Buildings and their Services*. BSRIA.

Latham, M. (1994) *Constructing the Team*. HMSO.

Environmental Protection Agency (1995) *Advice Notes on Current Practice in the Preparation of Environmental Impact Statements*. Ardcavan, EPA.

Halliday, S. P., Venables, R. K. and Newton, J. (1995) *A Client's Guide to Greener Construction*. CIRIA.

Halliday, S. P. (1996) *Feedback Case Studies*. BSRIA.

Tenner, E. (1996) *Why Things Bite Back – Technology and the revenge of unintended consequences*. Knopf.

Steingraber, S. (1997) *Living Downstream*. Virago Press.

Egan, J. (1998) *Rethinking Construction*. HMSO.

CIBSE Technical Memorandum 22 (1999) *Energy Assessment and Reporting Methodology: the Office Assessment Method*. CIBSE

Coventry, S. and Woolveridge, C. (1999) *Environmental Good Practice on Site*. CIRIA.

NBS (1999) *NBS Green Specification*. RIBA Publishing.

CIBSE Technical Memorandum 23 (2000) *Testing Buildings for Air Leakage*. CIBSE.

CIRIA (2000) Environmental Handbook for Building and Civil Engineering Projects: Construction Phase. CIRIA.

Halliday, S. P. (2000) *Green Guide to the Architect's Job Book*. RIBA Publications.

Bordass, W. (2002) *Learning more from our buildings – or just forgetting less?* Review for Building Research and Information Journal, Federal Facilities Council, Technical Report 145. *Learning from our buildings: a state-of-the-practice summary of post-occupancy evaluation*. National Academy Press, Washington.

Chapman, B., Liddell, H. L. and Halliday, S. P. (2005) *Design and Construction of Sustainable Schools*. Scottish Executive.

Liddell, H. (2006) Eco-minimalism – less is more. Green Building Bible Vol 1. Green Building Press, www.seda2.org/articles/Ecominimalism.html.

For downloadable POEs in the public domain, PROBE strategic papers and BUS questionnaires which may be obtained via license, visit www.usablebuildings.co.uk.

Landmarks in Post-Occupancy Evaluation

Building Performance Research Unit (1972) *Building Performance*. Applied Sci. Publ.

Boudon, P. (1972) *Lived-in Architecture*. Lund Humphries.

Newman, O. (1973) *Defensible Spaces: Crime Prevention Through Urban Design*. Colliers Books.

Ravetz, A. (1975) *Model Estate: planned housing at Quarry Hill, Leeds*. Croom Helm.

Zeisel, J. (1984) *Inquiry by Design, Tools for Environment-Behaviour Research*. CUP

Hedge, A. and Wilson, S. (1987) *The Office Environment Survey*. Building Use Studies.

Preiser, W., Rabinovitz, H. and White, E. (1988) *Post-occupancy Evaluation*. Van Nostrand Rheinhold.

Vischer, J. (1989) *Environmental Quality in Offices*. Van Nostran Rheinhold.

Baird, G. et al. (eds) (1996) *Building Evaluation Techniques*. McGraw-Hill

Bordass, W., Leaman, A. et al. (1997-2002) *Probe Studies* see Building Services Journal

Bordass, W., Leaman, A. et al. (2002) *Probe Studies* Building Research and Information Special Issue March 2002.

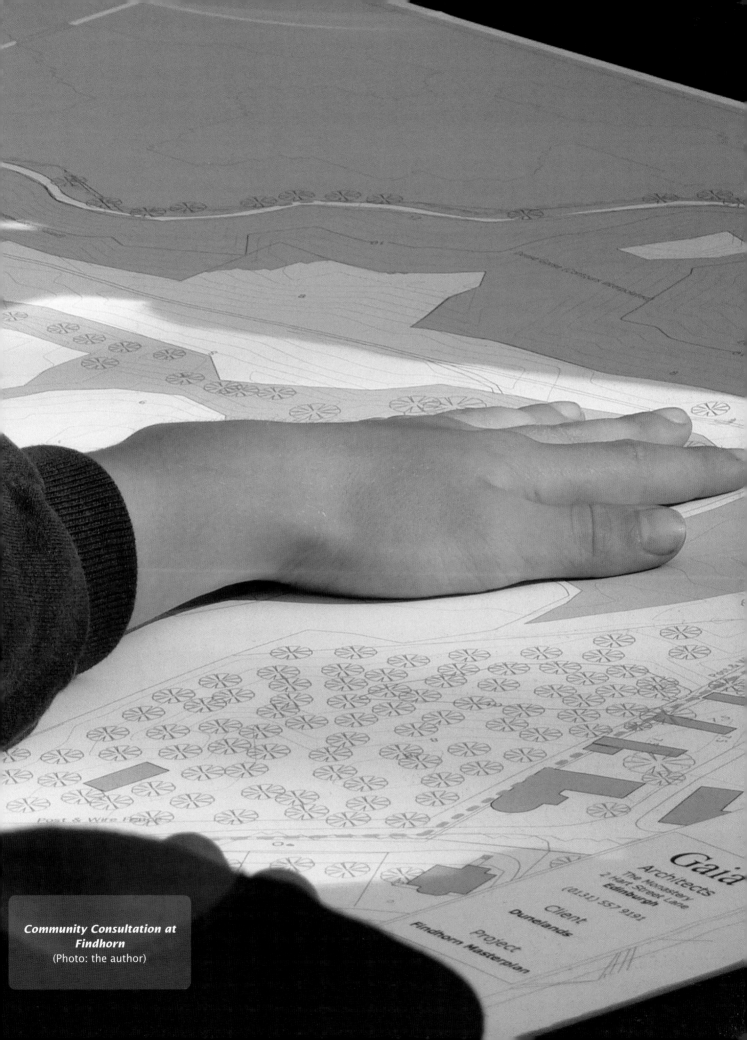

Community Consultation at Findhorn
(Photo: the author)

Gaia
Architects
The Monastery
1 Hart Street Lane
Edinburgh
(0131) 557 9191

Client
Dunelands

Project
Findhorn Masterplan

Post & Wire Fence

Chapter 14
Urban ecology

In which we look at innovative approaches to meeting building needs, such that community, environmental and economic concerns are interweaved for genuine benefit.

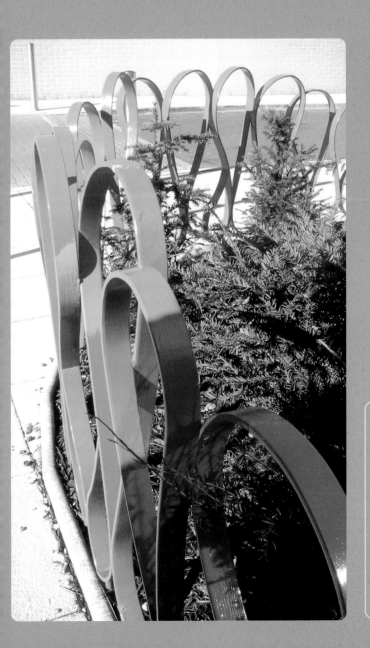

'To go to school with Nature and the old masters also in matters of town planning.'

Garden City Movement

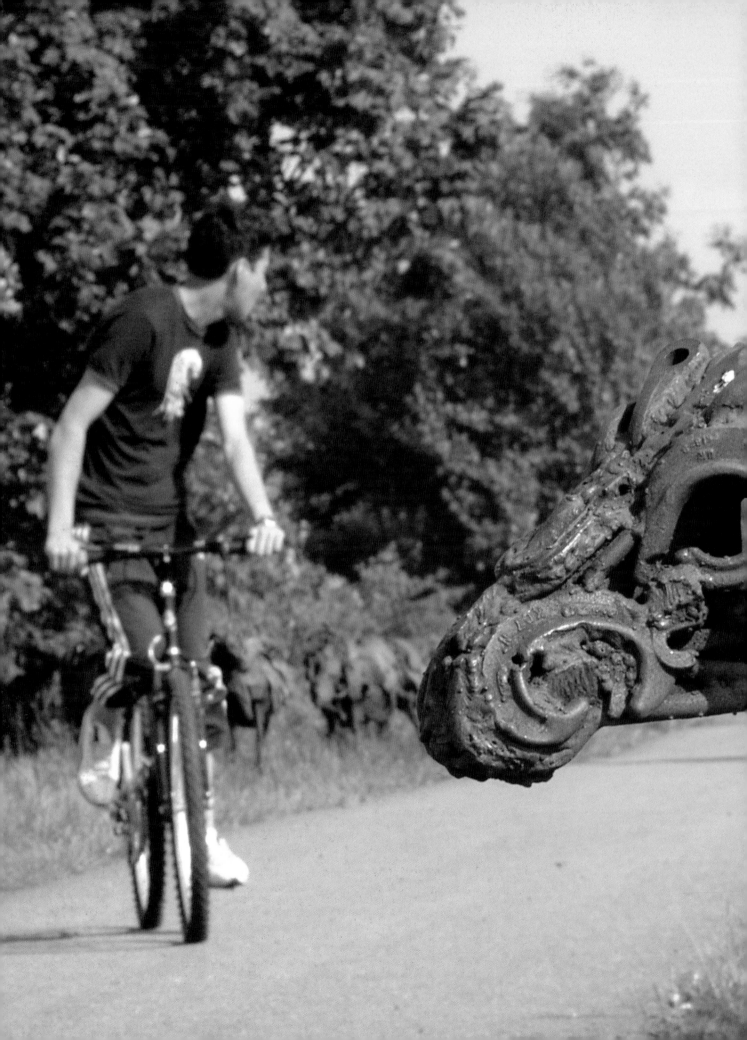

Contents

(Facing page)
Sustrans sculptures
(Photo: Jez Toogood; photo permission: Sustrans)

(Previous page)
Laurieston street furniture
(Photo: the author)

Case studies

Urban ecology

Introduction

This chapter is not a primer on urban design, on which a great deal of fascinating and absorbing material is available. It simply aims to look at the history of development concerns in relation to the city and to grasp some of the underlying principles that must accompany the best urban design if we are to be able to design truly sustainable cities.

Humans are now a predominantly urban species. The historic trend to urbanisation is accelerating and there is a need to recognise, and to mitigate, the significant pressures this places on the environment, including the rural hinterland that has to support the unsustainable resource flows through cities. Change is inevitable – by choice or necessity.

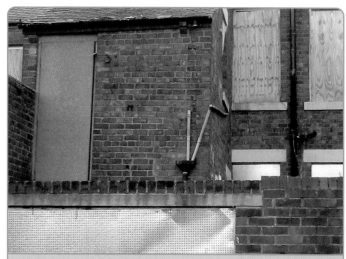

Failed communities are an ever-present feature in the UK
(Photo: the author)

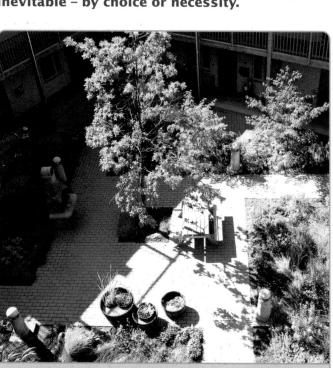

Integration of landscape into development
At Bo01 Malmö landscape was a fundamental aspect of the quality and community programme (Photo permission: Eva Dalman)

Only by serious attention to developing appropriate strategies, and real action at an urban scale, can pressures on the natural environment and on resources be alleviated, and some prospect of sustainable living be established for urban and rural communities. The benefits could be reaped immediately.

Previous chapters identify aspects of construction that must be part of our approach to sustainable design. This one asserts the crucial overarching need and opportunity to re-assert a balance between city and country, between human actions and ecology – and to develop the strategies that can resolve the current unsustainability of our demands and make better places.

This chapter investigates innovative approaches to meeting housing needs in northern Europe and beyond, such that community, environmental and economic concerns share equal priority. It identifies exemplar case studies including pioneer communities that are providing ecological, sustainable development solutions. These are early days in dealing with sustainability on a large scale. We must get beyond rhetoric and intent if we are really to meet the challenges that face us.

In the UK, the debate about built development has been heating up, with plans for large-scale developments in the south-east, in particular, proving challenging. The exemplars and information here provide good guidance on how to move forward, and the basis of frameworks that could enhance the quality and sustainability of communities.

What is urban ecology?

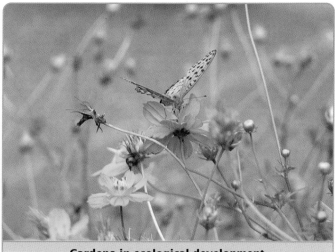

Gardens in ecological development
(Photo: Howard Liddell)

Two defining aspects of the twentieth century were the transition to a predominantly urban civilisation and the unsustainable exponential growth in human consumption of the earth's non-renewable resources. Fifty per cent of the world's people now live in cities, and this is increasing. The combined outcome has been to significantly change our communities, generate unprecedented waste and pollution, and create adverse effects on health and biodiversity. It need not be so.

Urban ecology is an attempt to develop strategies for living that allow us to fulfil social and community needs and aspirations whilst living within the carrying capacity of the earth. It is a response to the worldwide unsustainable patterns of growth that are now the norm, in a context of humankind as a predominantly urban species, dependent on the space around us.

Urban ecology seeks to develop long-term sustainable solutions to the critical problems that our contemporary living patterns generate. It aims to create a balance between urban and rural environments, and to provide for the real needs, requirements and aspirations of communities. The challenge of the development of settlements in the twenty-first century is to do much more with much less, to make less mess, to maintain connections to, and respect for, the natural systems that ultimately sustain us, and to retain, invent or rediscover social mechanisms that benefit our life quality.

There is much talk of sustainability as a combination of economic, environmental and social aspects. It is vital that we now find and show the linkages that can allow us to pursue appropriate development. There is a direct link between the appropriate design of our settlements and the impacts of our activities on the natural world. The contemporary understanding is that the situation we find ourselves in would be best resolved by an ecological approach.

Urban ecology represents a powerful example of the maturing of the environmental debate from technology issues to embrace quality, material, economic and social elements. There are a number of excellent flagship projects. They are recognisable, on the one hand, by the active engagement from the bottom up of collectives of committed individuals to design appropriate ways of living – the eco-city or eco-village; and on the other hand, and increasingly, by a strategic top-down approach, with strong objectives and clearly formulated programmes. They are underpinned by a genuine commitment to the benefits of community involvement, the use of quality control tools and environmental targets that exceed mandatory requirements and challenge contemporary norms such as extensive car ownership. The agenda is a wholly positive one that perceives the need for a radical change in our construction activity such that it is a force for better communities, economies and ecology.

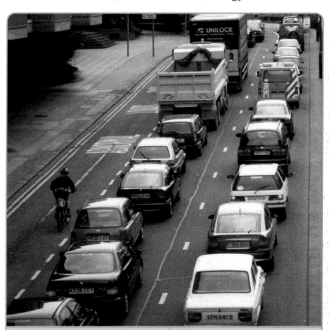

Extensive car ownership
Transport policy in the UK is beginning to reverse unsustainable trends in congestion, pollution and resource consumption but developing countries are heading in the opposite direction (Photo: Sustrans)

Case Study 14.1:

Blaabaerstien Housing Association

Nesodden, Norway, 1980s

The project, in Nesodden, a peninsula, opposite Oslo, consists of approximately 200 houses of various sizes, occupied by people of average income. It was designed in the 1980s. It is terraced housing of moderate to low density, integrated excellently into the rocky hillside terrain and backing onto a forest.

Cars are relegated to the perimeter in communal underground garages – an easy option in planning terms on a hillside. Access is available for deliveries with a common understanding that cars are not left. Schools and shops are a five-minute walk. The housing is subdivided into groups of about 20 units around courtyards/playgrounds. It is very social and an exemplar for private or social housing anywhere. It is recognised regionally as 'a really nice place to live', with a short boat ride separating it from Oslo waterfront. It also manages to remain affordable.

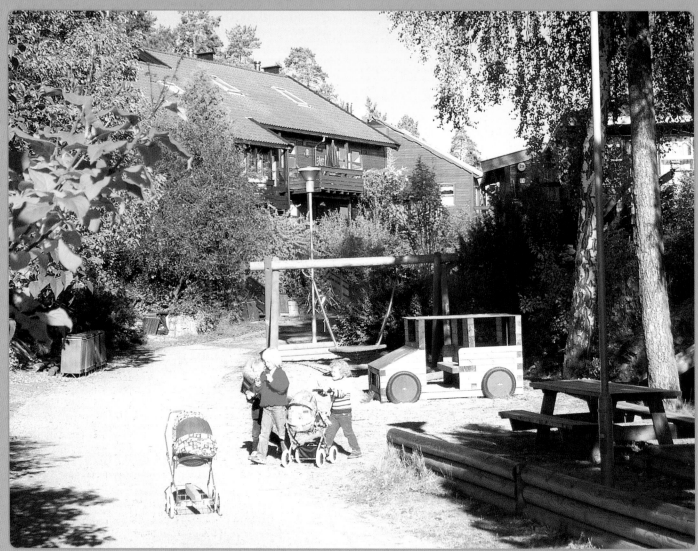

Photo: Chris Butters

Global context

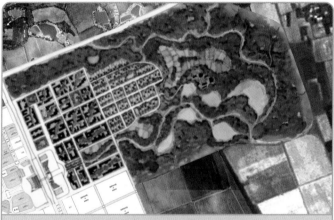

Gaia International: ecological masterplan, Tainan
(Drawing: Chris Butters)

The problems associated with human population pressure are not strictly urban or rural. Neither are they limited by continent or by income. Urban and rural poverty is a human tragedy. Rural poverty and strife imposes severe pressures on populations and the need to search further afield for resources. This has been the major driver of urban flow, a core issue raised by the Club of Rome and the Brundtland reports in the 1970s and 1980s.

Throughout the world industrialisation draws populations from the countryside with the promise of more opportunities for work and better wages – often weakening traditional social/family bonds and triggering concerns about breakdown of communities, citizenship and care of the most vulnerable. The countryside is stripped of its most able-bodied, depressing its economy even further, and accelerating migration to towns and cities. In the cities, this influx leads to overcrowding. Inadequate infrastructure combined with pollution, poor drainage, lack of good water supplies, poverty and slum conditions lead to disease. The resulting buildings are often resource intensive and have not traditionally responded to the natural environment. The wealthy invent the suburb. Gradually, public health legislation delivers improvements in water supply and drainage, and planning controls for buildings are introduced. However, the environmental health and pollution problems take generations to resolve.

Nothing has yet adequately addressed the problem of migration into cities. It remains unresolved despite decades of concern. Today, all over the world people travel significant distances on a daily basis – often between major conurbations – to pursue jobs and wages unavailable locally. Yet nearly 50% of the poorest people live in cities, confounding the original driver.

Wealth generation is also a fact of development. But wealth imposes different sorts of environmental, social and economic burdens. Notably, an abundance of wealth and international trade has decimated the global resource base. A spiral of escalating resource consumption also generates the need to search further afield for resources, but imposes additional problems of waste and pollution management. The issues of sources and sinks were discussed in Chapter 1. The widening recognition of the problems means that throughout the world there are now widespread initiatives to change unsustainable patterns of development.

Solutions are required that deliver living conditions and quality of life that are not just affordable and socially acceptable, but which generate continual improvement. Solutions must reflect the limits to growth and the opportunities for development through improved effectiveness in the use of resources. There is an undeniable moral imperative for a fairer distribution of resources.

The well-catalogued disturbance of ecosystems by humankind, in particular throughout the last century, and its impacts on climate and biodiversity are also evident. Viable solutions are needed that halt the current rate of destruction of natural habitats. We are in a position to reverse the trend and enhance natural biodiversity. To do so, it is necessary to pursue much better management of the built environment in a coordinated process that recognises the importance of using resources more effectively, supporting communities, enhancing biodiversity, creating healthy environments and minimising pollution.

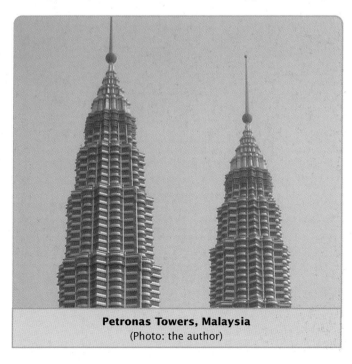

Petronas Towers, Malaysia
(Photo: the author)

Case Study 14.2:

Emscher Park, Germany

Various architects, late 1990s

Urbanisation is increasingly leading to the development of conurbations where adjacent towns, each with their expanding suburbia and road networks, can hardly be distinguished. Emscher Park is an initiative to overcome the problems associated with this kind of development in a major urban region centred on the Ems Kanal, running parallel and to the north of the Ruhr Valley and stretching between Dortmund and Düsseldorf. It encompasses a conurbation of 17 cities/towns.

The motivation was to green the area and give each city back its own identity. In a massive community participation exercise and with a plethora of architects, landscape designers and engineers, the 10-year initiative set about a mammoth redevelopment exercise.

It has involved a combination of enlightened and exciting infrastructural landscaping, including the imaginative use of old buildings and factories and a mix of refurbished and new buildings all focused on iconic structures and landmarks – at least one for each city area.

Initiatives include:

- A sub-aqua centre in disused mine works
- A new school, at Gelsenkirchen, designed by the children in a giant model
- Eco-housing at Kamen, based around community design workshops
- Water and plant landscape design generated by workshop participation
- Super-innovative building competitions resulting in projects such as the Herne city centre college under glass.

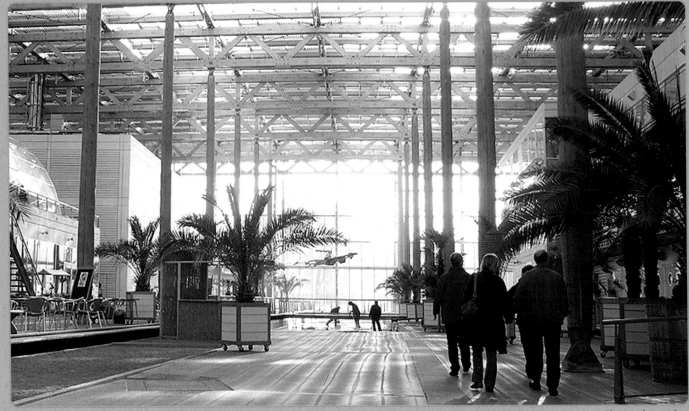

Photo: the author

Communities

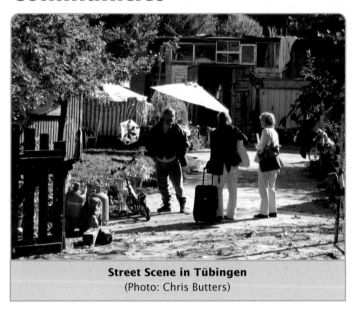

Street Scene in Tübingen
(Photo: Chris Butters)

Buildings and the built environment have a crucial impact on the physical and economic health and well-being of individuals, communities and organisations. Where the built environment contributes to ill-health and disaffection, to alienation and excessive financial liability, and where it undermines community, then it is unwelcome and undesirable. Given the evident problems in many communities, significant improvements are clearly possible and urgently necessary.

The UK planning framework and regulatory standard imposes little or no requirement on developers to address social or environmental needs or to look at economic factors beyond their own market forces/cost appraisals, and there is little joined-up thinking in planning and sustainability issues.

Approaches to housing provision in place in our neighbour countries are ahead of us in many respects. They are actively seeking to create sustainable communities by consideration of space use, interaction, intra-generational equity, the natural environment, resource effectiveness and flexibility. Those that place client involvement (including those in housing need) at the core of development strategies, rather than leaving decisions to a few centralised and private organisations, are proving extremely successful in building successful communities.

Urban environment

There is no universally agreed definition of a city or urban environment. Until recently, in England a city was a settlement with a cathedral. In Germany a city is defined simply by population size. Many modern cities would defy definition. No two cities are alike. For every common factor that can be drawn, another city will break the mould. Also, urban environments are in a constant and rapid flux of development, degeneration and regeneration.

Historically, people gathered for religion, trade, protection, relationships and resources. Settlements developed at distances defined by mode of transport and radius of travel – initially walking, then cart, horse, bicycle, train and car. The physical patterns of market towns are still visible in developed and developing countries.

In developed countries the car has now dominated for 50 years and the pattern is being reproduced across the globe. Perhaps a defining development in the growth of the settlement was when people no longer felt satisfied to travel to the local focal point of trade, romance, religion and resources, but instead bypassed these in search of ever more exotic alternatives and, perhaps, the city bypass exemplifies the change. The locus of activity is still largely defined by transport and in an age of cheap oil this is now global. But the change in communication technology is also important and beginning to define new communities. The gathering place of society has changed from tap and hearth to e-networks.

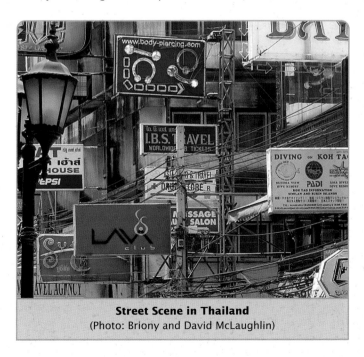

Street Scene in Thailand
(Photo: Briony and David McLaughlin)

Case Study 14.3:

Culemborg, Netherlands

Masterplan: Joachim Eble Architects, 2004-now

This high-density, low-rise development in eastern Netherlands was the brainchild of one individual, Marlene Kaptein. She has driven the project forward against some opposition and many funding difficulties. It is now two-thirds complete, and an exemplar of urban ecology.

Set in a city edge of mature trees and marginal agriculture, the development sits within a permaculture masterplan by Joachim Eble. It consists of a varied housing mix, a school, a library, theatre, workshops, offices and shops. The development sits adjacent to a main railway station and is car free.

The project exploits solar energy passively and actively throughout. The infrastructural use of water and trees is routine in the Netherlands and here successfully encourages productive gardening. There is a policy of environmentally sound materials and an interest in healthy building design, including innovative building techniques from self-build straw bale to terrace houses under glass and a series of sun-scoop courtyards.

As with many projects in the Netherlands, the democratic basis of the development is valued and locally determined policy-making is an integral part of the whole scheme.

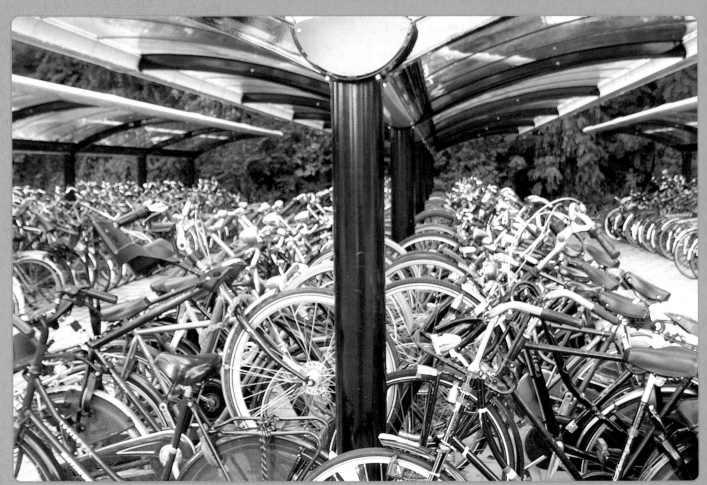

Case Study 14.4:

Tübingen, Germany

Various architects, Current

A development model adopted in the former French garrison of the town of Tübingen in southern Germany is empowering local people in the procurement of their own housing. The mixed-use development involves regeneration to accommodate housing for 10 000–15 000 people, as well as cafés, workshops and offices. An advisory service provides guidance on procuring architectural services and access to a network of other people seeking similar services.

There is generic development guidance related to landscaping, including external comfort, height of dwellings and minimum as well as maximum density. These are not particularly environmentally ambitious in terms of resources, especially within a German context, where there is far more ambition than in the UK. However, it is the procurement strategy and its cultural, social and economic implications that are inspiring, given the lack of choice in UK housing.

Elements of housing, including space allocation and running costs, are clearly costed. Clients are made aware of the financial implications of decisions such as single versus terraced or apartment dwellings, the provision of an attached garage or forecourt versus communal shared parking that leaves an equivalent area for landscaped recreational areas. Individually or as collectives they can assess their needs for flexibility, shared facilities and home office space versus local shared space serving similar purposes but in a social environment.

The result is architecturally diverse with a maturing landscape and has given rise to a thriving mixed-use community of cafés, restaurants, workshops and shared car use.

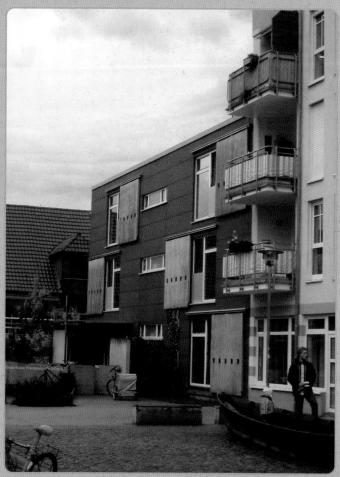

Photo: the author

Urban ecology in history

Rules and comments on city planning go back to ancient times, but self-conscious 'urbanism' is thought to be an invention of Ildefonso Cerdá, referring to Barcelona in the 1850s.

> **'A city should be designed so as to make its people secure and happy.'**
>
> Aristotle, *Book VII, Politics*

The onset of contagious diseases and epidemics in the nineteenth century led to engineering and infrastructure taking the ascendancy over architecture and landscape priorities in city planning. Stübben established rules that became the first modern town-planning tools and drove a reliance on solid building blocks, rather than the streets, planted public squares and private courtyards of seventeenth century London. Baumeister led a movement that made traffic the key to urban planning, and roads became synonymous with open space.

After Vitruvius and Alberti, Sitte is regarded as a major force in defining urban aesthetics and city planning. His thesis was 'to go to school with Nature and the old masters also in matters of town planning'.

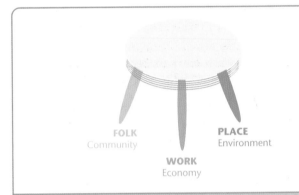

The three-legged stool
Geddes approached the issue of town planning from the perspective of the integration of work, folk and place which translates into the well-known tripos of sustainability represented here as the three legged stool. If one bit is unsupported it all falls down
(Image Howard Liddell, after Drew Mackie)

To Sitte, the issue was not mere sanitary drainage or traffic flows as his predecessors had insisted, but how to shape the city 'so that it would be psychologically and physiologically adequate for the needs of successive generations of city dwellers – specifically for their open-air assemblies and their promenading for the satisfaction of the individual contemplation'.

If Sitte is the father of city planning, then Patrick Geddes is arguably the father of urban ecology. The two met in 1909 and Geddes became convinced of the merits of ancient city planning. Geddes is widely believed to be the originator of the 'triple bottom line' of sustainable development. His planning analysis hinged on the tripos of 'folk–work–place', which translates directly into the sustainability parlance of 'society–economy–environment'.

We have forgotten how to design successful places
Siena's centre is a successful multi-functional space of immense character. Changing our transport choices could make the design of such places possible again. (Photo: the author)

> **'Ample space, well-built clean healthy housing, abundant garden space, preservation of natural landscape, pollution and litter free.'**
>
> William Morris

Post-industrial cities

The problems associated with human settlement have multiplied post-industrially. Many people have sought physical and social models and patterns of development as a consequence of disquiet about their environments. Solutions largely evade us.

The aspiration for the modern town began when industrialists, such as Lever, Cadbury and Rowntree, became interested in architecture and town planning. They were particularly interested in the provision of quality social housing for their workers that integrated town and country. Around the same time, the Arts and Craft Movement was promoting 'decency of surroundings'. Bournville's architect/planner designed terraces and semi-detached cottages with garden areas and allotments to allow families to grow their own fresh food. This approach was to develop into the Garden City Movement of the early twentieth century.

> **'A city is made by the social congregation of people, for business and pleasure and ceremony . . . A person is a citizen in the street. A city is not as Le Corbusier thinks, a machine for traffic to pass through, but a square for people to remain within.'**
>
> Goodman (1947)

Howard's theory of three 'magnets' and Unwin's *Town Planning in Practice* began an influential inter-war obsession with social engineering. The attempt to create a community blending the advantages of both the town and the country, with pleasant environment, plentiful local employment, peopled in Howard's words 'by a happy people' began. The individual garden city was perceived as only part of a much larger development, with a cluster of garden cities around a central city all interconnected and sharing leisure facilities and services.

The Le Corbusier-driven interest in urban form based on militaristic concerns – high-rise blocks presented a smaller target to aerial bombers – struck a chord after World War II and has influenced social housing worldwide ever since. A focus on physical planning and traffic from pre-World War I – with visions of multi-layered streets and flying machines – continued to influence city planning into the 1970s, with the idea that vehicles and pedestrians should be separated vertically. This is evidenced in Cumbernauld Town Centre and the former Bull Ring, Birmingham. However, the critique of this approach was forming as early as 1947.

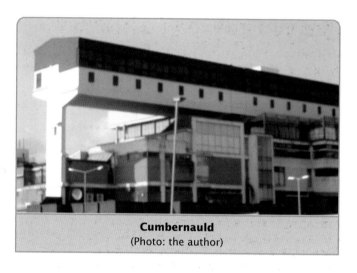

Cumbernauld
(Photo: the author)

In the 1950s in the UK, legislation and planning controls for buildings led to the rise of suburban housing around existing cities, and later slum clearances. This was responsible for some staggeringly ill-conceived examples of housing provision. There was a worthy attention to infrastructure, building controls and drainage, but with little attention to human/social needs, the local economy and the facilities that are provided by mixed-use environments that are typical of organic growth. Social and environmental problems were compounded as subsequent generations lost economic, physical and emotional connection with the natural environment once achieved through work, location or family. Serious concerns about the break-up of family and kinship in technically driven slum clearance programmes (Willmott and Young) and concepts such as the urban village (Jacobs) began to have strong influence and led to an embargo on building high-rise blocks for social housing in the UK. Security and community came to be drivers of social development in the 1970s.

The 1980s and 1990s saw a transformation of ownership patterns and a loosening of planning legislation. The major physical effects have been seen in the commercial areas of city centres and in the car-based periphery and suburbia. This left a vacuum in the residential sector and in mixed-use development in city centres and the inner core around this.

A defining aspect in the changing urban environment is the spread and scale of the 'downtown' syndrome, spaces alive during weekdays and otherwise desolate. Wealthy city workers retreat to the spacious suburbs, where they pay their taxes. The intermediate ring is increasingly characterised by a disaffected underclass in poorly constructed and under-resourced environments.

Case Study 14.5:

Halifax Children's EcoCity

Gaia Planning and TASC Agency, 2003

The Children's EcoCity exercise carried out in Halifax in 2003 was a commissioned integral element within the Yorkshire Towns Initiative. The Eco-City project involves children designing and creating part of a utopian city development either in their imagination or in a real context.

The EcoCity project started out in 1993 as a one-week workshop for 40 primary schoolchildren, from four countries, building their own ecotopian city. It has become a significant opportunity to engage both children and adults in sustainable community development.

The children build a 6mx6m scale 1:100 model covering a major urban area. At the end of the week they present their design to parents, friends, politicians and agencies in what is often a frenzy of wonderment that urban design along environmentally friendly lines can be 'child's play'. It does have a distinct and significant importance as a catalyst to involving adults in a mature debate on sustainable and unsustainable development. Projects have taken place in Belfast, Glasgow, Edinburgh, Halifax and Johannesburg.

In Halifax, the overlap between the children's proposed initiatives and those of adults engaged in a parallel process was 85%. This included proposals that the adults acknowledged would never have surfaced without the children promoting them.

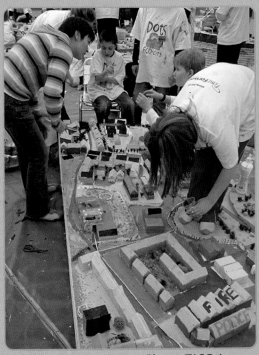

Photo: TASC Agency

The systems approach to cities

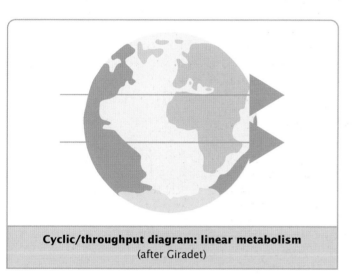

Cyclic/throughput diagram: linear metabolism
(after Giradet)

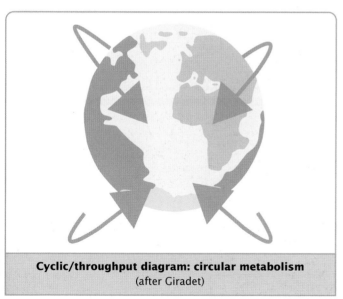

Cyclic/throughput diagram: circular metabolism
(after Giradet)

As long as the trend toward urban living continues, and it shows no sign of abating, it is crucially important that we reduce the burden cities impose to a level that can be sustainably managed in coexistence with the hinterland. Dense conurbations rely on drawing in resources from their surroundings, and need throughputs of food, water, energy and materials in excess of their capacity to produce or resource.

They generate waste and sewage in excess of what they manage and, because in densely populated areas waste is a hazard not a resource, are dependent on remote disposal. They are energy intensive due to the effort of moving resources and waste. They provide a one-way (linear) route for nutrients – nitrogen, phosphorus and potassium – which is mostly diluted and lost in sewage. Meanwhile, urban and rural communities increase their dependence on the manufacture and transport of energy-intensive farming, including expensive fertilisers to replenish the losses. Water is threatened in a number of conurbations, with pressure on aquifers threatening urban and rural communities. It is vital that efficiencies and clean processes are found to turn current 'linear' systems in cities to closed cycles approaching ever-increasing autonomous management. Giradet's book is an essential source of information.

Urban form

The traditional urban city block is well exemplified by Barcelona, with its six-storey, 100-m deep blocks with 50m internal courtyards. To replace housing with equivalent accommodation in the central courtyard would require a skyscraper of 36 storeys. Leslie Martin clearly demonstrated that the whole of Manhattan could be put into six storeys on its perimeter with better shelter and better mix of private and public outdoor area.

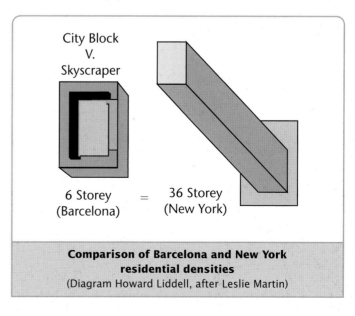

City Block
V.
Skyscraper

6 Storey (Barcelona) = 36 Storey (New York)

Comparison of Barcelona and New York residential densities
(Diagram Howard Liddell, after Leslie Martin)

Case Study 14.6:

Locus, Upper Tay Valley

Aberfeldy Community, Scotland, 1974

The Aberfeldy Self-Sufficiency Group – a collective of local business and professional people disenchanted with the effectiveness of government in dealing with rural areas – was formed in 1974 in the Highland town. Its aim was to determine a strategy for developing the area in a self-reliant and environmentally benign manner. Over a six-month period the six Local Community Councils in the Upper Tay Valley undertook a number of community workshops in which local aspirations were identified and prioritised. The resultant report was presented to the local planning office for inclusion in the area Local Plan.

In the period of 30 years since, the region has reversed the downward spiral of rural population decline and built up a vibrant and growing community. Many new companies have been established focused on development of skills and resources to generate, first and foremost, benefit to the local economy.

Evolving from the original initiative, the Locus Project fostered both a local development company and a major green tourism initiative (a Scottish Tourism Oscar winner). It was based on an integrated set of interpretative loop trails – called the 'overground'.

Visitors are guided from an introductory exhibition on a series of trails, where the emphasis is on present-day activities and people working in the scenic, historic setting of the Perthshire Highlands. The Locus Project has been through many changes in response to community need in and around Aberfeldy. The most recent £1M regeneration of the Locus building involved the provision of offices, cyber-studios and an all-purpose theatre space.

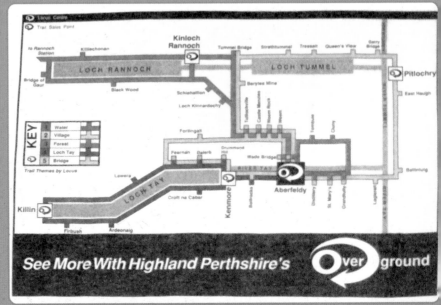

Image concept and design: Howard Liddell

Case Study 14.7:

Schafbrühl, Nr. Tübingen

Architects: Joachim Eble Architects, 1985

This development on the outskirts of Tübingen in south Germany was one of the very first major residential ecological design projects in the world and possibly stands as the first modern example of urban ecology. The project of 220 houses was completed in 1985.

It resulted from the desire of a group of families, interested in Rudolph Steiner's philosophy, to develop their own housing. The development, which takes its aesthetics from a nearby traditional village, represented a break from the tendency to high-rise development. Yet the four-storey, high-density scheme achieves the same density as the neighbouring 15-storey blocks, but with a sense of local vernacular architecture.

The houses are built from environmentally sound and healthy materials, and each has a winter garden as a focal point. It has vetted materials throughout – based on Baubiologie principles. The majority of the construction is of brick (lower walls and floors) and all finishes are of low-emission materials (lime plaster, organic paints, natural timber-board floor finish, etc.).

The landscape strategy is particularly impressive. The use of porous surfaces and the creative use of water within courtyards means that trees, bushes, flowers, vegetables and a thriving local composting initiative has built up over 20 years to provide a rich backdrop to the housing. There is 100% pedestrianisation of the whole project interior, with cars kept strictly to the periphery. Local initiatives such as a local cooperatively owned shop, a café, small offices and a nursery school have thrived.

This project is notable for the fact that it delivered a relatively high-density development with a very human scale, without resorting to the tower block layout of the neighbouring housing.

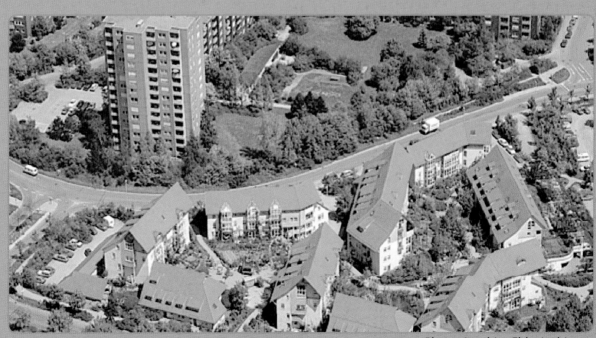

Photo: Joachim Eble Architects

Growth

Towns most commonly have developed at crossroads – transport nodes – where a significant building such as a church would be sited. The ancient Egyptian hieroglyph of a city is a crossed circle. Typically, the quadrants created between meeting routes develop their own identities and a circular route completes the sense of a distinct town. In most contemporary cities there is a core that then extends and sprawls until an outer ring road becomes necessary. Expansion has generally occurred along transport and utility service lines. Less than 1% of the building stock is renewed each year. Change occurs as a combination of, predominantly, evolution in a subtle manner and, to a lesser extent, but more dramatically, large-scale intervention. An aspect of the former is the intensification of activities in the outer ring of the American-style, car-based 'edge city' that in time could create the basis for an efficient perimeter public transport network and a pedestrianised core. Projects such as that in Hasselt, Belgium and Curitiba, Brazil are actively pursuing such models.

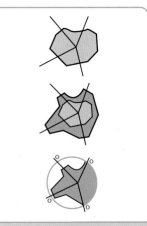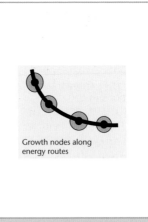

Growth nodes along energy routes

Towns most commonly have developed at crossroads
Typically, the quadrants created between meeting routes develop their own identities and a circular route completes the sense of a distinct town.

(From *Energy and Planning* by A. Mackie and H. Liddell)

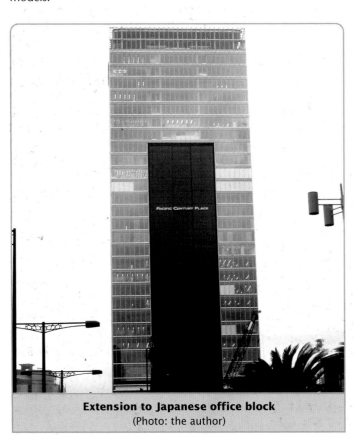

Extension to Japanese office block
(Photo: the author)

Density and compactness of cities proves to be a rich seam for debate and discussion. There are clearly no absolutes, although the 5 km radius is a recurrent theme in planning development. The 1990s saw the start of a move away from sprawl and back to densification, which offers benefits of supporting mixed-use, public transport and shared energy systems.

The 5 km radius:

- can be walked in under an hour
- is a comfortable bike ride
- can be covered by trams and buses at 20 km/h in 15 minutes
- any part of a 10-km-wide city can be reached in half an hour
- a city of 225 000 is enclosed within a 10 km diameter at a density of 30 p/ha
- this number is also used for the energy-efficient city.

Transport

The two major issues relating to the car and the city are pollution and congestion. A strict programme of fixes – both technical (efficiency, fuel economy, alternative fuels) and non-technical (a shift of freight and people to alternatives, reductions in speed, engine size and journey length) – could readily produce between 20% and 50% CO_2 reductions over a 10-year period, and improvements in health and efficiency. However, currently we still have a projected rapid growth in car ownership, with only marginal technical and non-technical improvements.

Victorian cities were compact and had mixed uses, but became separated (especially homes from workplaces) in the interests of public health. The railways and the car allowed for greater dispersal and separation accelerated.

In the 1890s, Sitte wrote that horse-drawn vehicles were taking the dominant role in the arrangement of streets and plazas, in laying out new towns and regularising old ones. In the 1930s, Mumford held that cars and electricity were the drivers in rapid deconcentration of cities. Average travel speeds in urban environments fell rapidly through the latter part of the twentieth century – in central London from 21 km/h in 1972 to 18 km/h in 1990 – less than the speed of a horse-drawn carriage or bicycle.

Sustainable solutions will involve the redesign of cities so that walking and cycling are feasible and enjoyable, and where high-quality public transport satisfies the bulk of journeys (in particular regular journeys) not carried out by bicycle or on foot.

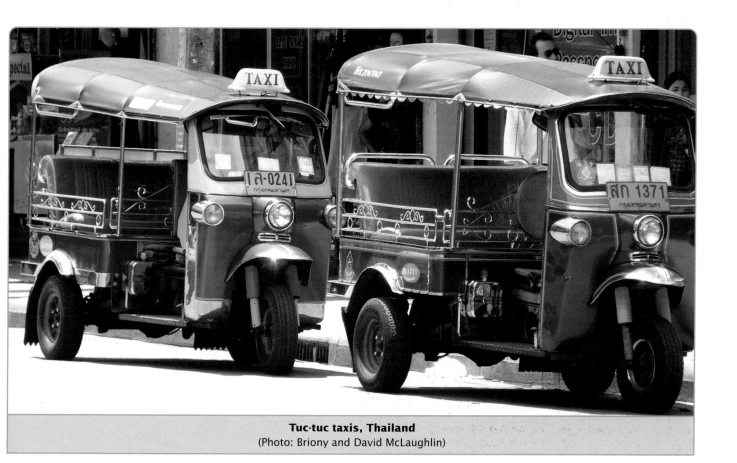

Tuc-tuc taxis, Thailand
(Photo: Briony and David McLaughlin)

Climate

Most buildings and cities up to the beginning of the twentieth century evolved in a manner responsive to climate and were geometrically efficient. Traditional cold climate settlements avoid windy hilltops or cold valleys, where there is an energy and comfort penalty, and vice versa in warm climates. Traditionally buildings were responsive to climate - protecting from sun or wind where necessary and opening up to sun where this was a benefit. Solar gain or shade, courtyards and openings, trees and shrubs were all commonly used to aid a favourable microclimate. Airflow was important. Streets perpendicular to rivers encouraged catabatic flow of airborne pollutants into river valleys. Much of this has been lost in the development of space and buildings that are independent of microclimate and increasingly reliant on artificial energy inputs.

Cities have a high proportion of surfaces with high solar absorbance – asphalt, tiles and concrete all retain solar heat.

Modern buildings are rarely responsive to climate
The "international style" has ignored the impact of form and orientation such as on this circular Tampa towerblock. All elevations are identical - the micro-climate context is not.
(Photo: the author)

Greenhouse gases trap heat and this is accentuated in cities, where pollution concentrations are greater. Energy generation creates waste heat – cars, people, fans and lights – and heat extraction from buildings and cars equivalent to 1–10% of solar heat. All this contributes to the creation of urban heat islands. The implications for building design are enormous. Urban buildings, sealed and mechanically serviced to avoid air and noise pollution, fight an increasingly warm environment largely generated by their own inefficiencies. We must start taking design in another direction.

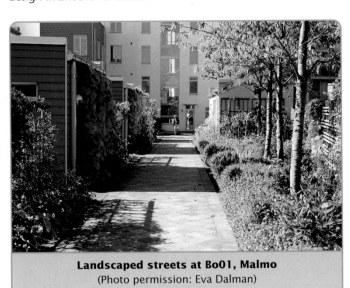

Landscaped streets at Bo01, Malmo
(Photo permission: Eva Dalman)

Landscape

There is growing understanding and respect for the potential of well-considered urban landscape. Often seen as mere amenity and add-on, it has the ability to fulfil very practical purposes and to add quality. It can toughen and soften, shelter and screen, lighten and clean.

It can support cultural, leisure, practical and commercial activity, provide delight, aid external comfort and contribute to enhancing biodiversity. Increasingly, the landscape in urban environments – once segregated to the edges of individual buildings – is being joined up.

This results, in part, from the converging drives to pedestrianisation and soft landscape. It provides real opportunity for integrated SuDS strategies and wildlife corridors – all of which can enhance the experience of moving through the city.

Permaculture

'Permaculture' was coined in 1978 by Bill Mollison, an Australian ecologist. It has developed many meanings but is intended to refer to permanent culture. It is the active integrated design of human habitats and food production systems to combine land use and community building in order to create sustainable living patterns. It embraces food production and resource efficiency, and extends to economic and social structures such as co-housing. The principles are applicable to all forms of urban and rural development and lifestyles.

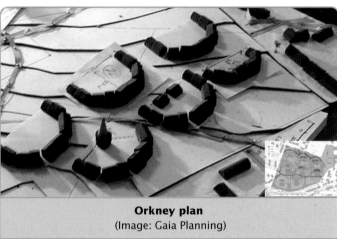

Orkney plan
(Image: Gaia Planning)

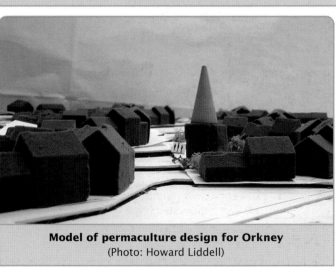

Model of permaculture design for Orkney
(Photo: Howard Liddell)

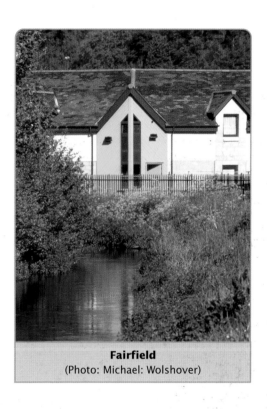

Fairfield
(Photo: Michael: Wolshover)

Regeneration

There has been a strong focus on the urban environment in the UK in recent years, and significant investment in a wide range of initiatives to promote better towns and cities. Northern England, in particular, has benefited from a range of relatively modest art and culture projects that have revitalised previously run-down regions and buildings. Walsall, Sheffield, Leeds, Manchester, Salford, Newcastle and Gateshead have all benefited from 'the Guggenheim effect'. These have attracted local and national interest, and driven demands for urban housing. This has brought jobs and provided local focal points. University estates have also recognised the value of iconic buildings to their ability to attract students and hence their status – leading to significant regeneration of run-down campus environments.

The revivals have been largely economic, adding value to urban property and bringing tax income and spending power back to run-down regions. The emphasis is on brownfield site development and often high density accords with aspirations of urban ecology, but many elements are missing. There is remarkably little attention to biodiversity, transport planning, materials, growing and resource effectiveness, which is common to a number of contemporary European projects.

Case Study 14.8:

Sustainable Design Framework: Laurieston, Glasgow

Gaia, 2005

Those involved in urban and rural development control are seeking ways to pursue sustainable developments and this project demonstrates some of the emerging strategies.

Gaia acted as sustainable design consultants for the mixed-use development in Laurieston aiming to be a "World Class City Quarter" incorporating around 1700 residential units and 300 000 sq. ft of commercial/retail space. This area of Glasgow had already successfully applied a strategy to support the quality of the architectural development, including the massing and use of materials. Gaia's role was to develop a framework for sustainable development for the Laurieston Masterplan/ Outline Planning Application, which can carry

through to appraisal of developers. The aim was to enable the development (which is in 12 phases) to take a step up in quality of design specification and implementation by showing evidence of real implementation of sustainable design.

Gaia worked with the client to determine the minimum standard for the 1st phase of the development and a series of enhanced targets that could be used to ratchet up the standards over time. These standards, which cover management tools, health, resources, pollution, community and bio-diversity, take the form of a brief for a best practice development underpinned by robust commitments to its implementation within an agreed timescale.

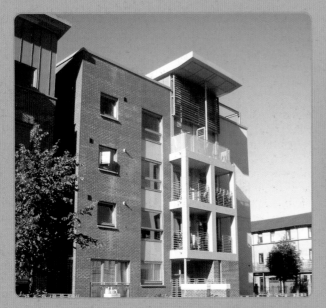

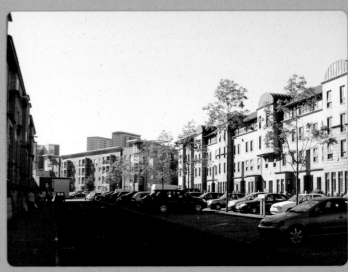

Photos: Howard Liddell

Pioneer communities

From little acorns . . .

The origin and principal drivers of sustainable construction lie in the efforts of individuals and small groups who have sought to identify and resolve problems of resource throughputs, work and social interaction. Hence the predominance of the 'eco-village' rather than the 'eco-town' or 'eco-city'. Many a civil servant has wandered the Centre for Alternative Technology (CAT) in Wales to learn about sustainability. Exploration and experimentation with lifestyles and technology led to the development of pioneer communities and exemplar solutions on small scales – appropriate to their impact.

What is an eco-village?

Eco-villages are urban, suburban or rural communities of people who are intentionally striving to develop vital and mutually supportive, healthy, low-impact lifestyles and social structures that reverse degradation of the environment and re-establish a sustainable relationship with the planet's ecosystems. Conscious of the breakdown of traditional support functions and marginalisation of weaker members of societies, they are aiming to integrate ecological design with political and social structures that can be successfully maintained into the future. They have a strong ecological and ethical dimension – supporting ecological and organic means of food production, local produce and small business, local materials for construction, renewable energy and energy efficiency, holistic, preventative medicine, lifelong learning, ecological business initiatives, minimising pollution, safeguarding the natural environment and supporting fair trade with less developed countries.

The eco-village initiative has been listed in the UN's top 100 listing of best practice.

There are examples of these small pioneer communities across the globe and they are rural, urban and suburban: Ithaca, Findhorn, Shafbrühl, Steyerberg, CAT, Arcosanti, Auroville, Crystal Waters, Christiania, New Alchemists, to name a few. Most make a strong link between their community and ecology, maximising natural energy systems and organic local food production, minimising waste and developing broad life skills. They are often criticised or marginalised as 'utopian'. There is a real sense in which they are successful because of the shared commitments and responsibility of members and the social structures they have put in place. Often perceived as giving up on 'society', they are of course a well-kept secret of very high life quality and social support. Their replicability is often questioned on the basis that many people subscribe to less rather than more personal involvement with their neighbours, although there is no evidence of this.

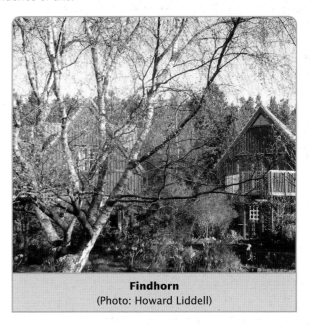

Findhorn
(Photo: Howard Liddell)

However, there is an ambition and need to replicate these solutions on a larger scale, where the opportunities and benefits might be greater. It is only as the problems of unsustainable development have become widely recognised, and the inability of conventional development planning to respond to political and consumer pressure to resolve the adverse impacts of our lifestyles, that it has been possible for these ecological models to be given consideration.

Case Study 14.9:

Lebensgarten, Steyerberg, Germany

The 60-house Lebensgarten (living garden) in north Germany is a pioneer eco-community that has developed an ex-wartime armaments work camp into a village operating on permaculture principles. It is one of many such projects across the globe and is a major centre for the worldwide eco-village movement. The project is managed through a weekly democratic forum of residents, which maintains the integrity of the environmental principles, and determines the practicalities of development and change. It is a car-free village with peripheral parking and a shared community solar-powered electric car for local journeys. It has a fully integrated energy policy that includes a CHP electricity and district heating scheme – supplemented by thermal and photovoltaic solar energy systems. All the houses are based on ecological design principles.

There are private (amenity) and communal (productive) permaculture gardens, which sit on the edge of mature woodland in a south-facing sun-scoop form.

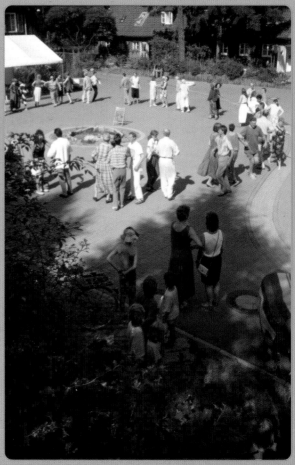

Photo: Howard Liddell

. . . Great big oaks do grow

Recent European projects, including a number comprising tens of thousands of new homes, have sought to establish new benchmarks in design by setting standards on a wide range of issues, which include mandatory considerations such as energy efficiency (but with much higher expectations) and also new parameters such as mixed-use planning, healthy indoor environments, techniques to encourage biodiversity and dedicated areas and landscaping for food production. Many are also tackling transportation and car management as fundamental aspects of improving environments and life quality.

The Hammarby model is intended as a prototype for future development – with an ambition to maximise resource economy in a sustainable residential development near Stockholm. Supply of electricity, cooling, heating and water is linked with waste, sewage and land management to provide for office, housing and other needs.

Water-conserving equipment minimises infrastructure and DHW. Wastewater is treated. Sewage sludge produces bio-soil for fertiliser and biogas for cookers and cars. Rainwater is drained where possible to ground locally – and polluted road run-off treated separately. Low-power electrical kit and ventilation systems reduce demand. CHP district heating is supplied from combustible waste- and sewage-driven heat pumps. District cooling is available for businesses. DHW is from solar panels and electricity from PVs. All combustible and organic waste is collected in a network of pipes linked to storage containers. An IT strategy aims to provide for individual metering, communications, alarms, etc.

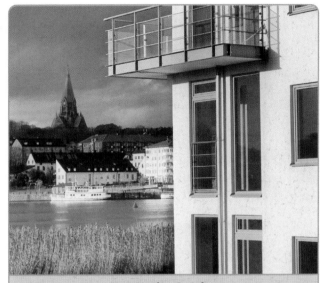

Hammarby, Sweden
The Hammarby model is a prototype for development that maximises resource economy

The water, sewage and garbage goals have been excellent, with separation into rain water, traffic water and sewage water to their own sewage works. Rainwater is kept clean and infiltrated into the ground. Traffic water is cleaned before it goes to the sea. Sewage water is cleaned, sludge is treated in a biogas plant, biogas is used in cars as fuel, and the treated biological material is so clean that it is used as fertiliser and humus. The energy reduction goal of 50% was not met.

The more sustainable city

- Maintenance of healthy neighbourhoods and communities
- Full involvement of all stakeholders in development issues
- Safe local environments for exercise and meeting
- Mixed-use development
- Presumption for keeping existing buildings
- A bio-diverse rich habitat
- Super-efficient, diverse, integrated transport system
- Design for external comfort
- Reclaim, reuse and recycling of resources and nutrients
- Safe, clean water and drainage infrastructure
- Resourcing of local, non-toxic, natural, low-embodied-energy materials
- Water conservation, capture and storage, and efficient treatment
- Energy-efficient form
- Energy capture and storage
- Radical reduction in power requirements
- Radical reduction in energy consumption of appliances
- Super-efficient energy systems (mixed use, diverse, CHP and district heating)
- Rapid move to carbon neutrality and renewable fuels.

Case Study 14.10:

The Green City of Tomorrow, Malmö, Sweden

City of Malmö, 2001

Vastra Hamnen is a harbour industrial area consisting of open ground with sparse vegetation. It is being redeveloped as a city district with dwellings, shops and offices in a process that involves major reclamation. The aim is for the district to be an international flagship of environmentally sound dense urban development.

The first phase, Bo01, was completed in late 2001. It includes 100% renewable energy supply, quality targets on building performance, a site-wide waste management strategy and clean transport. A special focus was placed on the ecological value of the site and this has generated many attractive landscape designs.

- *Quality programme.* Good and varied buildings provided by a diverse range of architects with provision for social interaction and functionality as the underpinning element. All the houses are built to pre-agreed standards for building performance, including materials that exclude dangerous substances and good energy efficiency.
- *100% renewable energy.* From sun, wind, water and biogas from local refuge. A minor part is played by photovoltaics. Much of the heating is supplied from aquifers and solar collectors. The network exchanges energy with the city grid and is in net balance.
- *Waste treatment.* Collecting stations for recyclable goods are placed throughout. Organic waste, including sewage, goes to the biogas plant, where it generates fuel for cars or is put into the gas grid. The remaining waste is burned for heat.
- *Rainwater management.* Run-off is that element of the rain that does not evaporate or seep into the ground and so has to be managed. The intention at Bo01 was to have minimum ground compaction to facilitate ground seepage alongside landscaping – sedum roofs and a network of ponds in courtyards and squares slow down the run-off and reduce the flow into drains. The remainder flows to open canals and thence to the existing open water.
- *Biodiversity.* The aim is to create a diverse range of natural life with parks and green spaces. The area, which is a breeding ground for avocets, little terns and common terns, has an ecologist working with the builders, landscape architects and other contractors. The aim is for the ecologist to have a long-term educational role in the community.
- *Green space.* A green space factor is used to integrate the design of the buildings with the natural environment. The building contractors are required to compensate the developed areas by providing green spaces such as plant beds, foliage on walls, green roofs, ponds, trees and bushes. Surfaces are quantified (0) for hard surfaces on roofs and courtyards, 0.8 green roofs. A total factor of no less then 0.5 was required. This use of green factors is increasingly common practice in Germany.
- *Green points* are given to elements that benefit biodiversity – bird nesting boxes, bat boxes, natural areas. The contractors are allowed to choose from a range of items to achieve a minimum of 10 points.
- *Traffic.* The area is planned around high quality cycleways and footpaths to make these attractive for short journeys, with an integrated public bus service planned. A mobility office provides information on transport. Sweden's public transport runs on green fuels, car pools have electric- and gas-powered vehicles, and maintenance vehicles are planned to be electrically powered.
- *IT and environment.* The area is supplied with cable connections, a local web-TV is planned and there is the facility to monitor resource use in the houses.

Case Study 14.10 (Continued):

The Green City of Tomorrow, Malmö, Sweden

City of Malmö, 2001

Targets

- Water consumption to be reduced by 50% compared to new inner city development
- Heavy metals and other pollutants to sewage water to be reduced by 50%
- Drainage water to be linked to water network
- All surface water to be managed locally
- Nitrogen content of treated sewage water not to exceed 6 mg/l and phosphorus not to exceed 0.15 mg/l (95% of phosphorus in greywater, urine and faecal matter to be recovered for agricultural use)
- Maximum of 60 kWh/m^2 and more than one-third to be electricity
- 80% of energy recovered from waste and sewage to be used

- Totally renewable energy
- 20% reduction in recyclable materials and waste (by weight)
- 60% reduction in landfill (by weight)
- 50% reduction in harmful or hazardous waste (by weight)
- Expansion of sorting at source: organic, combustible, electrical and electronic, hazardous, textiles, packaging, bulk items
- Waste transport to be reduced by 60%.

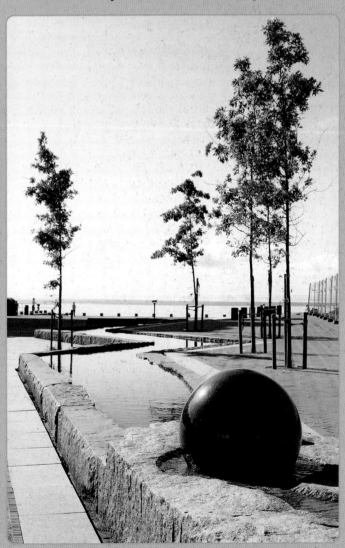

Photo permission: Eva Dalman

Bibliography

Texts

Geddes, P. (1931) *Sciences in General*. Life.

Mumford, L. (1961) *The City in History*. Penguin.

Collins, C. and Crasemann Collins, C. (1965) *Camillo Sitte and the Birth of Modern Planning*. Phaidon.

Jacobs, J. (1965) *The Death and Life of Great American Cities*. Penguin.

McHarg, I. (1968) *Design with Nature*. MIT Press.

Kohr, L. (1971) *The Inner City*. Y. Lolfa.

Martin, L. (ed.) (1976) *The Architecture of Form*. Cambridge University Press.

Kennedy, M. (1986) *Oko-Stadt: Band 1 – Prinzipien einer Stadtokologie. Oko-Stadt: Band 2 – Mit der Natur die Stadt planen*. Fischer.

Bartlett, S. et al. (1991) *Cities for Children*. UNICEF, Earthscan.

Littlefair, P. J. (1991) *Site Layout Planning for Daylight and Sunlight*. BRE.

Girardet, H. (1992) *The Gaia Atlas of Cities*. Gaia Books Ltd.

Blowers, A. (ed.) (1993) *Planning for a Sustainable Environment*. Earthscan.

Whitelegg, J. (1993) *Transport for a Sustainable Future – The Case for Europe*. Bellhaven Press.

Brand, S. (1994) *How Buildings Learn*. Viking.

Cote, R. P. et al. (1994) *Designing and Operating Industrial Parks as Ecosystems*. Dalhousie University.

Liddell, H. and Mackie, A. (1994) *Energy Conservation and Planning*. Scottish Office.

Barton, H. et al. (1995) *Sustainable Settlements – A Guide for Planners, Designers and Developers*. UoWE.

Beatley, T. and Manning, K. (1997) *The Ecology of Place*. Island Press.

BSRIA (1997) *Sustainable Housing – Options for independent energy, water supply and sewerage*.

Rogers, R. et al. (1999) *Urban Renaissance: Sharing the Vision*. Urban Task Force.

Corbett, J. M. (2000) *Designing Sustainable Communities*. Island Press.

Mitchell, W. J. (2000) *E-Topia*. MIT Press.

Santouris, M. (ed.) (2000) *Energy and Climate in the Urban Built Environment*. James & James.

UK Round Table on Sustainable Development (2000) *Planning for Sustainable Development in the 21st Century*. RCEP.

EEBPP (2002) *The Road to More Efficient Transport* (www.energy-efficiency.gov.uk/transport).

Hendriks, Ch. F. and Duijvestein, C. A. J. (eds) (2002) *The Ecological City*. Impressions Aeneas.

Dreiseitl, H., Grau, D. and Ludwig, K. H. C. (2003) *Waterscapes Planning, Building and Designing with Water*. Birkhauser.

Projects

Helsinki Planning Department (1998) Ecological Building Criteria for Viikki.

KUKA and City of Hanover (1998) Hanover Kronsberg Model of a Sustainable New Urban Community.

Finnish Association of Architects (2000) Towards a Sustainable City – The Viikki Eco-Neighbourhood Blocks.

Dalman, E. (Ed)., (2001) *Bo01 Staden, Byggnaderna, Planen Processen, Hållbarheten*. Svenskbyggtjanst.

NABU (2001) *Urban Ecology, Newsletter No. 6, Sustainable Development and the Road from Rio*.

NABU (2002) *Urban Ecology – Projects in Europe – Visions for Oslo?*

Index

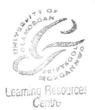